BODY TIME®
707 B Heinz Ave.
Berkeley, CA 94710

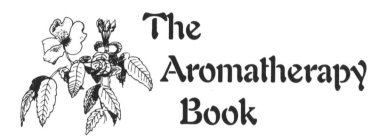

The Aromatherapy Book

The Aromatherapy Book

Applications & Inhalations

Jeanne Rose

With illustrations by
John Hulburd

Herbal Studies Course / Jeanne Rose
San Francisco, California

North Atlantic Books
Berkeley, California

ISBN 1-55643-073-6

Published by
Herbal Studies Course/Jeanne Rose
San Francisco, California
and
North Atlantic Books
P.O. Box 12327
Berkeley, CA 94712

Cover art: "Egypt" by George Barbier, from *The Romance of Perfume* by Richard Le Galliene, published by Richard Hudnut, New York and Paris, 1928.

Tables Six, Seven, and Ten are from *Aromatherapy: To Heal And Tend The Body* by Robert Tisserand, published by Lotus Press, 1988, and are reproduced with the permission of the author.

Cover and book design by Paula Morrison.

Printed in the United States of America

The Aromatherapy Book: Applications & Inhalations is sponsored by the Society for the Study of Native Arts and Sciences, a nonprofit educational corporation whose goals are to develop an educational and crosscultural perspective linking various scientific, social, and artistic fields; to nurture a holistic view of the arts, sciences, humanities, and healing; and to publish and distribute literature on the relationship of mind, body, and nature.

Our motto:
"Moderation in all things is all that counts!"
—J. Rose

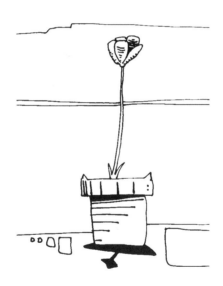

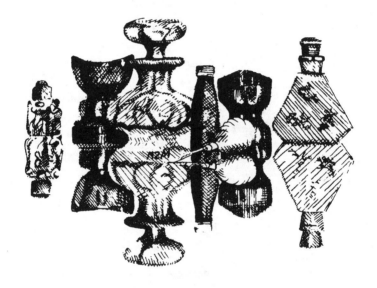

Dedication

To the women who have made the word *Aromatherapy*
known and used throughout the world:

VictoriaEdwards
SusanLeigh
AlexandraAvery
ChristineMalcolm
MindyGreen
KathyKeville
PatriciaDunn-Serota
JuliaMeadows
DianeRaimundo
ZiaWesley-Hosford
KathrynMcCarthy
DebraNuzzi
ColleenKDodt
SharonAckland
SusunWeed
SusanChavis
BarbaraBobo
RaeDunphy
ShirleyPrice
ValerieWorwood
JoniLoughran
CeslieRossi
AmberRose
MargueriteMaury
DanièleRyman
DorenePetersen
AnnBerwick
MichellineArcier
KathrynDeGraff

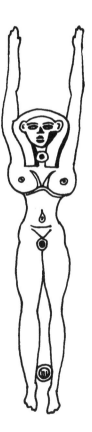

Especially to
Annette Green
Executive Director, Fragrance Foundation

Acknowledgements

Victoria Edwards, owner of a wonderful line of Aromatherapy products called Leydet, was very helpful in adding some important facts to some of the lesser known and little-used essential oils. She also allowed me to incorporate her table of oils and their uses that in this work is called Table 2. Thank you, Victoria.

John Steele was gracious and allowed me to use the information that he and Avraham Sand have put together and called the Tiferet-Lifetree Aromatherapy Treatment Kit. This is an easily used, complete combination of essential oils and the directions to use them. It includes twelve treatment blends and can be carried by the traveler and will supply all your aromatherapy needs.

Jennifer Meyer, a friend indeed, and the best when it comes to turning poorly written sentences into word-rich wonders.

Ginger Ashworth, who put this text onto my son's Mac SE/30 and in the process taught me a bit about computers.

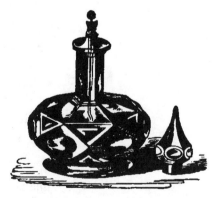

PERFUME LAMP

Table of Contents

PART II • THE RECIPES

PART III • AROMATHERAPY MAGIC

PART IV • SURVEY ON THE SENSE OF SMELL

PART V • THE END

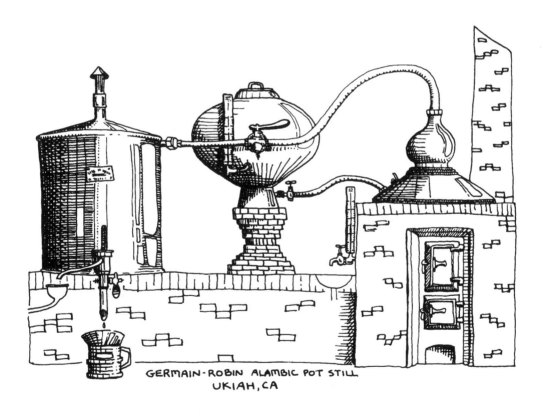

GERMAIN-ROBIN ALAMBIC POT STILL
UKIAH, CA

Publisher's Note

All plants and their essential oils, like all medicines, may be harmful and dangerous if used improperly—if they are taken internally when prescribed for external use, if they are taken in excess, or if they are taken for too long a time. Allergic reactions and unpredictable sensitivities or illness may develop. There are other factors to consider as well—since the strength of wild herbs and various essential oils varies, knowledge of their growing conditions and distillation methods is helpful. Be sure your herbs are fresh and whole and your essential oils are not contaminated with foreign objects like melting rubber stoppers. Keep conditions of use as sterile as possible.

We do not advocate, endorse or guarantee the curative effects of any of the substances listed in this book. We have made every effort to see that any botanical that is dangerous or potentially dangerous has been noted as such. When you use plants and their essential oils, recognize their potency and use them with care. Medical consultation is recommended for those recipes marked as dangerous.

The botanical names listed under each herb and essential oil do not always refer to one species only, but also to others, which in herbal medicine have been recognized as substitutes.

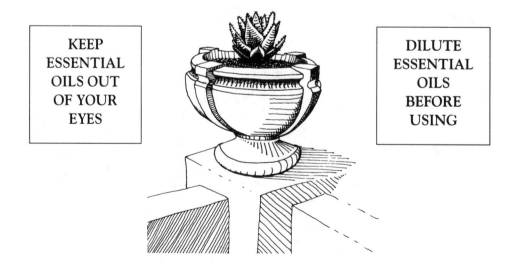

KEEP
ESSENTIAL
OILS OUT
OF YOUR
EYES

DILUTE
ESSENTIAL
OILS
BEFORE
USING

AUTHOR'S PREFACE

*A*romatherapy, or healing with essential oils through the sense of smell by inhalation and through application of these therapeutic volatile substances, like many other valuable therapies now being rediscovered, dates back to ancient times. Aromatic oils were used by the Egyptians, Greeks and Romans. Stills, in which volatile substances are distilled, were in use at least since 400 B.C. The beauteous Cleopatra used scented oils to entice Antony. She inhaled these luscious substances, she had expensive, rare oils rubbed upon her body by her servants, and she bathed in romantic essences.

In early Egypt many thousands of years ago, cones of scent were placed in headdresses and the scentual unguents would slowly melt in the warm Egyptian atmosphere. As the person moved through the day, lovely vapours of scent would waft slowly along with them.

CLEOPATRA HAD THE SCENT

In the Newe Worlde, stone houses or *temez-cals* were used by the Toltecs and the Aztecs to treat physical and mental problems. These were small rooms of adobe or stone built adjacent to the temples. Opposite the tiny entrance was a section that contained a little lake of hot water and stones. The lake was covered over with all manner of fragrant flowers and herbs. As the water heated, the steamy vapours passed through the layer of flowers, heating them and releasing their essential oils into the heated atmosphere. The hot scented air had a stimulating effect on circulation and the metabolism, and one's skin and complexion became soft and clean through the absorption of the sweet healthful vapours.

Today, *aromatherapy*, which we define as the treatment with volatile or essential oils from plants (and sometimes animal secretions, as with musk and civet), is undergoing a strong revival. But what is this elusive essence of plant material called *essential oil?* It is the heart and soul of the plant. It is the essence that deters bugs from eating the plant. It is the fragrant, aromatic heart of the plant that attracts bees and pollinating insects. It is the chemical component contained in tiny plant cells that is liberated during the distillation process. Many scientists throughout Europe and the United

States are exploring the power of these essential oils, looking into the once-forgotten recipes and formulations that were popular in the late '30s.

Aromatherapy is a way of treating mental and physical illness through inhalation and through the external application of essential oils with pressure-point therapy or simple massage. Body massage and inhalations with essential oils treat mental problems, while massage and the internal use of these concentrated essences treat physical problems. Problems of the skin are treated by external applications of essential oils in aromatherapy products.

The sense of smell is one of the most powerful of the senses. Scents and smells have a deep influence on men and women. In the act of smelling something we renounce our own individuality even more completely than when we touch. We allow scent to enter ourselves and we open ourselves to scent. To paraphrase Patrick Susskind* who wrote the novel *Perfume*, "Scent is the relative of breath. Together with breath it enters human beings, who cannot defend themselves against it, not if they want to live. And scent enters into one's very core, goes directly to the heart and decides for good and all between affection and contempt, disgust and lust, love and hate. (S)He who rules scent rules the hearts of men."

The use of the essential oils of flowers and plants stimulates and uplifts our spirits. When you feel melancholy or lethargic, for example, the simple inhalation of a Jasmine or Orange blossom acts on your spirit. The direct inhalation of the odors generally affects the mind psychologically, although inhalation can also have direct physiological effect via the limbic system in the brain and the blood circulation. For example, rubbing oil of Jasmine on the temples, pressing firmly and rubbing in a circular motion will definitely ease away a headache. The Jasmine enters into the body both through the skin as well as through the nasal mucosa.

Essential oils can also be used during seasonal changes. Jasmine, Rose Geranium and Rose essential oils are perfect for use during the winter season as they stimulate and revitalize and help ease us from the lethargy of winter to the warmer time of spring. Use Peppermint oil during the warm summer months for cooling and Lemon Verbena oil as an autumn oil and for relaxation.

Essential oil from leaves such as that from Lemon Verbena or Eucalyptus acts generally upon the metabolism to balance and tone. We can use

---

Perfume, by Patrick Susskind. New York: Alfred A. Knopf, 1986

these by inhalation when we are unable to concentrate on a difficult problem: they help concentrate mental energy and they balance all bodily functions. Inhaling the scent of Eucalyptus helps to clear and revitalize the respiratory system. Who can forget the comforting warm rubs on the chest during childhood or the scent of this oil in the humidifier when you were young and sick? Does Eucalyptus oil remind you of your youth and home?

Essential oils from flowers act on the spirit and are used to treat lethargy or lack of interest.

Essential oils from roots and barks act on the mucous membranes and are used to treat conditions of long standing.

There are several ways to use the essential oils. You can simply put some oils into a pan of boiling water and inhale the vapors—but this is a wasteful use of valuable oils. You can put oils into your bathtub to beautify your skin and to heal skin problems as well as for the healthful effects of the scent—this is also a bit expensive. One of the best ways is to use an aromatic diffusor that is especially made for the purpose of volatizing oils. This equipment is available via mail order from most sources of essential oils, which are listed in Chapter VI. It uses a few drops of oil, a tiny amount, and breaks the drops up into a fine mist of micro-droplets that gently disperses the natural therapeutic scent into the room. These micro-particles stay suspended for several hours and revitalize the air through their healing, antiseptic and deodorant action.

Essential oils have so many uses. Chapter I will give you a sense of which oil to use for any specific purpose. Geranium is considered a cellular stimulant and is good for oily and inflamed skin. Jasmine and Orange blossom as well are considered rejuvenating for the skin and body and especially effective for women. Jasmine, as well as having a rejuvenative effect, is considered aphrodisiacal and relaxing. It is a very special scent to diffuse throughout the room when you have romantic company or wish to get romantic. Orange blossom and Lemon Verbena in the diffusor is good for the complexion and in the evening to help you sleep. With these oils you would probably dream of pleasant social situations.

Essential oils can be used in many different ways, and for a hint of the thousands of formulas available and that you could make for yourself, see Part II of this book.

This is a very brief description of aromatherapy and its application. The use of aromata is just one part of a path that leads to total health and beauty. There is more . . .

The Path of Health, Beauty and a Peaceful Mind

1. **Good Nutrition and Clean Water and Fresh Air**
   For Your Cellular Structure, the Inner Self

2. **Exercise**
   For the Muscular Self and to Improve Circulation

3. **Hydrotherapy with Herbs**
   Lots of Healing Baths for the Physical Self, the Outer Self

4. **Massage/Acupuncture/Hugs**
   For the Circulation and to Balance the Electrical Forces in the Body

5. **Aromatherapy**—Inhalations for the Mind/Applications Externally
   For the Entire Body and the Subconscious Self

So keep smiling, work hard and take care of yourself.

—Jeanne Rose, Winter 1992
San Francisco

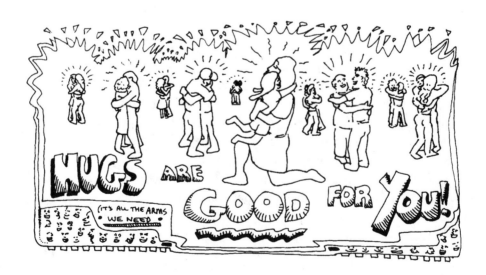

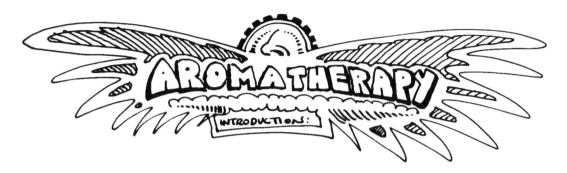

INTRODUCTION

by Victoria Edwards

When I first heard that Jeanne Rose was writing a definitive book on Aromatherapy, I was excited. When I studied with her twenty years ago she was writing *Herbs & Things*, which sparked renewed interest in the uses of herbs. Previously very little had been written on herbs since the 1930s. *Herbs & Things* changed that, and inspired others to create and experiment. A whole field of books, companies and products became established in the eighties, which taught decorators, gardeners, cooks, and all kinds of people involved in healthful living—including body care and natural cosmetics—how to make use of and grow herbs.

The Aromatherapy Book will be solid gold in the array of aromatherapy books that have appeared in the last five years. It is innovative and full of new information. Here as in all her books, Jeanne Rose is a quirky, engaging story-teller—warm-hearted and humorous.

As you read the stories and recipes, you will be led down the same fascinating road I travelled twenty years ago, when Jeanne Rose, my first aromatherapy teacher, began to enthrall me with what different scents could do for the mind, body and spirit. Even more now than then, attending to this wisdom brings us closer to valuing the natural wisdom of the planet—which we must do in order to care for it.

Victoria Edwards
Leydet Aromatics
Fair Oaks, California

Part I

The Directions

"Ah, I see! You are creating a new scent."
—*Perfume*
by Patrick Susskind

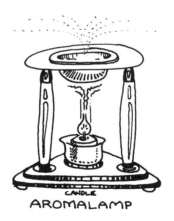

CANDLE
AROMALAMP

Perfume, by Patrick Susskind. New York: Alfred A. Knopf, 1986

Chapter I

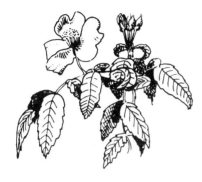

Choose
the Correct Oil

Spring Night
> Nasturtium flowers glowing orange on the darkened fence.
> Sumptuous Jasmine weaving a wicked scentual spell on the breeze
> Pink stars on purplish evening quilt
> The mating scream of the city cat
> Touches my soul. Tickles me with delight.
> —Jeanne Rose, May 1991

Essential oils are the essence of the plant, its heart and its soul. This essence is not oil as Olive oil is oil. Essential oils have little to no fatty substance. Push steam or boiling water through twenty pounds of plant material and you release the essential oil that is trapped in the cellular substance, the glands of the leaf, root, bark, seed or flower, which constitutes only a smidgeon of the entire plant.

To use an essential oil you must first know what your problem is. Read Table 1. Locate the problem or situation and then look on your essential oil shelf. Which of the oils do you actually have on hand? Define your terminology in Chapter II and then look up the oil in Chapter III. Now you will be ready to learn the secrets and wonderful uses of these concentrated fragrant essences.

Table 1.
. . . What Is the Problem? Which Oil to Use?

This may be the most important table in this book. With this table you can choose the essential oil that you prefer to use for each problem. You can choose from your existing supplies rather than go shopping for a very particular oil that only exists on the dark side of the moon. Find the situation that you are trying to treat. Choose one of the oils you already have or at least shop for an oil that is reasonably priced from the selection given.

We, Victoria Edwards or Jeanne Rose, have marked with a star (*) the essential oil that is the best or is a favorite.

You may well ask why so many oils are listed for each condition. My response would be that each of us is a unique individual with separate and diverse preference as to scent and individual and unique memories triggered by each scent.

Essential oils have both physiological as well as psychological use. Find the oil that works for you.

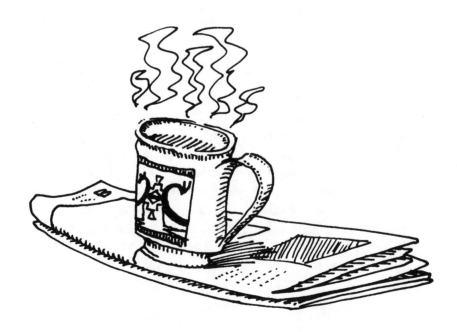

TABLE 1

Abortive Agents
  Carrot Seed oil
  Juniper oil
  Marjoram oil
  *Mugwort oil
  *Pennyroyal oil
  Sage oil

Abscess, *cold*
  Bergamot oil
  Chamomile oils
  Garlic oil
  Lavender oil
  *Tea Tree oil

Abscess, *warm*
  Onion oil
  *Onion poultice

Acne
  Almond, Bitter oil
  Ammi visnaga oil
  Anise oil
  Bergamot oil
  Cajeput oil
  Camphor oil
  Cedarwood oil
  Chamomile oils
  Immortelle oil
  Juniper oil
  Lavender oil
  Lemon oil
  Neroli oil
  Niaouli oil
  Peppermint oil
  Rosemary oil
  Sandalwood oil
  *Tea Tree oil
  Thyme oil

Adrenal Gland
  Ambretta oil
  Chamomile oil
  Pinus sp. oil
  Piscea alba oil

Aging
  Garlic oil
  Lemon oil
  Onion oil
  Thyme oil
  Spikenard oil

AIDS
(see Immune System, *to strengthen*)
  Air Cleansers &
    Refreshers
  Cinnamon oil
  Fir oil
  Lemon oil
  *Orange oil
  Peppermint oil
  Pine oil

Air or Room Disinfectants
  Bergamot oil
  Cinnamon oil
  Clove oil
  Eucalyptus oil
  Juniper oil
  Lemon oil
  Lime oil
  Pine oil
  Sage oil
  Thyme oil

Albuminuria
(*albumin in the urine*)
  Juniper oil

Alcoholism
(*detoxification from*)
  Fennel oil

Allergies, *general*
  Immortelle oil
  Melissa oil
  Yarrow oil

Allergies, *skin*
  Artemisia arborescens oil
  German Chamomile
    oil
  Melissa oil
  Rose oil

Analgesic, *reduces pain*
(see Pain)
  Bergamot oil
  Chamomile oil
  Lavender oil
  Marjoram oil
  Rosemary oil
  Ylang-Ylang oil

Anaphrodisiac
(*reduces sexual desire*)
  Marjoram oil

Anemia
  Lemon oil
  Roman Chamomile oil
  Thyme oil

Angina
  Bergamot oil
  Ginger oil
  Lemon oil
  Thyme oil

Anorgasmia
(unable to orgasm)
Anise oil
Black Pepper oil
Cardamom oil
Clary Sage oil
Coriander oil
Fir oil
Jasmine oil
Juniper oil
Onion oil
Patchouli oil
Rose oil
Sandalwood oil
 (hormonal)
Savory oil *(physical)*
Ylang-Ylang oil
 (emotional)

Anti-Allergenic
Ammi visnaga oil

Antibiotic
(combats infection)
*Garlic oil
Lavender oil
MQV (Niaouli) oil
Myrrh oil
Tea Tree oil

Antidepressants
Basil oil
Bergamot oil
Clary Sage oil
Geranium oil
Grapefruit oil
Jasmine oil
Lavender oil
Melissa oil
*Neroli oil
Orange oil
Patchouli oil
Petitgrain oil
Rose oil
Sandalwood oil
Verbena, Lemon, oil
Ylang-Ylang oil

Anti-Fungal
Cinnamon oil
Marjoram oil
Myrrh oil
Savory oil
Tagetes oil
Tea Tree oil

Anti-Inflammatory
Bergamot oil
Calendula oil
German Chamomile
 oil
Lavender oil
Myrrh oil

Antiseptics
*(All essential oils inhibit
 the growth of organisms
 [bacteria, germs] but
 some are more effective)*
*Bergamot oil
Cajeput oil
Cinnamon oil
*Eucalyptus oil
Fir oil
Garlic oil
Immortelle oil
 *(Helichrysum italicum
 oil)*
*Juniper oil
*Lavender oil
Niaouli oil
Onion oil
Pine oil
Rose oil
*Rosemary oil
*Sandalwood oil
Savory oil
*Tea Tree oil
Thyme oil

Antiviral Agents
(kill viruses)
 Artemisia annua oil
 Bergamot oil
 Eucalyptus oil
*Garlic oil
 Geranium oil
 Helichrysum oil
 Lemon oil
 Melissa oil
 Rose, Bulgarian, oil
*Tea Tree oil
 Thyme oil

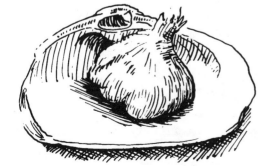

TABLE 1

Anxiety
Benzoin oil
Bergamot oil
Citronella oil
Clary Sage oil
Frankincense oil
Geranium oil
Grapefruit oil
Heliotrope flowers
Jasmine oil
Juniper oil
Lavender oil
Lemon oil
Lemongrass oil
*Marjoram oil
Melissa oil
Mugwort oil
Neroli oil
Orange oil
Patchouli oil
Rose oil
Sandalwood oil
Vanilla oil
Verbena, Lemon oil
Vetiver oil
Ylang-Ylang oil

Apathy
Bergamot oil
Cajeput oil
Clary Sage oil
Jasmine oil
Patchouli oil

Aphrodisiacs
(to stimulate the sex drive)
Black Pepper oil
Cardamom oil
Cinnamon oil
*Clary Sage oil
*Jasmine oil
*Neroli oil
Patchouli oil
*Rose oil
*Sandalwood oil
*Ylang-Ylang oil
  *(psycho-somatic
  problems)*

Appetite, *to increase*
Black Pepper oil
Caraway oil
Cardamom oil
Coriander oil
Garlic oil
Ginger oil
Grapefruit oil
Hyssop oil
Lemon oil
Myrrh oil
Oregano oil
Sage oil
Tangerine oil
Tarragon oil *(anorexia
  & bulimia & digestion
  disturbance caused
  by emotions)*
Vetiver oil

Appetite, *to reduce*
Bergamot oil
Juniper oil *(balance
  appetite)*
*Lavender oil
Onion oil *(reduce
  hunger)*

Arterial Infection
Garlic oil
Lemon oil
Marjoram oil
Onion oil

Arteriosclerosis
Garlic oil
Juniper oil
Lemon oil
Onion oil
Rosemary oil

Arthritis
(see Rheumatism)

Asthma
Ammi visnaga oil
Benzoin oil
Cajeput oil
Eucalyptus globulus oil
Eucalyptus polybractea
  oil
Garlic oil
Hyssop oil
Inula graveolens oil
Lavender oil
Rosemary oil

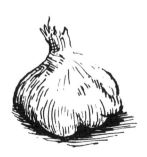

Astringents
(tighten tissues, reduce fluid loss)
Basil oil
Bay oil
*Cedarwood oil
*Cypress oil
*Frankincense oil
Geranium oil
*Juniper oil
Lemon oil
*Myrrh oil
Oakmoss oil
Patchouli oil
Rosemary oil
*Sandalwood oil

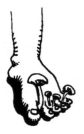

Athlete's Foot
(see Fungicides)
Sage oil
*Tea Tree oil

Back Pain
(see also Lumbago; Pain)
Birch oil
Black Pepper oil
Lavender oil
Marjoram oil
Rosemary oil
Ylang-Ylang oil

Bactericides
(Most PEO)
Bergamot oil
Cajeput oil
Eucalyptus oil
Garlic oil
Juniper oil
Lavender oil
Niaouli oil
Rosemary oil
Tea Tree oil

Baldness
Birch oil
Clary Sage oil
*Jojoba oil
Lavender oil
Rosemary oil

Bed-Wetting
Cypress oil

Birthing
(induction, ease pain)
Clary Sage oil
Jasmine oil
Lavender oil
Pennyroyal oil

Blackheads
Cajeput oil
Tea Tree oil

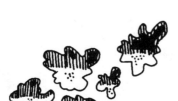

Bladder, *infection of*
Bergamot oil
Cajeput oil
Eucalyptus oil
Fennel oil
Juniper oil
Lavender oil
Myrrh oil
Myrtle oil
*Sandalwood oil
Thyme oil
Thuja oil (Cedar leaf oil)

Bladder, *inflammation or cystitis*
Bergamot oil
Cedarwood oil
Eucalyptus oil
Garlic oil
Juniper oil
Lavender oil
*Sandalwood oil

Bladder, *inflammation of mucous membrane*
Bergamot oil
Cedarwood oil
Eucalyptus oil
Garlic oil
*Juniper oil
Lavender oil
Roman Chamomile oil
Sandalwood oil

Bladder, *painful urination*
Cedarwood oil
Juniper oil

8

TABLE 1

Bleeding
(see Blood, *arresting*)

Blepharitis (*eyelid inflammation*)
(see Eyes, *conjunctivitis*)

Blisters
Eucalyptus oil
Lavender oil

Blood, *arresting bleeding*
Cistus oil (hemostatic)
Cypress oil
Geranium oil
Lemon oil
Rose oil

Blood, *to cleanse & purify*
Artemisia tridentata oil
Eucalyptus oil
Garlic oil
Juniper oil
Rose oil
Rosemary oil

Blood, *excessive loss (menstruation)*
Cinnamon oil
Cypress oil
Frankincense oil
Rose oil

Blood, *lack of*
(*to build up*)
Lemon oil
Onion oil
Roman Chamomile oil
Thyme oil

Blood, *to thin*
Lemon oil

Blood Pressure, *to lower*
German Chamomile oil
Lavender oil
Marjoram oil
Melissa oil
*Nutmeg oil (*systolic*)
Ylang-Ylang oil

Blood Pressure, *to raise*
Clary Sage oil
Hyssop oil
Jasmine oil
Rosemary oil

Blood Sugar, *for low*
(*hypoglycemia*)
Eucalyptus oil
Fennel oil

Boils
Artemisia arborescens oil
Bergamot oil
Clary Sage oil
Lavender oil
Lemon oil
Onion oil
Niaouli oil
Roman Chamomile oil
Tea Tree oil
Thyme oil
Yarrow oil

Boredom & Lethargy
Cardamom oil
Juniper oil
Lemongrass oil
Rosemary oil

Brain Strokes
Sage oil

Breasts, *engorgement of*
Geranium oil
Peppermint oil

Breasts, *insufficient milk from*
Anise oil
*Fennel oil
Jasmine oil

Breasts, *stimulating growth of*
Geranium oil
Ladies Mantle dew
Vetiver oil
Ylang-Ylang oil

Bronchitis
Benzoin extract
Camphor oil
*Eucalyptus oil
Fir oil
Garlic oil
*Hyssop oil
Immortelle oil
Inula oil
Lemon oil
*Peppermint oil
Sage oil
Sandalwood oil
Spruce oil
Thyme oil
Turpentine oil
Violet oil

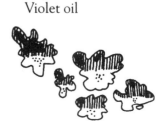

Bruises
*Bruise Juice (See Ch. VI, CA: Herbal BodyWorks)
Helichrysum oil
Mugwort oil
Parsley oil
Rosemary oil
Sage oil

Burns
Chamomile oils
Geranium oil
Helichrysum oil
*Lavender oil
Tea Tree oil

Calluses
Clove oil
Garlic oil
Orange oil

Cancer, *supportive treatment*
(see also Immune System)
Borneol oil
Carrot Seed oil
Clove oil
Cypress oil
Eucalyptus oil
Garlic oil
Geranium oil
Hyssop oil
Onion oil
Parsley oil
Tarragon oil
Tea Tree oil
Thuja oil
Violet oil

Carbuncles
Bergamot oil
Lavender oil

Cell Regenerator
Lavender oil
Neroli oil
Tea Tree oil

Cellulite
Caraway oil
Cypress oil
Fennel oil
Juniper oil
Lavender oil
Orange oil
Oregano oil
Rosemary oil

Cephalic
(*clears mind, stimulates mental process*)
Basil oil
Rosemary oil

Cholagogue
Chamomile oil
Lavender oil
Rosemary oil
Sage oil

Cholesterol, *too high*
Rosemary oil

Cholera
Camphor oil
Eucalyptus oil
Peppermint oil

Circulation, *reducing*
(*for hypertension*)
Clary Sage oil
Garlic oil
Lavender oil
Marjoram oil
Melissa oil
Ylang-Ylang oil

Circulation, *stimulating*
(*for hypotension*)
Camphor oil
Cinnamon oil
Cumin oil
Hyssop oil
Pine oil
Rosemary oil

Circulation, *unbalanced or irritated*
Cypress oil
Garlic oil
Hyssop oil
Thyme oil

Cirrhosis
(see Liver, *inflammation*)

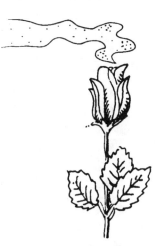

TABLE 1

Colds
Black Pepper oil
Cajeput oil
Camphor oil
Cinnamon oil
Eucalyptus oil
Garlic oil
Ginger oil
Hyssop oil
Immortelle oil
Lavender oil
Melissa oil
Oregano oil
Pennyroyal oil
Peppermint oil
Pine oil
Rosemary oil
Sage oil
Thyme oil

Colic
Anise oil
Cumin oil
Dill oil
*Fennel oil
Lavender oil
Marjoram oil
Melissa oil
*Peppermint oil
Roman Chamomile oil

Colitis
Bergamot oil
Dill oil
Lavender oil
Neroli oil
Roman Chamomile oil
Tarragon oil
Ylang-Ylang oil

Conjunctivitis
(see Eyes, *conjunctivitis*)
*Fennel Seed, Comfrey
  root wash

Connective Tissue, *weakness of*
Rose oil
Rosewood oil

Constipation
(see Intestines,
  constipation)
Cumin oil

Convalescence
(see Regeneration, *after
  illness*)

Convulsions
Clary Sage oil
Lavender oil
Neroli oil
Roman Chamomile oil
Rose oil
Ylang-Ylang oil

Corns
Garlic oil
Fennel oil
Thuja oil

Cough
Anise oil
Benzoin extract
Cardamom oil
Cinnamon oil
Eucalyptus oil
Fir oil
Frankincense oil
Hyssop oil
Jasmine oil
Juniper oil
Marjoram oil
Myrrh oil
Niaouli oil
Pennyroyal oil
Pepper oil
Peppermint oil
Rosemary oil
Sandalwood oil
Thyme oil

Cough, *whooping*
Basil oil
Cypress oil
Hyssop oil
Lavender oil
Myrtle oil
Pennyroyal oil
Rosemary oil
Thyme oil
Violet oil

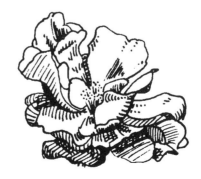

Cramps
Basil oil
Bergamot oil
Camphor oil
Cardamom oil
*Clary Sage oil
Coriander oil
Cypress oil
Eucalyptus oil
Fennel oil
Hyssop oil
Juniper oil
Lavender oil
Marjoram oil
Pennyroyal oil
Pepper oil
Peppermint oil
Roman Chamomile oil
Rose oil
Rosemary oil
Sandalwood oil

Cystitis
(see Urinary Tract)

Dandruff
MQV oil
Rosemary oil
Tea Tree oil

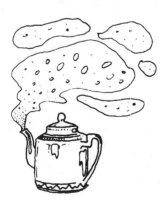

Deodorants
(*to reduce odor*)
*Benzoin tincture
*Bergamot oil
  Cilantro wash
*Coriander oil
*Clary Sage oil
  Cypress oil (*for feet*)
  Eucalyptus oil
  Fir oil (*for feet*)
*Lavender oil
  Melissa oil
  Patchouli oil
  Petitgrain oil
  Pine oil
*Rose oil
*Rosewood oil
*Sage oil
*Tea Tree oil

Depression
(see Antidepressants)

Dermatitis
(see Skin Care,
  dermatitis)

Detoxify
Fennel oil
Garlic oil
Geranium oil
Helichrysum oil
Lime oil
Juniper oil
Lemon oil
Parsley oil

Diabetes
Cedar oil
Eucalyptus oil
Geranium oil
Juniper oil
Onion oil

Diarrhea
Black Pepper oil
Camphor oil
Clove oil
Cypress oil
Eucalyptus oil
Garlic oil
Geranium oil
Ginger oil
Lavender oil
Melissa oil
Myrrh oil
*Neroli oil
Onion oil
Orange oil
Peppermint oil
Roman Chamomile oil
Rosemary oil
Sandalwood oil
Savory oil

Digestive Aids
Anise oil
Basil oil
Bergamot oil
Black Pepper oil
Cardamom oil
Dill oil
Fennel oil
Frankincense oil
Hyssop oil
Marjoram oil
Melissa oil
Rosemary oil

Digestive Problems
(see Stomach, *digestive*)

Diphtheria
Bergamot oil
Eucalyptus oil
Lavender oil

TABLE 1

Disinfectant
(see Air or Room
 Disinfectants)
 Citrus oils

Diuretics
 Anise oil
 Benzoin tincture
 Black Pepper oil
 Camphor oil
 Cardamom oil
 Cedarwood oil
 Cypress oil
 Fennel oil
 Garlic oil
 Juniper oil
 Onion oil
 Parsley oil
 Rosemary oil
 Sage oil
 Sandalwood oil

Dizziness
(see Fainting)
 Camphor oil
 Lavender oil
 Peppermint oil

Dyspepsia
(see Stomach, *digestive*)

**Earaches,
inflammation**
(*otitis*)
 Basil oil
 Cajeput oil
 Chamomile oils
 Hyssop oil
 Lavender oil
 Myrtle oil
 Tea Tree oil

Eczema
 Artemisia arborescens oil
 Bergamot oil
 German Chamomile
  oil
 Hyssop oil
 Lavender oil
 Neroli oil
 Tea Tree oil

Edema
 Garlic oil
 Geranium oil
 Onion oil
 Rosemary oil

Emmenagogue
 Angelica oil
 Basil oil
 Clary Sage oil
 Hyssop oil
 Juniper oil
 Lavender oil
 Marjoram oil
 Rose oil
 Rosemary oil

Emotional Coldness
 Black Pepper oil
 Clary Sage oil
 Ginger oil
 Grapefruit oil
 Jasmine oil
 Orange oil
 Patchouli oil
 Ylang-Ylang oil

**Emotional Trauma &
Fatigue**
 Geranium oil
 Grapefruit oil
 Lavender oil
 MQV oil
 Neroli oil
 Niaouli oil
 Rose oil
 Rosemary oil

Epilepsy
 Basil oil
 Lavender oil
 Rosemary oil
  Contraindicated:
   Camphor oil
   Hyssop oil
   Sage oil
   Thuja oil

Euphoriants
*Clary Sage oil
 Grapefruit oil
 Jasmine oil
 Rose oil
 Ylang-Ylang oil

Expectorants
 Benzoin tincture
 Bergamot oil
 Eucalyptus oil
 Fir oil
 Marjoram oil
 Myrrh oil
 Pine oil
 Sandalwood oil
 Spruce oil

Eyes, *conjunctivitis*
Clary Sage oil
Lavender oil
Roman Chamomile oil
Rose oil
Fennel Seed &
  Comfrey root wash

Eyes, *fogginess*
Clary Sage oil
Myrtle hydrosol
Rosemary hydrosol
Fennel Seed &
  Comfrey root wash

Eyes, *infection of lids*
Clary Sage oil
Geranium oil
Lemon oil
Myrtle hydrosol
Roman Chamomile oil
Fennel Seed &
  Comfrey root wash

Eyes, *tired*
Clary Sage oil
Lavender oil
Myrtle hydrosol
Roman Chamomile oil
Rose oil

Fainting
Basil oil
Bergamot oil
*Camphor oil
Fir oil
Lavender oil
Melissa oil
Peppermint oil
Pine oil
Roman Chamomile oil
Rosemary oil
Savory oil

Fear
(see Anxiety)

Febrifuge,
(see Fever reducer)

Feet, *stinky*
Sage oil
Tea Tree oil

Fever Reducer
Bergamot oil
Black Pepper oil
Camphor oil
Chamomile oil
Eucalyptus oil
Hyssop oil
Lemon oil
Melissa oil
Pennyroyal oil
*Peppermint oil
Roman Chamomile oil
Sassafras oil
Tea Tree oil

Fingernails
Castor oil
Cypress oil
Lavender oil
Sandalwood oil

Fingernails, *brittle*
Biotin tablets
Lemon oil
Onion oil
Rosemary Verbenon oil

Fistula
*(abnormal passage
  from abscess to skin
  surface)*
*Lavender oil
Myrrh oil
*Tea Tree oil

Flatulence
Anise oil
Bergamot oil
Black Pepper oil
Caraway oil
Cinnamon oil
Clary Sage oil
Clove oil
Fennel oil
Hyssop oil
Juniper oil
Lavender oil
Lemon oil
Marjoram oil
Myrrh oil
Nutmeg oil
Orange oil
Oregano oil
Pennyroyal oil
Peppermint oil
Roman Chamomile oil
Rosemary oil
Sandalwood oil
Savory oil

Fleas, *to repel*
Eucalyptus oil
Geranium oil
Lavender oil
Lemon oil
Pennyroyal oil
Rosemary oil
Tea Tree oil

Foot Odor
(see Deodorants)
Sage oil
Tea Tree oil

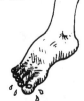

14

TABLE 1

Fungicides
(kill yeasts and molds)
Angelica oil
Camphor oil
Cilantro oil
Cinnamon oil
Citronella oil
Coriander oil
Fennel oil
Immortelle oil
Lavender oil
Myrrh oil
Nutmeg oil
Tagetes oil
Tea Tree oil
Thyme oil

Gall Bladder, *to stimulate function*
Carrot Seed oil
Grapefruit oil
Lavender oil
Rose oil
Rosemary oil
Rosemary Verbenon oil
Sage oil

Gall Bladder, *infection or inflammation*
Fir oil
Parsley oil
Rose oil
Rosemary oil

Gall Bladder, *stimulation of bile flow*
Pennyroyal oil
Peppermint oil
Roman Chamomile oil
Rosemary oil
Sage oil

Gallstones
Chamomile oil
Eucalyptus oil
Lavender oil
Onion oil
Parsley oil
Peppermint oil
Rosemary oil
Turpentine oil

Gastralgia
(see Stomach, *gastralgia*, etc.)

Genitals, *gonorrhea effects*
Benzoin extract
Bergamot oil
Cedarwood oil
Eucalyptus oil
Frankincense oil
Garlic oil
Jasmine oil
Lavender oil
Lemon oil
Parsley oil
Sandalwood oil

Genitals, *itching*
(pruritus)
Bergamot oil
Clary Sage oil
Lavender oil
Roman Chamomile oil
Tea Tree oil

Genitals, *lack of erection*
Fir oil
Jasmine oil
Juniper oil
Savory oil
Thuja oil

Genitals, *mucus discharge from*
Bergamot oil
Cedarwood oil
Eucalyptus oil
Frankincense oil
Geranium oil
Juniper oil
Lavender oil
Myrrh oil
Patchouli oil
Sandalwood oil
Tea Tree oil

Genitals, *syphilis*
Lemon oil
Parsley oil
Sassafras oil

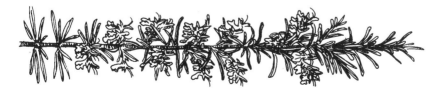

Genitals, *vaginal discharge from*
Benzoin tincture, diluted
Bergamot oil
Clary Sage oil
Eucalyptus oil
Frankincense oil
Hyssop oil
Lavender oil
Marjoram oil
Myrrh oil
Rose oil
Rosemary oil
Sage oil
Sandalwood oil
Tea Tree oil
Thyme oil

Genital Herpes
(see Herpes)

Germicides
(see Antiseptics)

Gout
Cajeput oil
Camphor oil
Fir oil
Garlic oil
Juniper oil
Lemon oil
Rosemary oil
Sassafras oil
Thyme oil
Turpentine oil

Grief
(see Antidepressants)

Gums, *bleeding and/or inflammation*
Clove oil
Cypress oil
Lemon oil
*Myrrh oil
Sage oil
Thyme oil

Gums, *care of*
Fennel oil
Lemon oil
Myrrh oil
Sage oil
Tea Tree oil
Thyme oil

Hair, *brittle*
*Jojoba oil
*Rosemary oil

Hair, *dandruff*
Clary Sage oil
Eucalyptus oil
Frankincense oil
*Jojoba oil
Patchouli oil
*Rosemary oil
*Tea Tree oil

Hair, *dry*
Carrot Seed oil
Chamomile oil
Frankincense oil
Geranium oil
Lavender oil

Hair, *falling out*
*Lavender oil
*Rosemary oil

Hair, *general care*
Cedarwood oil
Chamomile oil *(blonds only)*
Clary Sage oil
Cypress oil
Juniper oil
Lavender oil
Lemon oil *(blonds only)*
Patchouli oil
Roman Chamomile oil
*Rosemary oil
Rosewood oil
*Sage oil

Hair, *stimulate growth*
*Jojoba oil
*Rosemary oil

Hair, *loss*
Birch oil
Cajeput oil
Cedarwood oil
Clary Sage oil
Juniper oil
Lavender oil
Rosemary oil
Sage oil
Tea Tree oil
Thyme oil

Hair, *oily*
Bergamot oil
Cypress oil
Juniper oil
*Lavender oil
*Lemon oil
*Lemongrass oil
Rosemary oil
Sage oil
Thyme oil

TABLE 1

Hair, *to make shiny*
*Rosemary Verbenon oil

Hair, *split ends*
*Rosemary oil

Hay Fever
(see Allergies, *general*)

Headache
Eucalyptus oil
*Jasmine oil
Lavender oil (fever
  headache)
Lemon oil
Marjoram oil
Melissa oil
Peppermint oil
Roman Chamomile oil
Rose oil
Rosemary oil
Sage oil

Heart, *aching*
*Angelica oil
Champa oil
*Marjoram oil
Rose oil

Heart, *flutter or palpitations*
(*to quiet or sedate*)
Caraway oil
Lavender oil
*Melissa oil
Neroli oil
Peppermint oil
Roman Chamomile oil
Rose oil
*Ylang-Ylang oil (in
  dilution)

Heartburn
(see Stomach, *heartburn*)

Heart Failure
Camphor oil
Cumin oil
Rosemary oil

Heart Stimulant
Angelica oil
Anise oil
Camphor oil
*Citronella oil
Cumin oil
Hyssop oil
Rosemary oil

Heart Tonic
Angelica oil
Anise oil
Cumin oil
Garlic oil
Hyssop oil
Lavender oil
Marjoram oil
Melissa oil
Neroli oil
Peppermint oil
Rose oil
Rosemary oil

Hæmorrhagia
(see Blood, *arresting
  bleeding*)

Hemorrhoids
Cypress oil
Garlic oil
Frankincense oil
Juniper oil
Myrrh oil
Tea Tree oil

Hepatic
(*helps the liver*)
Chamomile oils
Lemon oil
Peppermint oil
Rosemary Verbenon oil
Thyme oil

Herpes
*Basil oil
Bergamot oil
Camphor oil
Citriodora globulus oil
Eucalyptus oil
Geranium oil
Grapefruit oil
Melissa oil
*Rose, Bulgarian, oil
Tea Tree oil

Hiccups
Caraway oil
Fennel oil
Tarragon oil

Hoarseness
Cypress oil
Jasmine oil
Lemon oil
Myrrh oil
Thyme oil

Hormones, *balancing estrogen*
Clary Sage oil
Fennel oil
Geranium oil
Sage oil

Hydration of the Skin
Rose oil

Hypertension

(see Circulation,
 reducing)

Hyperventilation

Frankincense oil
Ylang-Ylang oil (in
 dilution)

Hypnotic

(sleep aid)
 Chamomile oil
 Lavender oil
 Marjoram oil
*Neroli oil
 Ylang-Ylang oil

Hysteria

(see Nerves)

Immune System, *to strengthen*

Angelica oil
 Artemisia oils
 Cajeput oil
 Eucalyptus oil
*Garlic oil
*Lavender oil
*MQV oil
 Niaouli oil
*Tea Tree oil

Impotence

Anise oil
 Black Pepper oil
 Cardamom oil
 Cinnamon oil
 Clary Sage oil
 Coriander oil
 Fir oil
 Jasmine oil
 Juniper oil
 Onion oil
 Patchouli oil
 Rose oil
 Sandalwood oil
 (hormonal)
 Savory oil *(physical)*
 Thuja oil
 Ylang-Ylang oil
 (emotional)

Infection

Garlic oil
 Immortelle oil
 Lemon oil
 MQV oil
 Niaouli oil
 Tea Tree oil
 Thyme oil

Inflammation

Chamomile oils
 Clary Sage oil
 Eucalyptus oil
 Immortelle oil
 Lavender oil
 Myrrh oil
 Peppermint oil
 Rose oil
 Sandalwood oil

Insect Bites

Chilé Pepper oil
 Clove oil
 Garlic oil
 Lavender oil
 Lemon oil
 Onion oil
 Pennyroyal oil
 Peppermint oil
 Sage oil
 Sassafras oil
 Savory oil
 Tea Tree oil

Insect Repellants

Artemisia oils
 Basil oil
 Bay Laurel oil
 Cedarwood oil
 Citronella oil
 Clove oil
 Eucalyptus oil
 Geranium oil
 Lemon oil
 Lemongrass oil
 Mugwort oil
 Onion oil
 Orange oil
 Pennyroyal oil
 Peppermint oil

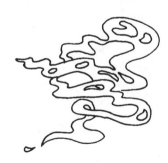

TABLE 1

Insomnia
(see also Nerves)
 Basil oil
 Bergamot oil
 Camphor oil
 Lavender oil
*Marjoram oil
*Neroli oil
 Orange oil
 Roman Chamomile oil
 Rose oil
 Sandalwood oil
 Verbena oil
 Ylang-Ylang oil

Intestines, *colic in*
 Anise oil
 Benzoin extract
 Bergamot oil
 Cardamom oil
 Dill oil
 Fennel oil
 Juniper oil
 Lavender oil
 Peppermint oil

Intestines, *colon infection*
 Garlic oil
 Immortelle oil
 Onion oil
 Myrtle oil
 Tea Tree oil
 Thyme oil

Intestines, *constipation*
 Basil oil
 Cumin oil
 Fennel oil
 Lavender oil
 Marjoram oil
 Pepper oil
 Roman Chamomile oil
 Rose oil

Intestines, *infection*
 Bergamot oil
 Black Pepper oil
 Garlic oil
 Lavender oil
 Roman Chamomile oil
 Rosemary oil
 Tea Tree oil

Intestines, *putrefaction*
 Cardamom oil
 Cinnamon oil
 Coriander oil
*Garlic oil
 Lemon oil
 Marjoram oil
 Onion oil
 Tea Tree oil

Intestines, *worms*
(*vermifuge*)
 Bergamot oil
 Caraway oil
 Eucalyptus oil
 Hyssop oil
 Juniper oil
 Lemon oil
 Onion oil
 Peppermint oil
 Roman Chamomile oil
 Savory oil
 Tarragon oil
 Thuja oil
*Turpentine oil

Invigoration
 Cardamom oil
 Coriander oil
 Juniper oil
 Lemongrass oil
 Rosemary oil
 Savory oil

Irritability
 Benzoin, inhale
 Frankincense oil
 Lavender oil
 Roman Chamomile oil
 Rose oil
 Ylang-Ylang oil

Itching
(see Skin Care, *itching*)
 Tea Tree oil

Kidney, *inflammation*
 Cedarwood oil
 Eucalyptus oil
 Frankincense oil
 Roman Chamomile oil
 Sandalwood oil

Kidney, *inflammation of nearby area*
Cedarwood oil
Eucalyptus oil
Frankincense oil
Juniper oil
Roman Chamomile oil

Kidney, *tonic*
Cedarwood oil
Clary Sage oil
Eucalyptus oil
Juniper oil
*Sandalwood oil

Kidney Stones
Fennel oil
Geranium oil
Juniper oil
Roman Chamomile oil

Laryngitis
Benzoin, inhale
Frankincense oil
*Melissa oil
Sandalwood oil
Thyme oil

Laxative
Caraway oil
Cumin oil
Fennel oil
Juniper oil
Marjoram oil
Sage oil
Violet oil

Lethargy
(see Euphoriants; Mind, *mental fatigue*; Stimulants, *body*)

Leukocytosis, *stimulants for*
All oils, especially:
Bergamot oil
Lavender oil
Roman Chamomile oil

Lice
Cinnamon oil
Clove oil
Eucalyptus oil
Geranium oil
Lavender oil
Lemon oil
Lemongrass oil
Oregano oil
*Pennyroyal oil
Rosemary oil
Thyme oil
*Turpentine oil

Liver, *congestion of*
Cypress oil
Roman Chamomile oil
Rose oil
Rosemary Verbenon oil

Liver, *detoxifying*
Helichrysum oil
juniper oil
Lemon oil
Lime oil
Roman Chamomile oil

Liver, *hepatitis*
Rosemary oil

Liver, *inflammation*
(*cirrhosis*)
Lemon oil
Juniper oil
Rosemary oil

Liver, *irritation*
Cypress oil
Lemon oil
Lime oil
Roman Chamomile oil
Rose oil
Rosemary oil
Sage oil
Thyme oil

Liver, *jaundice*
Cypress oil
Geranium oil
Lemon oil
Lime oil
Roman Chamomile oil
Rosemary oil
Thyme oil

Liver, *tonic for*
Carrot Seed oil
Fennel oil
Helichrysum oil
Lemon oil
Lime oil
Tangerine oil

Lumbago
(see also Back Pain)
Birch oil
Ginger oil
Ylang-Ylang oil

Lymphatic System, *inflammation of nodes*
Eucalyptus oil
Juniper oil
Lavender oil
Onion oil
Sage oil

20

TABLE 1

Lymphatic System, *stimulant*
Caraway oil
Cumin oil
Cypress oil
Fennel oil
Immortelle oil
Lemon oil
Oregano oil
Rosemary oil
Tarragon oil

Malaria
Artemesia annua oil

Measles
Chamomile oils
Eucalyptus oil
Tea Tree oil

Memory
(see Mind)
*Basil oil
*Rosemary oil

Menopause Disorders, *hot flashes & sweating*
*Clary Sage oil *(hot flashes)*
Fennel oil
Geranium oil
*Melissa oil
Roman Chamomile oil *(hormonal balance)*
Sage oil *(sweating)*

Menstruation, *excessive blood loss*
(menorrhagia)
Cypress oil
Rose oil

Menstruation, *irregular*
Clary Sage oil
Melissa oil
Mugwort oil
Rose oil

Menstruation, *painful*
(menstrual cramps)
Anise oil
Bergamot oil
Caraway oil
Carrot Seed oil
Clary Sage oil
Cypress oil
Ginger oil
Jasmine oil
Marjoram oil
Melissa oil
Pennyroyal oil
Peppermint oil
Rose oil
Rosemary oil

Menstruation, *scanty or late*
(amenorrhea)
Anise oil
Caraway oil
Carrot Seed oil
Cinnamon oil
Clary Sage oil
Clove oil
Cypress oil
Fennel oil
Hyssop oil
Jasmine oil
Juniper oil
Lavender oil
Melissa oil
Mugwort oil
Myrrh oil
Nutmeg oil
Oregano oil
Pennyroyal oil
Roman Chamomile oil
Rosemary oil
Sage oil
Sassafras oil
Tarragon oil

Migraine
Anise oil
Basil oil
Chamomile oils
Eucalyptus oil
Jasmine oil
Lavender oil
Lemon oil
Marjoram oil
Melissa oil
Onion oil
Rosemary oil

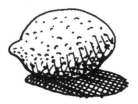

Mind, *mental fatigue*
(loss of concentration or
poor memory)
*Basil oil
Cardamom oil
Citronella oil
Lemon oil
Lemongrass oil
Peppermint oil
*Rosemary oil
Verbena oil

Mood Swings
Benzoin, inhale
Bergamot oil
Clary Sage oil
Fennel oil
Frankincense oil
Geranium oil
Jasmine oil
Rosewood oil

Mouth, *bad breath*
Bergamot oil
Cardamom oil
Clove buds (chew)
Eucalyptus oil
Fennel oil
Peppermint oil
Thyme oil (diluted)

**Mouth, *inflammation
of mucous membranes***
Geranium oil
Lemon oil
Myrrh oil
Sage oil
Tea Tree oil

Mouth, *thrush*
Cinnamon oil
Geranium oil
*Myrrh oil
Savory oil
*Tea Tree oil
Thyme oil

Mouth, *ulcers*
Camphor oil
Myrrh oil
Pennyroyal oil
Sage oil
Tea Tree oil

**Muscles, *aching or
sore***
Birch oil
Cajeput oil
Eucalyptus citriodora oil
Ginger oil
Juniper oil
Lavender oil
Lemon oil
Pepper oils
Pine oil
Roman Chamomile oil
Rosemary oil
Tangerine oil

**Muscles, *tension or
stiffness***
Chamomile oils
Eucalyptus oil
Lavender oil
Pepper oils
Tangerine oil

Muscles, *tonic for*
(see Tonic, *body*)

Nausea
Cardamom oil
Cinnamon oil *(in
pregnancy)*
*Fennel oil
*Ginger oil
Lavender oil
Melissa oil
*Peppermint oil

**Nerves, *to ease
nervous tension &
stress***
Angelica oil
Basil oil
Bergamot oil
Camphor oil
Carrot Seed oil
*Chamomile oils
Cypress oil
Galbanum oil
Geranium oil
Grapefruit oil
Jasmine oil
*Lavender oil
Lemon oil
Lemongrass oil
Lime oil
*Marjoram oil
*Melissa oil
Orange oil
Neroli oil
Patchouli oil
Petitgrain oil
Pine oil
Roman Chamomile oil
Rose oil
*Rosemary oil
Rosewood oil
Sandalwood oil
Tangerine oil
Vetiver oil
Ylang-Ylang oil

22

TABLE 1

Nerves, *tonic for*
Clary Sage oil
Cypress oil
Lavender oil
Marjoram oil
Onion oil
Petitgrain oil
Rosemary oil
Sage oil
Thyme oil

Nervousness
Benzoin, inhale
Bergamot oil
Camphor oil
Chamomile oils
Lavender oil
Lemon oil
Marjoram oil
Myrrh oil
Neroli oil
Orange oil
Roman Chamomile oil
Tangerine oil

Neuralgia
Eucalyptus oil
Geranium oil
Pennyroyal oil
Peppermint oil
Roman Chamomile oil
Turpentine oil

Neurasthenia
(*mental fatigue*)
Basil oil
Clary Sage oil
Lavender oil
Marjoram oil
Rosemary oil

Nightmares
(see Anxiety; Nerves)

Nosebleed
Cypress oil
Frankincense oil
Lemon oil

Obesity
Juniper oil
Lemon oil

Overexcitement
(see Nerves)

Oxidation, *to inhibit in food & cosmetics*
Benzoin or Benzoic acid
Ginger oil
Grapefruit oil

Pain
(*analgesics*)
Bergamot oil
Birch oil
Camphor oil
Eucalyptus oil
Geranium oil
Lavender oil
Marjoram oil
Peppermint oil
Roman Chamomile oil
Rosemary oil
Wintergreen oil

Paralysis
Basil oil
Lavender oil
Peppermint oil
Rosemary oil
Sage oil

Phobia
(see also Anxiety)
Jasmine oil
Melissa oil
Neroli oil

Pimples
Cedar oil
Helichrysum oil
Tea Tree oil

PMS, *moodiness and*
Bergamot oil
*Clary Sage oil
Galbanum oil
Geranium oil
Jasmine oil
Neroli oil
Patchouli oil
Rose oil
Rosewood oil
Tangerine oil
Ylang-Ylang oil

PMS, *water retention and*
Agnus castus tincture
Cypress oil
Fennel oil
Geranium oil
Juniper oil
Rosemary oil
Spruce oil

Pneumonia
Camphor oil
Fir oil

Poisoning, *food*
Apple cider vinegar
Garlic oil
Lavender oil
Pepper oils
Thyme oil

Polyps, *nose*
Calendula oil

Prostatitis
Fir oil
Jasmine oil
Onion oil
Thuja oil

Pruritus
(see Genitals, *itching of*)
Tea Tree oil

Psoriasis
(see Skin, *psoriasis*)

Regeneration after Illness
Basil oil
Clary Sage oil
Clove oil
Eucalyptus citriodora oil
Ginseng
Hyssop oil
Lemon oil
Rosemary oil
Thyme oil

Respiratory System, *inflammation of mucous membrane of*
Cajeput oil
Cedarwood oil
Hyssop oil
Inula oil
Lavender oil
Myrrh oil
Sandalwood oil

Respiratory System, *removing secretion and mucus*
(*expectorant*)
Basil oil
Benzoin, inhale
Bergamot oil
Cedarwood oil
Eucalyptus oil
Hyssop oil
Inula oil
Marjoram oil
Myrrh oil
Pennyroyal oil
Peppermint oil
Rosemary oil
Sandalwood oil
Spruce oil

Rheumatism
Camphor oil
Citronella oil
Coriander oil
Cypress oil
Eucalyptus oil
Fir oil
Garlic oil
Ginger oil
Juniper oil
*Lavender oil
Lemon oil
Lemongrass oil
Marjoram oil
Nutmeg oil
Onion oil
Oregano oil
Pepper oils
*Rosemary oil
Sage oil
Sassafras oil
Thuja oil
Thyme oil
Turpentine oil

Ringworm
Bergamot oil
Cinnamon oil
Clove oil
Lavender oil
Neem oil
Peppermint oil
Tea Tree oil
Thyme oil
Turpentine oil

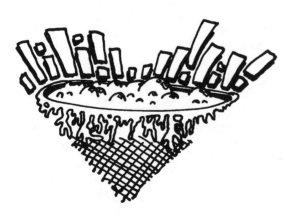

TABLE 1

Rubefacient
(produces warmth and redness when externally applied)
Eucalyptus oil
Ginger oil
Juniper oil
Marjoram oil
Pepper oils
Rosemary oil

Scabies
Bergamot oil
Birch tar
Lavender oil
Peppermint oil
Pine oil
Rosemary oil

Scarlet Fever
Eucalyptus oil

Scars, *to minimize*
Helichrysum italicum
  plus
  Rosa rubinginosa oils
Malva-infused oil

Sedatives *(calming)*
Chamomile oils
Clary Sage oil
Frankincense oil
*Lavender oil
Linden blossom tea
Marjoram oil
Melissa oil
Neroli oil
Rose oil
Sandalwood oil
Spikenard oil
Valerian oil

Shock
Camphor oil
Melissa oil
Peppermint oil

Sinusitis
Cajeput oil
Eucalyptus oil
Fir oil
*Garlic oil
Inula oil
Lavender oil
Lemon oil
Peppermint oil
Tea Tree oil
Thyme oil

Skin, *acne*
Bergamot oil
Cajeput oil
Camphor oil
Cedarwood oil
Galbanum oil
Geranium oil
Helichrysum oil
Jasmine oil
Juniper oil
Lavender oil
Lavender Spike oil
Myrtle oil
Patchouli oil
Peppermint oil
Roman Chamomile oil
Rose oil
Sandalwood oil
Sweet Thyme oil
*Tea Tree oil

Skin, *astringent oils*
Bergamot oil
Cedarwood oil
Cypress oil
Frankincense oil
Geranium oil
Immortelle oil
Juniper oil
Lemon oil
Myrrh oil
Myrtle oil
Rosemary oil
Sandalwood oil

Skin, *bathing*
Dill oil ⎫
Lavender oil ⎬ stimulating
Rosemary oil ⎭
Thyme oil ⎫
Sandalwood oil ⎬ relaxing
Ylang-Ylang oil ⎭

Skin, *broken veins*
Cypress oil
Parsley oil
Roman Chamomile oil
*Rose oil

Skin, *calluses, horny skin*
Benzoin tincture
Clove oil
Garlic oil
Orange oil
Rosehip Seed oil

Skin, *chapped*
Benzoin tincture
Blue Chamomile oil
Carrot Seed oil
Geranium oil
Immortelle oil
Lavender oil
Lemon oil
Myrrh oil
Onion oil
Patchouli oil
Rose oil
Sandalwood oil

Skin, *to cleanse*
Basil oil
Juniper oil
Lemon oil
Niaouli oil
Peppermint oil

Skin, *congested*
Basil oil
Juniper oil
Lemon oil
Niaouli oil
Peppermint oil

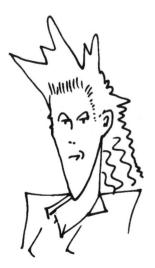

Skin, *dermatitis, inflammations and diseases of*
Blue Chamomile oil
Cajeput oil
Carrot Seed oil
Cedarwood oil
Cinnamon oil
Clove oil
Eucalyptus oil
Hyssop oil
Immortelle oil
Juniper oil
Myrrh oil
Onion oil
Peppermint oil
Rosehip Seed oil
Sage oil
Sandalwood oil
Thyme oil

Skin, *dry*
Carrot Seed oil
Cedarwood oil
Geranium oil
Immortelle oil
Jasmine oil
Lavender oil
Lemon Verbena oil
Niaouli oil
Orange oil
Rose oil
Rosewood oil
Sandalwood oil
Ylang-Ylang oil

Skin, *freckles*
Lemon oil
Onion oil

Skin, *infections*
Blue Chamomile oil
Eucalyptus oil
Garlic oil
Lavender oil
Myrrh oil
Roman Chamomile oil
Rosemary oil
Spikenard oil
Tea Tree oil

Skin, *inflammation*
Benzoin extract
Bergamot oil
Blue Chamomile oil
Carrot Seed oil
Cedarwood oil
Eucalyptus oil
Geranium oil
Hyssop oil
Immortelle oil
Jasmine oil
Lavender oil
Myrrh oil
Niaouli oil
Patchouli oil
Peppermint oil
Roman Chamomile oil
Rose oil
Sandalwood oil
Tea Tree oil

Skin, *irritated*
(for sensitive skin)
Artemisia arborescens oil
Geranium oil
Helichrysum oil
Inula oil
Lavender oil
Myrrh oil
Roman Chamomile oil
Rose oil

TABLE 1

Skin, *itching*
Benzoin tincture
Jasmine oil
Lavender oil
Peppermint oil
Roman Chamomile oil

**Skin, *mature,*
*rejuvenating oils for***
Cypress oil
Fennel oil
Frankincense oil
Lavender oil
Myrrh oil
Neroli oil
Orange oil
Patchouli oil
Rose oil
Rosehip Seed oil
Sandalwood oil
Spikenard oil
Vetiver oil

Skin, *normal*
Bergamot oil
Cedarwood oil
Geranium oil
Jasmine oil
Lavender oil
Neroli oil
Roman Chamomile oil
Rose oil
Rosewood oil
Ylang-Ylang oil

Skin, *oily*
Bergamot oil
Cajeput oil
Camphor oil
Cedarwood oil
Cypress oil
Eucalyptus oil
Frankincense oil
Geranium oil
Juniper oil
Lavender oil
Lemon oil
Lemongrass oil
Orange oil
Peppermint oil
Rose oil
Rosemary oil
Sandalwood oil
Ylang-Ylang oil

**Skin, *pimples or*
*blemished***
Galbanum oil
Immortelle oil
Lavender oil
Lemon oil
Rosemary oil
Sage oil
Tea Tree oil
Thyme oil

Skin, *psoriasis*
Bergamot oil
Galbanum oil
Lavender oil

Skin, *to regenerate*
Frankincense oil
Lavender oil
Neroli oil
Patchouli oil
Rose oil
Rosemary oil
Sandalwood oil
Tea Tree oil

Skin, *sensitive*
Jasmine oil
Neroli oil
Orange oil
Roman Chamomile oil
Rose oil

Skin, *to tone*
Calendula oil
Chamomile oils
Lavender oil
Neroli oil
Orange oil
Rose oil
Rosemary oil
Thyme oil

Skin, *wrinkles*
Anise oil
Carrot Seed oil
Cypress oil
Fennel oil
Frankincense oil
Myrrh oil
Neroli oil
Rose oil
Rosehip Seed oil

Sleep Aids
Heliotrope oil
Vanilla oil

Spasms, antispasmodics
Basil oil
Bergamot oil
Camphor oil
Cardamom oil
Clary Sage oil
Coriander oil
Cypress oil
Eucalyptus oil
Fennel oil
Hyssop oil
Juniper oil
Lavender oil
Marjoram oil
Pennyroyal oil
Peppermint oil
Roman Chamomile oil
Rose oil
Rosemary oil

Spleen, tonic
(splenetic)
Black Pepper oil
Fennel oil
Kewda oil
Parsley oil
Roman Chamomile oil
Rose oil

Sprains
Birch oil
Camphor oil
Eucalyptus oil
Lavender oil
Rosemary oil

Sterility, in women
Geranium oil
Jasmine oil
Rose oil

Stimulants, body
Black Pepper oil
Camphor oil
Cardamom oil
Coriander oil
Eucalyptus oil
Garlic oil
Geranium oil
Juniper oil
Lemon oil
Onion oil
*Peppermint oil
*Rosemary oil
Sage oil
Thyme oil

Stomach, digestive & dyspepsia
Anise oil
Basil oil
Bergamot oil
Caraway oil
Cardamom oil
Dill oil
Eucalyptus oil
Fennel oil
Frankincense oil
Juniper oil
Lavender oil
Marjoram oil
Pepper oils
Peppermint oil
Roman Chamomile oil
Rosemary oil

Stomach, gastralgia or gastritis
Roman Chamomile oil

Stomach, heartburn
Cardamom oil
Pepper oils

Stomach, highly acidic
Lemon oil
Peppermint oil

Stomach, infection
Immortelle oil

Stomach, inflammation of mucous membranes
Lemon oil
Pennyroyal oil
Roman Chamomile oil

Stomach, tonic
Basil oil
Cardamom oil
Fennel oil
Juniper oil
Lemongrass oil
Lemon Verbena oil
Melissa oil
Myrrh oil
Oregano oil
Pepper oils
Peppermint oil
Roman Chamomile oil
Rose oil
Savory oil
Tangerine oil

Stress
Chamomile oils
Eucalyptus oil
Geranium oil
Grapefruit oil
Lavender oil
Pine oil
Spearmint oil

TABLE 1

Stretch Marks
Carnation oil
Helichrysum oil
Jasmine oil

Sudorific
(see Sweat)

Sunburn
Aloe vera gel
Immortelle oil
Lavender oil
Lemon oil
Peppermint oil
Roman Chamomile oil

Sunstroke
Lavender oil
Lemon oil
Melissa oil
Peppermint oil
Rose oil

Suprarenal Gland, tonic
(see also Adrenal
  Gland)
Fir oil
Geranium oil
Sage oil

Sweat, *to induce*
Camphor oil
Juniper oil
Pennyroyal oil
Peppermint oil
Rosemary oil
Sassafras oil
Yarrow oil

Sweat, *to reduce*
(see Deodorants)
Clary Sage oil
Rose oil
Sage oil

Teeth, *aching*
Cajeput oil
Clove oil
Nutmeg oil
Pennyroyal oil
Peppermint oil
Roman Chamomile oil
Sage oil

Teeth & Teething
Roman Chamomile oil

Tendonitis
(see also Rheumatism)
Birch oil
Rosemary oil

Throat, *sore*
Clary Sage oil
Eucalyptus oil
Geranium oil
Lavender oil
Melissa oil
Tea Tree oil
Thyme oil

Thrush
Myrrh oil
Tea Tree oil

Thyroid
Lemon oil
Palmarosa oil

Tissue, *fatty*
(*reducing*)
Juniper oil
Lemon oil

Tonic, *body strengthener*
Basil oil
Black Pepper oil
Cardamom oil
Coriander oil
Fennel oil
Frankincense oil
Geranium oil
Hyssop oil
Jasmine oil
Juniper oil
Lavender oil
Marjoram oil
Melissa oil
Myrrh oil
Neroli oil
Nutmeg oil
Roman Chamomile oil
Rose oil
Sandalwood oil
Tea Tree oil

Tonsilitis
Bergamot oil
Violet oil

Tuberculosis
Bergamot oil
Camphor oil
Eucalyptus oil
Hyssop oil
Lavender oil
Myrrh oil

Tumors
Cajeput oil
Eucalyptus oil
Tea Tree oil

Typhus
Lavender oil (*fever*)
Lemon oil

Urinary Stones
Fennel oil
Geranium oil
Hyssop oil
Juniper oil
Lemon oil
Roman Chamomile oil

Urinary Tract, *infection or inflammation of*
Bergamot oil
Cedarwood oil
Eucalyptus oil
Juniper oil
Lavender oil
Myrrh oil
Onion oil
Sandalwood oil
Tea Tree oil
Turpentine oil

Urine, *to stimulate secretion*
Anise oil
Benzoin extract
Camphor oil
Cardamom oil
Eucalyptus oil
Fennel oil
Garlic oil
Geranium oil
Juniper oil
Lavender oil
Onion oil
Pepper oils
Rosemary oil
Sage oil

Uterus, *tonic for*
Frankincense oil
Jasmine oil
Melissa oil
Myrrh oil
Rose oil

Vaginal Discharge
(see Genitals, *vaginal discharge from*)

Vaginitis
Roman Chamomile oil
Tea Tree oil

Varicose Veins
Bergamot oil
Cypress oil
Garlic oil
Juniper oil
Lemon oil

Vasoconstrictor
(constriction of capillaries)
Camphor oil
Chamomile oils
Cypress oil
Peppermint oil
Rose oil

Vasodilator
(small blood vessels expand)
Marjoram oil

Veins, *broken*
(see Skin, *broken veins*)

Viral Infection
Bergamot oil
Eucalyptus oil
Garlic oil
Rose oil
Tea Tree oil
Thyme oil

Voice, *loss*
Cypress oil
Lavender oil
Lemon oil
Melissa oil
Thyme oil

Vomiting
Basil oil
*Ginger oil
Lavender oil
Melissa oil
Peppermint oil
Roman Chamomile oil
Rose oil
Sandalwood oil

Vulnerary, *helps wounds heal*
Benzoin tincture
Calendula oil
Chamomile oils
*Lavender oil
Myrrh oil
*Tea Tree oil

Wake Up
Coumarin scent
*Jasmine oil
Peppermint scent
*Rosemary oil

TABLE 1

Warts
  Castor oil
  Clove oil
  Garlic oil
  Lavender oil
  Lemon oil
  Onion oil
  Thuja oil

Weight Loss
(see Appetite, *reducing*)
  Bergamot oil
  Fennel oil
  *Lavender oil
  Onion oil

Whooping Cough
(see Cough, *whooping*)

Worms
(see Intestines, *worms*)
  Hyssop oil
  Onion oil
  Tarragon oil
  Thuja oil
  *Turpentine oil

Wounds, *healing of*
(*formation of scar tissue*)
  Benzoin tincture
  Bergamot oil
  Camphor oil
  Clary Sage oil
  Eucalyptus oil
  Frankincense oil
  Geranium oil
  Helichrysum oil
  Hyssop oil
  Juniper oil
  *Lavender oil
  Marjoram oil
  Myrrh oil
  Patchouli oil
  Roman Chamomile oil
  Rosemary oil
  Sage oil
  Savory oil
  *Tea Tree oil

Wrinkles
(see Skin, *wrinkles*)
  Neroli oil
  Rose oil

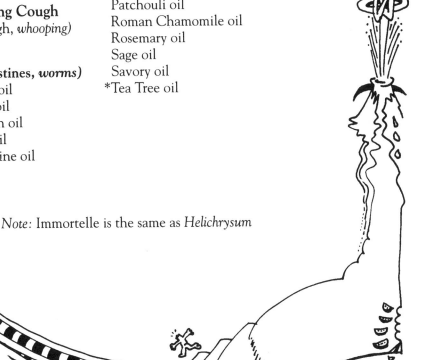

Note: Immortelle is the same as *Helichrysum*

31

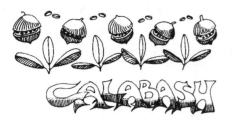

Table 2.
Essential Oils . . .
Healing Powers and
Uses

by Victoria Edwards*

We have marked with a star (*) the strongest or most appropriate.
⬗ denotes a warning.

Allspice oil
Gives added
  determination
Stimulant
Stomach tonic
Very vitalizing

Angelica oil
Anorexia
Asthma
Heart and Lung
  problems, apply 1
  drop above each
  breast
Legendary scent of the
  angels
Stomach ulcers
Perfume

Anise seed oil
1 drop: 8 oz. water, sip
Asthma
Colic
Coughs
Flatulence
Gland stimulant
Heartbeat, irregular
Impotence
Indigestion
Migraine
Painful periods

Aspic oil
A variety of Lavender
Usage similar to
  Lavender
Also called Spike
  Lavender

Basil oil
Bath and hair oil
*Brain and memory
  stimulant
*Depression
Insect bites
*Intellectual overwork
Sinus
*Soothes nerves
Stomach cramps
*Stress
•Inhale: A drop in
  palms of hand, rub
  together briskly and
  inhale

Bay Laurel oil
Insect repellent
Masculine scent
Sinus headaches
Stimulating
Uplifting

*used by permission of Victoria Edwards, Leydet Oils, P. O. Box 2354, Fair
Oaks, CA 95628

TABLE 2

Benzoin
  Euphoric
  Fixative in perfumes
  Seductive
  Sensual
  •Inhale: Uplifting for
    tired mind

Bergamot oil
  Acne
  Antiseptic
  Cold sores
  Depression
  Eczema
  External infections
  Gallstones
  Herpes
  Intestinal parasites
  Nervousness
  Psoriasis
  Soothes nerves
  Used in perfumery (do
    not use on skin prior
    to sun exposure)

**Birch oil
(Sweet Birch oil)**
  Astringent
  Counter-irritant
  Flavoring agent
  Similar to Wintergreen
    oil
  Sore, stiff muscles and
    joints

⬧ Bitter Almond oil
  Flavoring and scenting
    agent
  Can cause skin rash
  Not recommended

Black Pepper oil
  (add a few drops to
    bath or massage oil)
  *Frigidity
  Good for cold
    conditions
  *Impotency
  Restores tone to lax
    muscles
  Stimulates digestive
    system
  Stimulates respiratory
    system
  Stimulates urinary
    system
  •Inhale: Stimulating to
    the mind

Bois de Rose oil
  Acne
  Kidneys (5 drops in a
    bath)
  Perfume
  Skin care
  Substituted for Rose oil
  Used for making the
    finest-sounding
    musical instruments

Borneol Camphor oil
  Acne
  Chapped skin
  Cold sores
  Disinfects the
    alimentary canal
  Combats infectious
    diseases (has dual
    action of heating and
    cooling the skin)
  Interferes with
    homeopathic remedies
  Moth repellent
  ~~Only use white
    camphor, the yellow
    and brown are too
    toxic
  Strengthens the heart
  Warming liniment

Cajeput oil
  Asthma
  Bronchitis
  Earache
  Laryngitis
  Skin diseases
  Toothache
  •Inhale: To improve
    mental concentration

**Calendula (Marigold)
oil**
  Heals wounds, bruises,
    burns

Camphor oil
  Bruises and sprains—
    as compresses

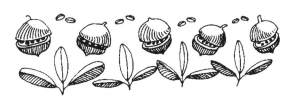

Caraway oil
Circulation
Digestive aid
Flavoring agent
Intestinal parasites
Mange in dogs
Scabies
Stimulant and
  carminative
Stimulates lymphatic
  system
Toothache
•Inhale: Refreshing to
  the conscious mind
•Inhale: To enhance
  alertness

Cardamom oil
Colic
Digestive aid
Mental fatigue
Nervousness
Pregnancy nausea
Vomiting, after-effect
  of
•Inhale: Aphrodisiac
•Inhale: Clears
  conscious mind
•Inhale: Stimulates
  appetite
•Inhale: Uplifting

Carrot Seed oil
Aging skin
Aids in retention of
  urine
Contains Vitamin A
Dry skin
Hepatic
Skin diseases
Wrinkles

Celery Seed oil
Bronchitis
Calming
Carminative
Diuretic
Good for nervousness
Good for swollen
  glands
Sedative
Stimulant
•Inhale: Awaken
  psychic awareness
•Inhale: Restful sleep

Cedarwood oil
Acne
Antiseptic for skin
  conditions
Astringent
Dandruff
Oily skin
Respiratory infections
Sedative
Urinary infections
The first known oil
  ever extracted
•Inhale: Balance
•Inhale: Calming
•Inhale: Promotes
  spirituality
⬦ **Note:** Not to be used
  in pregnancy.

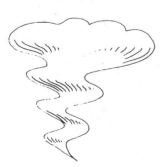

Chamomile oil
Acne
Calming
Headache
Liver problems
Migraines
Pains anywhere in the
  body
Soothing to
  inflammations of the
  skin (good for
  hyperallergenic and/or
  hypersensitivity)
Soothing to the nerves
Stress reducer
•Inhale: Peaceful
  feelings
•Inhale: Relaxing agent

Cinnamon leaf oil
Colds
Coughs
Digestion

Cinnamon oil
Antiseptic
Bath and massage oil
Dry heaves
Foot fungus
Sexual stimulant
Stimulant
Warming
•Inhale: Tap into
  psychic minds
⬦ **Note:** Must be
  diluted, can cause skin
  irritation if applied
  directly.

TABLE 2

Citronella oil
Hair oil
Heart stimulant
Insect repellent
Massage oil
Perfumery

Cistus oil
Insomnia
Musky scent
Nervousness
Perfumery
Skin conditions
Tonic

Clary Sage oil
Adrenal stimulant
Aids childbirth
Depression
Emotional stress
Encourages labor
(birthing)
Gargle for sore throat
Helps mother relax
Mildly intoxicating
Menopause
Nervousness
Perfumery
PMS
Relaxant
Soft, sweet herbaceous
note
Strengthens kidneys
Strengthens stomach
•Inhale: Euphoric

◊ Clove oil
Analgesic
Anti-cancerous
Antiseptic
Aphrodisiac
Mouthwash
Sores
Stimulant
Toothache remedy
Ulcers
Uterine tonic in labor
•Inhale: Facilitates
retrieval of long-
buried memories
•Inhale: Helps your
ability to memorize
Note: Needs to be
diluted or will burn
the skin.

Cumin oil
Exotic
Good for poor
circulation (massage)
Oriental
Stimulating spice note
in cooking and
perfumery
•Ritual: Protects the
home and for internal
protection

Cypress oil
Balsamic
Hemorrhoids
Menopause
Menstrual problems
Refreshing
Respiratory sedative
Spasmodic coughs
Sweet and balsamic
Varicose veins
Vasoconstrictor
•Inhale: For loss of
friends
•Inhale: For smoothing
transitions

Dill Weed oil
Carminative
Colic in babies
Dry heaves
Flavoring agent
•Inhale: Clears the
mind
•Inhale: Sharpens your
awareness

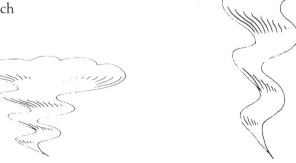

Eucalyptus oil
Bronchitis
Coughs
Diabetes
Disinfectant
Herpes
Influenza
Malaria
Measles
Respiratory tract
 infections
Sinuses
Sore muscles
Tuberculosis
Typhoid Fever
•Inhale: Heals
 respiratory system
•Ritual: Purifies, heals
 room of negative
 conflict

Eucalyptus citriodora oil
Herpes
Joint pain
Soothing and calming
 in baths and massage
 oil
Recuperating from long
 illness

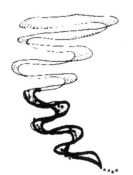

Evening Primrose oil
The oil is high in
 GLA-GAMA-
 Linolenic acid.
Used successfully to
 treat:
Arthritis
Asthma
Breast tenderness
Depression
Eczema
Hangovers
High blood pressure
Overweight
PMS

Fennel oil
Alcohol withdrawal
Antidote for poisonous
 mushrooms
Aperitif
Colic in babies
Dentifrice
Diuretic
Expectorant
Flatulence
Flu prevention
Increases breast milk
Indigestion
Laxative
Nervous vomiting
Relieves nausea
Stimulates estrogen
Tonic
•Inhale: Thought to
 increase lifespan
•Inhale: Thought to
 produce courage

Fir oil
Bronchitis
Nervous system
Respiratory
Stomach cramps
Urinary tract
•Inhale: Has elevating
 and grounding effect
 on mind and emotions

Frankincense oil
Antiseptic
Astringent (uterine,
 mucous membranes)
Digestive aid
Elevating
Expectorant
Hemorrhages
Infections of urinary
 tract
Leprosy
Sedative
Warming
•Inhale: Calms and
 awakens higher
 consciousness
•Inhale: Soothing effect
 on the mind and
 emotions
•Ritual: Burned in the
 Catholic Church for
 protection from evil
 spirits
•Ritual: Meditation

Galbanum oil
Perfumery
Rejuvenates aging skin
Represents the
 elements of air
Very bitter, blends well
 with sweet florals

TABLE 2

Geranium oil
(Rose Geranium)
Anxiety states
Balances adrenals
Balances hormones
Blends well with other
  oils
Diarrhea
Dry or oily skin
Gallstones
Jaundice
Massage or bath oils
Menopause
Sedative
Uplifting
• Inhale: Harmonious
  effect, calms and
  refreshes the body and
  psyche

Ginger oil
Antiseptic
Appetite stimulant
Breaks up congestion
  as a massage oil
Laxative
Rheumatic pains
Stomachic
Tonic
• Inhale: Promotes
  courage, confidence,
  also aggression
• Ritual: Purification and
  success

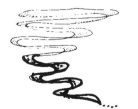

Grapefruit oil
Acts upon gall bladder
Astringent
Cellulitis
Digestive aid
Facial toner
Lymphatic stimulant
Obesity
Water retention
• Inhale: Induces
  euphoria

Honeysuckle oil
Asthma
Helps relieve nostalgia
Perfumery
Respiratory
Skin beautifier
• Inhale: Strengthen
  psychic awareness
• Ritual: Used in
  visualizing an increase
  in money flow

Hyssop oil
Asthma
Cancerous growths
Coughs
Eczema
Hay fever
Hypotension
  (hypertensive)
Parasites
Sore throat
Stimulates the medulla
  oblongata
• Inhale: Clears the head
  and vision
• Ritual: Heighten
  spirituality prior to
  religious rituals

Jasmine oil
Aphrodisiac
Childbirthing
Emotionally soothing
Frigidity
King of Flowers
Relaxing
Traditionally sacred to
  the spiritual use of the
  generative process
• Inhale: Emotionally
  soothing
• Inhale: Dispels
  depression
• Ritual: Affects on the
  emotional centers; for
  love rituals
• Ritual: Capable of
  leading us into
  brighter worlds of
  fantasy and sensuality

Juniper oil
Antiseptic
Arthritis
Astringent
Baths are invigorating
Cystitis
Diabetes
Diuretic
Paralysis
Specific for depleted
  kidney and bladder
  energy (bath)
• Inhale: Visualize being
  guarded from
  negativity and danger

Labdanum oil

Heals wounds
Insomnia
Nervousness
Perfumery
Sedative
Spinal degeneration (as
a massage oil)
•Ritual: Meditation

Lavender oil

Acne
Bath oil
Brain stimulant
Burns
Childbirth
Depression
Diverse applications
Douche
Hair and scalp
Headaches
Migraines
Nervous tension
Relaxation
Scalds
Skin care
•Inhale: Lightens
energy when we are
agitated, over-excited
or over-wrought

Lemon oil

Bactericidal
Chilblains
Detoxification
Infectious diseases
Liver stimulant and
cleanser
Oily skin
Purification
Wrinkles
•Inhale: Dispels
sluggishness
•Inhale: Stimulates
CNS

Lemongrass oil

Bath and massage oil
Indigestion
Oily skin
Perfumery
Purifier
Uplifting
•Inhale: Stimulates
psychic awareness

Lemon Verbena oil

Fever
Perfumery
Purifier
Sedative
Skin care
•Ritual: To excite
spiritual love

Lemon Thyme oil

Same as Thyme; see
Thyme

Lime oil

Astringent
Bronchitis
Deodorant
Liver pains
Stomach cramps

Linden Flower oil

Colds
Headache
Healing
Honey-like fragrance
Hysteria
Nervine
Perfumery
Promotes perspiration
Relaxing
Tonic
•Inhale: For high-
anxiety emotional
states
•Inhale: Quieting and
soothing effect

Mace oil

Carminative
Perfumery
Soap scenting
•Ritual: Enhance
psychic awareness
•Ritual: Lead you to
deep consciousness

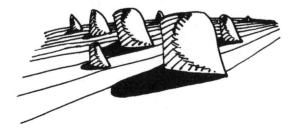

TABLE 2

Marjoram oil
Arthritis
Asthma
Bruises
Colds
Colic
Douches
Excessive sexuality
Insomnia
*Migraine
Muscle spasms
Nervous tension
Rheumatic pain
Sedative
Sprains
• Inhale: To allay
  anxiety and grief or
  love-obsession
• Inhale: To halt the
  desire for sexual
  contact

Melissa oil
Allergies
*Cold sores
Depression
Fevers
General tonic
*Herpes
Indigestion
Infertility
Menstrual irregularities
Nausea
Nervous tension
Rejuvenates
Shock
Vertigo
• Inhale: Brings peace of
  mind
• Inhale: Emotional
  serenity (a woman's
  oil)

Mimosa oil
Perfumery
Sensitivity
• Ritual: Anoint
  forehead before bed
  for prophetic dreams
• Ritual: With
  visualization to bring
  love

Mugwort oil
Bronchitis
Calming
Colds
Moxibustion
Nervousness
Poison Oak remedy
Regulates the female
  cycle
Sore muscles
• Inhale: With herbs in
  "dream pillows"
⚬ **Note:** Not to be used
  during pregnancy or
  lactation.

Mullein (infused) oil
Earache
Sore joints
Stretch marks
Sunburn

Myrrh oil
Cools the skin
Cuts
Embalming
Laryngitis
Preserves flesh
Purification
Reduces inflammation
Reduces wrinkles
Ulcers
Uterine disorders
Wasting degenerative
  diseases (massage), for
Wounds
Youthful complexion
• Inhale: Expands
  awareness
• Inhale: Calms fears
  about the future
• Ritual: For past-life
  regression

Myrtle oil
Antiseptic
Diarrhea
Douche
Emblem of love
Respiratory system
Skin wash
Tonic
• Inhale: Balances
  energy system

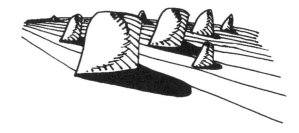

Narcissus oil
Narcotic effect
Soothes the nerves
Sweet floral
- Inhale: Relaxes the mind
- Ritual: To enrich love already shared with another
- Ritual: To manifest new relationships
- ⬡ **Note:** Do not take internally.

Niaouli oil
Antiseptic
Bronchitis
Burns
Earache
Infection
Influenza
Laryngitis
Protects immune system from virus
Wounds
- Inhale: To raise the energy and form a shield against negative energy
- Ritual: To combat a psychic attack from another

Neroli oil
*Antidepressant
Aphrodisiac
Deodorant
Diarrhea
Facial softener
*Insomnia
Light and woody backnote
Perfumery
Sedative
- Inhale: Joyous and uplifting

⬡ Nutmeg oil
Carminative
Diarrhea (rubbed in diluted form)
Digestive stimulant
Rheumatism
Strong psycho-stimulant
- Ritual: Bring money into one's life
Note: Toxic in large doses.

Oakmoss oil
Congested sinus
Earthy bass note
Headache
Perfumery
Used in chypre blends
- Ritual: Increase cash flow
- Ritual: Increase personal prosperity
- Ritual: For visualization

Opopanax oil
Musty balsamic smell
Perfumery
Similar to Myrrh and Frankincense

Orange oil, Sweet Orange
Anxiety states
Baths
Calming
Colds
Expels gas from intestines
Insomnia
Nervousness
Revives wrinkled skin
Skin care

Oregano oil
Analgesic
*Antiseptic
Expectorant
Infections
Lowers cholesterol levels in blood
Muscle relaxant
Stimulant
- Inhale: Energizes, helps you to accomplish household tasks

TABLE 2

Orris oil
Colic
Cosmetics
Coughs
Dentifrices
Diuretic
Hoarseness
Perfumery
Stomachic
• Ritual: Spread on bed
  sheets to induce
  amorous feelings
  Ritual: Used in love
  rituals

Parsley oil
Benefits nerve centers
  in head and spine
Soothing to stomach,
  kidneys, spleen and
  intestines
◌ **Note:** Toxic in large
  doses

Patchouli oil
Cures apathy
Dry skin
Eases confusion and
  indecision
Endocrine glands
Nerve stimulant
Peace of mind
Scent of '60s hippies
Seductive
Stimulant
Rejuvenating
• Inhale: Relieve
  confusion

Palmarosa oil
Acne
Cellular stimulant
Hydrating
Perfumery
Refreshing (lemony
  rose scent)
Skin care
Wrinkles
• Ritual: Inhale for
  attracting love

Peppermint oil
Analgesic
Antiseptic
Children's oil
Colds
Cooling
Digestive disorders
Fevers
Flu
Headaches
Kidney and gallstones
Menstrual cramps
Nausea
Respiratory disorders
Sedative
• Inhale: To halt
  negative thoughts

◌Pennyroyal oil
Causes abortion
Headache
Insect repellent
Liver and spleen tonic
Nervous disturbances
Reduces fevers
Relieves seasickness
Rids fleas
Toothache
Used for female
  disorders
• Ritual: For protection

Petitgrain of Orange oil
(Made from leaves)
Bitter
Digestive aid
Floral
Fresh
Invigorating
Perfumery
Tonic
Used to sharpen
  awareness

Peru Balsam oil
Disinfectant
Expectorant
Perfumery
Ringworm
Stimulant
Stomachic
Used externally on
  sores
Used for stomach
  ulcers

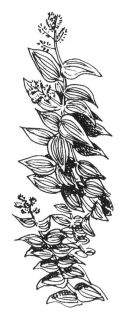

Pine oil
Aches and pains
Antiseptic for
  respiratory tract
Baths
Fatigue
Flu
Gout
Joint pains
Kidney and bladder
Male stimulant
Male restorative
Massage oil
Sinus
Stimulant of the
  adrenal cortex
•Ritual: Protection
•Ritual: To attract
  money

Rose oil
Acts upon the liver,
  stomach and blood
Cleansing and
  regulating
Cooling
Depression
Drives away
  melancholy
Female sex organs (the
  physical aspect of the
  female symbol)
Increases semen
Laxative
Mature dry skin
Perfumery
Sedative
Sensitive skin
Skin care
Soothing
Tonic (psychological
  impotence)
•Inhale: To calm
  domestic strife
•Ritual: The power to
  unite physical and
  spiritual love, the
  source of beauty, joy
  and happiness

Rose Geranium oil
(See also Geranium)
Calms and refreshes
  the psyche and body
Massage oil
Perfumery
Potpourris
Skin oil for aged,
  wrinkled skin

Rosemary oil
A universal aid
Arthritis
General weakness
Hair and skin
Hair tonic
Liver and gall bladder
  stimulant
Loss of memory
Mental fatigue
Stimulates mind and
  body

Rosemary Verbenon oil
Dry skin
Liver and gall bladder
  disorders

Sage oil
Aches and pains
Dries up milk when
  nursing
Gargle for sore throat
Menopause
Nerve and adrenal
  stimulant
Restores the energy of
  the whole organism
Used to reduce labor
  pains

TABLE 2

St. John's Wort oil
Burns
Nerve and spinal
  trauma
Ulcers
Whiplash injuries
Wounds
•Ritual: Balances all
  chakras
•Ritual: Heals
  emotional pain in the
  sensitive

Sandalwood oil
Acne
Aphrodisiac
Bladder infections
Depression
Diarrhea
Dry skin
Gonorrhea
Massage oils
Nervous tension
Sedative
Strep and staph
  infections
Sweet, woody scent

Savory oil
Antiseptic
Digestive and mental
  stimulant
Fungus infections
Insect bites
Intestinal parasites
Nervous and other
  stomachaches
Sexual debility

Sassafras oil
Arthritis
Exhaustion
Poison Oak or Ivy
Perfumery
Rheumatism
Skin diseases

Spearmint oil
Appetite stimulant
Douching
Flavoring agent
Massage and bath oils
Refreshing to skin and
  muscles
Stimulating
Women's complaints

Spikenard (Nard) oil
Anti-aging
Incurable skin
  problems
Ritual plus Anointing
  oil

Spruce oil
Expectorant
Lung congestion
Respiratory antiseptic
Tightens watery tissue

Styrax oil
(See Benzoin)
  Mixed with Labdanum
  to make Amber oil
Perfumery

Tarragon oil
Anorexia
Balances the nervous
  system
Digestive problems
  caused by emotions
Painful or irregular
  periods

Tangerine oil
Laxative
Peripheral circulatory
  system,
  especially teenagers
  and children
  (complexion
  problems)
Stomachic

Tea Tree oil
Acne
Cancer
Chicken Pox
Cold sores
Dental abscesses
Energy stimulant
Infections
Pimples
Skin cancer
Staph infections
Strep throat
Surface infections
Tinea

Terebinth oil
Analgesic
Antiseptic
Baths
Colitis
Constipation
Dissolves gallstones
Genito-urinary
  antiseptic
Loosens bronchial
  phlegm
Parasites
Pulmonary

Thuja Cedar oil
Diuretic
Prostate hypertrophy
Relaxing
Soothing for skin in
  baths
Tonic for impotency
Urinary sedative
Venereal warts
Warts

⚬ **Thyme oil**
Acne
Candida albicans
Fatigue
General stimulant
Infectious diseases
Mental exhaustion
Respiratory diseases
Skin antiseptic
Sore throats
Yeast infections
• Inhale: Stimulates
  intelligence
⚬ **Note:** Needs to be
  diluted.

Tolu Balsam oil
Cough syrups
Expectorant
Perfumery (used by
  Aztecs)
Stimulant
Tonic

Vervain oil
Colognes and soaps
Expectorant for coughs
  and colds
Stimulates creativity
Tranquilizer

Vetiver oil
Bath oil
Blends with
  Sandalwood and Rose
Moth repellent
Perfumery

White Thyme oil
(see also Thyme)
  Antiseptic
  Colds
  Sinus

⚬ **Wintergreen oil**
*Analgesic
Antiseptic
Flavoring agent
Relieves sore muscles
  and joints

Yarrow oil
Headache
Protection from
  radiation poisoning
Respiratory system
Severe wounds and
  boils

Ylang-Ylang oil
Aphrodisiac
Calms nerves
Depression
Euphoric
Exotic bath and body
  oil
Frigidity
Impotence
Insomnia
Oily skin
Perfumery
Regulates cardiac and
  respiratory rhythm
Relaxes
Sedative
Soothes anger and
  intense physical pain
Voluptuous scent

Chapter II

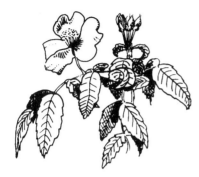

An Aromatic Glossary of Useful Terms

Warm Winter
Glistening strands of web among the Lilac
Iridescent green hummer flashing near the Fuchsia
Fragrance of freshly warmed earth
Smooth strong feel of the Oak banister
And the wholehearted croak of the invisible frog.
—Jeanne Rose, January 16, 1991

AT = Aromatherapy
EO = Essential Oil
PEO = Pure Essential Oil

Absolute • An absolute is not a raw material, but a prepared perfume material. These substances are highly concentrated, completely alcohol-soluble and are usually liquid. Absolutes are obtained by the alcohol extraction of a concrète (see *concrète)* or from the fatty extracts of plants. Occasionally absolutes are solid or semi-solid (Clary Sage). Absolutes can also be obtained from the water of a distillation process, such as Lavender water-absolute or Rose water-absolute. Absolutes from pommades are often considered essential oils; they are "volatile oils" (see *volatile oil).* The part of an Absolute one can steam-distill is called an Absolute oil.

Acid • This refers to a substance with a pH below 7.0 (normally hair and skin have a pH between 4.0 and 6.0) used to control bacteria on the skin and keep the skin healthy. Acid is the opposite of alkaline. Even though some of the best-made soaps are slightly alkaline, this alkalinity helps to temporarily reduce skin pH so that dirt and grease can be stripped or washed away, and then the skin returns very quickly to its normal slightly acid pH. Strongly alkaline cosmetics and strong alkaline soaps can upset normal skin pH level (especially for those who are unhealthy).

Acidophilus • There are several varieties of bacteria that thrive in acid environments. These include *Bifidus* (mother's milk bacteria) and *Acidophilus* (healthy intestinal bacteria). These are helpful in digestive upsets, as treatments for certain vaginal disorders, and as treatments in skin care. For instance, yogurt can be thinned with water, certain essential oils added (such as Tea Tree), and a cleansing "skin milk" or vaginal douche is the result.

Adulteration • Essential oils are often adulterated, that is, changed, cut, diluted or mixed with synthetic scents. Some essential oils are extended, that is, diluted with pure fruit kernel or nut oils (Hazelnut oil, Almond oil or Apricot kernel oil). This is done to increase the profit of the manufacturer or seller of the product. If a cheap volatile or synthetic oil has been added to an essential oil and called *pure* or PEO, then this is a case of adulteration and not to be tolerated. Go to any store and price some Rose oil. It should cost about $1000 an ounce or $10 a milliliter. If it costs less it is definitely a victim of adulteration or is simply *synthetic* (that is, made from non-plant sources). [I have seen PEO Rose for sale at $15/ml=20 drops.] As Stefan Arctander says in *Perfume and Flavor Materials of Natural Origin*, ". . . Adulteration . . . the intention of acquiring the business [order] through a devaluation of the oil in relation to the labelling of its container. The consumers of perfume oils are buying odor, not certain physico-chemical data . . ." Essential oils are expensive however and should probably not be used "straight" or "neat" (directly out of the bottle and onto the skin).

Aesthetician • A licensed professional who recommends and practices skin care and the use of treatments for beauty and health.

Alcohol • Usually refers to the substance produced by a fermentation of sugars, starch and other carbohydrates (Potato fermentation=vodka, Corn fermentation=bourbon, Sugar-cane fermentation=rum). Alcohol is used in cosmetics as an antiseptic. Since it dissolves fat it can be used as a carrier for essential oils, to incorporate them, to scent shampoo or other water-based products or to provide a medium for therapeutics. Alcohol dissolves fat so it should not be used in products for dry skin or hair. In the cosmetic (industry) sense alcohol refers to the hydroxyl compound [–OH] as a functional part of a cosmetic formula. In this form it is a good emollient and is said to provide protection for skin moisture.

Algin, Alginate, Alginic Acid • These names refer to a gelatinous precipitate that is extracted from brown algae and absorbs up to 300 times its weight in water. Used externally it is a cosmetic thickener and stabilizer. Used internally, algin has the capability of combining with heavy toxic metals in food in the body and allowing them to be passed harmlessly out with the feces.

Alkaline • A substance or solution with a pH of 7.0 or above. Most soaps and detergents are alkaline.

Allantoin • This is an organic compound that occurs naturally in Comfrey plants, and can be synthetically made from urea. Allantoin is a cellular regenerative, so it is useful in any product used to promote healing in cuts or burns, including sunburn. In home-made cosmetics Comfrey root, ground or blended, or Comfrey root or leaf tincture can easily be added to your products.

Amino Acids • These make up a large group of organic compounds that represent the end product of protein metabolism. They are necessary for growth of all parts of the body, skin, hair and nails.

Ammonia • Found in many products, especially fertilizers, cleaning products, bleaches and hair permanents. Extremely harmful and irritating, especially to the eyes and to any mucous membrane. Can cause permanent allergenic response in some individuals.

Amphoteric • A substance that can act either as an acid or a base. (Wool can absorb both acid and alkaline dyes.) Proteins are amphoteric as are their building blocks—amino acids.

Anhydrous Lanolin • A=without, and hydrous=water; Lanolin is the fat from the sheep's skin that goes into the wool. (The wool is sheared and the lanolin is extracted without harming the animal.) Anhydrous lanolin or lanolin is very protective and absorbs water to keep skin nice and soft and is used for this purpose in cosmetics (see also *lanolin*).

Antioxidant • A substance that inhibits the oxidation that turns cosmetics rancid. Antioxidants include vitamin E and BHA (butylated hydroxyanisole), enzymes and some oils such as Grapefruit seed extract.

Apple Cider Vinegar • A natural solvent in oils and creams. It acidifies products. When used in shampoos and rinses, it separates individual hairs so they can be thoroughly cleansed. Sounds like a great addition to the shampoo of bears, hairy men and Husky dogs.

Argil • A type of clay used in products to absorb skin impurities.

Aroma • The fragrance of something; what a particular plant product smells like. Our language does not have a real vocabulary for the 10,000 odors that we can perceive (in contrast to the only 2,000 or so colors), and so we must do our best by describing aromas by other subject matter, such as "smells like ripe Cantaloupe," "Eglantine Rose leaves have the aroma of green Apples," "he eats so much sugar, he has the aroma (odor) of rotten fruit."

Aromachology • A word coined by the Doyenne of the Fragrance Foundation, Executive Director Annette Green, meaning a new science that combines the interrelationship of psychology and the latest in fragrance technology to transmit through odor a variety of specific feelings—relaxation, exhilaration, sensuality, happiness and achievement—directly to the pleasure center of the brain (the seat of emotions, memory, creativity and sensuality).

Aromatherapy • The use of essential oils from aromatic plants to restore and enhance health and beauty as defined by the American Aromatherapy Association. Aromatherapy uses as its basic ingredients essential oils, which represent the highest herbal energy. Essential oils are highly concentrated, volatile extracts retrieved from aromatic herbs, flowers, seeds and trees; they contain hormone-like properties, vitamins, minerals and natural antiseptics.

Ascorbic Acid • This is vitamin C. It is used in nutrition and cosmetics. It is often used in cosmetics to enhance acid balance of a product, to retard oxidation, as a preservative, to fix colors and to stabilize creams.

Baking Soda • This is sodium bicarbonate, a soft, ultra-fine powder used as a dentifrice with sea salt. It prevents mold when an open box is placed in the fridge and keeps the interior sweet-smelling. It acts as a cleansing agent, is used as a mouthwash and is sprinkled on smelly carpets to absorb unpleasant odors. Baking soda also has use in creams and lotions to add smooth texture.

Balsam • This is a natural raw material exuded from a tree or a plant. Balsams are either physiological or pathological products, in that they are either naturally occurring or a result of injury to the plant. Balsams are insoluble in water and usually completely soluble in alcohol. They act as preservatives, are used to treat skin problems and are generally sweetly fragrant.

Barrier Agents • A substance used to protect the skin from harmful agents such as detergents, irritants or even water. These are generally oily substances derived from vegetable (oils), animal (lanolin from sheep wool) or petroleum (which is not recommended). They are used in commercial products, industrial preparations and cosmetics.

Beeswax • A natural product made by bees, especially used to thicken creams and lotions.

Bentonite • A naturally occurring clay from volcanic ash that forms a gel when mixed with water. It is used externally to "draw" in facials and packs. It is used internally to "cleanse" the digestive tract and as a laxative as well.

Benzoic Acid • A preservative derived from gum Benzoin and other substances used to preserve foods and cosmetics. A tincture of Benzoin is used to harden sensitive skin such as the "elbows" of large dogs that become abraded and sore from lying down. It is anti-fungal and has use in deodorants, dentifrices and other products.

Biotin • A white crystalline substance called one of the B vitamins, sometimes called vitamin H for hair, and used in creams to lend texture. It is necessary in the body for fat metabolism, health and growth. It has also been found to be one of the only substances that when taken consistently actually stimulates fingernail growth.

Boric Acid • A water-soluble, white crystalline substance found throughout the living and inanimate world and concentrated in certain minerals. It is a mild antiseptic and is used in body powders, in salves and bandages for burns and wounds, and in eye lotions for soothing. It lends a shiny glassy look to certain cosmetics. No longer in use internally. Acts as an antiseptic and astringent externally. It is anti-fungal. In years past the only commercial source of boric acid was the volcanic waters of the hot springs in Tuscany, Italy.

Calcium Carbonate (Chalk) • This is a very fine white powder that is easily scented and used in tooth powder as a whitening abrasive. It occurs naturally in oyster shell, limestone and in other material. This substance is also used in nutrition as an antacid and as a cosmetic filler. In *Jeanne Rose's Herbs & Things* there are several useful and well-known recipes including my favorite:

Rosemary Tooth Powder: Mix together ½ oz powdered Orris root, 1 oz powdered Rosemary charcoal,* ½ oz powdered chalk, ½ oz powdered Peppermint herb and 10 drops essential oil of Peppermint. Sieve to remove any pieces and bottle the powder in a container.

Carotene • BetaCarotene is pro-vitamin A and occurs naturally in plants and animal tissue and is readily available in Carrots. It is used in cosmetics primarily as a coloring agent but is also considered by cosmetic makers to be a particularly good addition to nourish the skin and aid cell regeneration.

Carrageenan • A substance found in red algae that is extracted primarily from Irish Moss. It is soluble in hot water and used as an emulsifier in cos-

---

*To make Rosemary charcoal, char several cups of dried Rosemary in a dry cast-iron skillet. When it begins to char or blacken, turn off the heat and stir vigorously. If you toast it too long, it begins to gray and you will have ash instead of charcoal.

metic products including toothpaste. It is found sometimes in foods, especially creamy foods such as Chocolate milk. No toxicity has been reported.

Castor Oil • An herbal oil extracted from the Castor bean and used in masks, night creams, lipsticks and other cosmetic products.

Chalk • See Calcium Carbonate.

Chelating Agents • These are substances that can form bonds with metals. Chlorophyll is one, as well as the "heme" part of hemoglobin. These substances are useful when dyeing fabrics, as deactivators of enzymes and for water softening, etc.

Chemotype • A plant that is cloned and therefore identical in every way with the "mother" plant. It is not grown from seed. The same plant can produce its essential oil with several different chemical components, depending upon whether it is grown from seed or cloned, or depending on the time it is left in the still. Certain chemotypes are desirable because the chemical components are different (more gentle, less toxic, softer scent, different plant hormones). But a chemotype from one year's planting may be dramatically different from another year's because of weather changes or varying soil conditions. Certain chemotypes are dependent on altitude and the mineral composition of the soil. To date, chemotypes are incompletely labelled and command a very high price.

Chlorophyll • The natural green part of a plant important in photosynthesis. As chloro=green color is to phyll=plant, so is heme=red or iron to globin=blood.

Cider Vinegar • A sour liquid made from cider by fermentation and used to clarify and acidify hair products. Used as well in various body-care products to preserve them. See also *Apple cider vinegar*.

Cocoa Butter • A solid fat that is obtained from seeds of *Theobroma cacao*, the Chocolate plant. Is used as an emollient in creams and lotions, melts at body temperature and is sometimes allergenic.

Coconut Oil • An oil obtained from the Coconut and used as a moisturizer in various products. Goes rancid easily. It is used to make soap but often the pure Coconut oil soap is drying and generally of low quality. Cheap to buy. Sometimes causes allergic reactions.

Collagen • A protein found in the connective tissue of animals and used in plastic surgery to plump up tissues so that people look young and unwrinkled. Soluble collagens are used in all sorts of body-care products for that smooth, unwrinkled look.

Concrète • A French word referring to a particular perfume basic material and how it is prepared. For example, with Jasmine the freshly picked flowers prepared by the cold-process method of enfleurage becomes a pommade that is extracted with alcohol and the alcohol then evaporated. The perfume material is now called the concrète pommade of Jasmine. Concrètes are also produced by extracting plant tissue with hydrocarbon solvents or petroleum ether and then removing the solvent. Pronounced con – cret (rhymes with fret).

Cordial • An invigorating medicine, food or drink that comforts, gladdens and exhilarates. Often made with herbs and spirits, or can be made with herbs, essential oils and spirits. Try making a Peppermint herb tea and adding 1 cup tea to 1 cup of white wine in which you have dissolved 1–2 drops of Peppermint oil. This would be called a digestive cordial.

Decoctions • A liquid extract of the hard parts of plants such as the bark, root, rhizome or seed. One to four ounces of the plant material is added to twenty ounces of water and then boiled or simmered for five to twenty minutes. This is then cooled and strained and used for cosmetic or medicinal purposes. Makes 16 ounces decoction, with the herbs left over to be used in poultices or baths.

Demineralized Water • Water that has had the minerals and ions removed. Considered necessary for high-end body-care products.

Detergent •A type of cleanser, usually synthetic, that reduces water surface tension and emulsifies soil or dirt so that they can be removed. Some detergents are bio-degradable.

Diatomaceous Earth • A type of earth made up of the fossil deposits of siliceous skeletons of diatoms. This earth has an irritating surface (glasslike and sharp) and can be used to clean carpets and rid them of fleas and mites. Absorbs oil and water and is used in abrasive agents, cleansers for the face or for environmental uses. Very cheap. Irritating if inhaled.

Distillation • The process of driving off gas or vapor (water) from liquids or solids by heating. In aromatherapy, water and herb or plant material are heated, the water turns to steam, and the steam passes through the plant cells or glands that contain the essential oils, bursting them and releasing the volatile oils. The steam and volatile oil are then passed through a cooling chamber where the steam turns to water, releasing the essential oil, which remains on the surface of the water. This is then decanted or poured off. Distillation usually occurs in a still (see *still*).

Diuretic • Something that causes an increase in the production of urine.

Dolomite • A mineral that contains calcium magnesium carbonate and is used as an abrasive and whitener in products for the teeth. Occasionally used in skin cleansers.

Emollient • A substance that is soothing to the external surface of the body and moisturizes by preventing water loss. Some emollients are Comfrey root, Marshmallow root, lanolin, etc. Some emollients cause allergic reactions.

Emulsifier • A substance that allows two disparate substances to merge, such as the egg in mayonnaise that binds the Lemon juice to the oil. Emulsifiers are useful in cosmetics to create smooth creams and lotions. Sometimes allergenic.

Emulsion • A mixture of oil and water. Most creams and lotions are emulsions. "An emulsion is a colloidal system in which one liquid is dispersed in the form of fine droplets throughout another liquid with which it cannot evenly mix . . ." from *On Food and Cooking* by Harold McGee, Charles Scribner, 1984.

EO • These initials refer to Essential Oil. It is usually identical with PEO.

Essence • Has various meanings depending on context: (1) a substance considered to possess in high degree the predominant quality of the plant, (2) the basic underlying quality, (3) the essential oil, (4) the volatile matter that constitutes a perfume, and (5) also an alcoholic solution of an essential oil such as 1 ounce of vodka in which has been dissolved 1 drop of Peppermint oil.

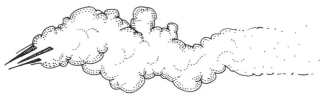

Essential Oil • A volatile material that is contained within plant cells and derived by physical process (such as distillation) from the plant. Some essential oils are not in the living tissue but are formed during destruction of the living tissue. Certain botanical species have little scent but they produce a volatile or essential oil when macerated that starts a fermentation (destructive) process—the macerate is then distilled and the volatile oil comes off. See also Stefan Arctander, *Perfume and Flavor Materials of Natural Origin*, pages 13–17.

Expectorant • Something that causes one to cough up or spit up phlegm.

Extract • A prepared perfume material or the alcoholic solution of the odorous part of a pommade or something that is obtained by distillation.

Fixative • Something that holds or "fixes" the scent. It usually slows down evaporation of the odorous material. Some fixatives exalt or improve the scent; some are odorless and simply "hold" the main scent intact.

Glucose • A type of sugar from Grape or Corn and used in cosmetics and medicine. Soothes irritated or burnt skin.

Grape Seed Oil • An ultra-fine oil expressed from the seeds of Grapes and used as a carrier oil in aromatherapy. Nonallergenic.

Grapefruit Seed Extract • An extract derived from Grapefruit seeds that has preservative and anti-bacterial qualities. A good stabilizer for aromatherapy products.

Gum • A sticky substance secreted by some trees and shrubs.

Gum Arabic • A gum from *Acacia senegal* that is slowly soluble in water and provides a gelatinous acid base for nonoily cosmetics. Makes a demulcent and emollient base and is very soothing to all skin surfaces. Has been known to cause allergic or irritant reactions. See also *Jeanne Rose Herbs & Things*, Chapter 3: Acacia, gum.

Gum Tragacanth • An emollient and demulcent, yields a thick mucilage that when combined with water is useful in lotions and creams.

Herb • (1) A seed-producing annual, biannual or herbaceous perennial that does not develop persistent woody tissue but dies down at the end of the growing season—this is a botanist's definition; (2) A plant *or* plant part valued for its medicinal, savory, cosmetic or aromatic qualities—this is the definition that was used by the ancients as well as by modern herbalists and which includes *any* part of *any* shrub, tree, flower, seed, fern, algae, lichen, etc., any plant; (3) The leafy top of an herbaceous plant considered separately from its root—generally a cook's definition. Compare Celery, Celery root, Celery seed, Celery oil.

Honey • A delicious food produced by bees, it tests on the acid side but is soothing and is used as an emollient or preservative in some body-care products. Sometimes causes allergic reactions.

Hormone Creams • Contain synthetic estrogens and are used as firming creams. Only temporarily firms, smooths and plumps up the skin.

Humectant • Added to creams and lotions to help the skin retain moisture. Draws moisture from the air. Glycerine is a good example. Sometimes causes allergic reaction depending upon the specific ingredients.

Hydrate • The ability to restore or maintain the normal fluid proportion in the skin or body. Hydrating agents are used in cosmetics to keep the skin natural, moist, firm and young-looking.

Infused Oil • Results when an herb or plant part is soaked or macerated in oil, then heated gently and the oil strained out. The resulting oil is called *infused*. This process is used for Calendula-infused oil and others, which are generally used as carrier oils in aromatherapy products.

Infusion • Boiling water is poured over an herb and the herb is soaked or "infused" for a period of time and then strained. The resultant liquid is the infusion and the herb leftovers can be used in poulticing. Essential oils can be added to the infusion for increased efficacy in facial steams, lung lubrications, hair steams, etc.

An example for a *Healing Facial Steam:* Bring 1 quart of water to a boil, turn off the heat, and add 1 ounce of mixed herbs (for normal skin use a mixture of Peppermint, Camomile and Rose). Steep, soak, infuse for 5 minutes. Add 2 drops of PEO of Rose or Chamomile. Put your face over pot, cover with towel, inhale the steam and let steam play about the face for 5–10 minutes. Now you may strain out the herbs and use them to poultice or to make a facial or hair pack, and the infusion can be poured into your bath for a fragrant, healing bath.

Inhalation • A method of treating mental and physical problems through the inhalation of the volatile, essential oils of aromatic and medicinal plants rather than the drinking of the herbal tea or the injection of the oils. Inhalations can be used to stimulate the brain. The inhaled essential oils reach the body through the lungs and bloodstream or through the nose—then to the limbic system of the brain—with a release of hormones and neurochemicals to create mental/emotional effects. See Chapter IV for a diagram of pathways.

Example: Use 3 drops of PEO in a diffusor. Use Chapter I to find out which oils to use for which problems.

Irritant • A substance that irritates, such as Poison Oak or Nettles or some essential oils such as Clove oil when used on open sores.

Jojoba Oil • A vegetable wax that is extracted from *Simmondsia chinensis*. We call this an oil because it comes in a liquid form from the plant, but chemists have determined that the beans actually produce a wax. This is now a substitute for the banned whale oil and spermaceti that was once used to produce sparkling white, smooth cosmetics and fine-grade machine oil. Jojoba oil does not go rancid and is used to dissolve the sebum in plugged hair pores. This encourages fresh new hair growth. Jojoba is an excellent carrier "oil" for aromatherapy products. See also Chapter III.

Kaolin • A type of clay. When used in products it aids the absorption of excess oil secreted by the skin. Best for oily or problem skin. This is a very fine particle powder that is often applied to draining wounds and fistulas to absorb the moisture from these secretions.

Kukui Nut Oil • From a Hawaiian plant considered to be very soothing, emollient and good for damaged or slow-growing hair. Considered a scalp and hair restorative.

Lanolin • A wax that is produced by oil glands in sheep to waterproof their wool. After the sheep is sheared the lanolin is extracted or separated from the wool and used in cosmetics and ointments to smooth and soothe. Lanolin is yellow, sticky and unctuous and is easily absorbed by human and pet skin. Can cause allergies in those who are sensitive (see also *anhydrous lanolin*).

Lecithin • Derived from a phospho-lipid that makes up 30% of egg yolks, lecithin is an excellent emulsifier and is used in creams and lotions as an anti-oxidant to prevent rancidity.

Lotion • A smooth liquid applied externally to hands or body for softening, soothing. Made as a medicinal, cosmetic, cleanser or astringent depending on the herbs or essential oils used. Some lotions in addition are oily. A creamy liquid used as a cosmetic is also called a lotion.

Maceration • A process of extracting fragrant oils from the plant material. It is similar to enfleurage but uses hot fat rather than cold fat to immerse the petals and achieve the goal. *To macerate* is to soften or soak in warm fluid for a time to separate the solid matter from its elements.

Medicinal • A remedy used in treating physical or mental ailments.

Menthol • A naturally occurring substance in certain kinds of Mints, usually M. *arvensis* or Peppermint herb. An essential oil used in drug and cosmetic products because it is a counter-irritant, is cooling and has soothing properties.

Mineral Oil • A heavy oil derived from petroleum. Not recommended for use in body-care products because it leaves a nasty residue on skin and hair and if used internally has the ability to be absorbed and drag along oil-soluble vitamins and minerals from the body that are then excreted in the feces. Not recommended for babies or children.

Moisturizer • Something that helps the skin retain its natural moisture or adds moisture. Some herbs have moisturizing capabilities, and certain essential oils such as Jasmine oil and Rose oil when added to lotions and creams can increase the moisturizing capability of these products.

Mucilage • A substance that swells up in water and dissolves in the process. Forms a sticky, slimy, gelatinous mass that can be used as an emollient in cosmetics.

Odor Description • How do you describe the 10,000 odors? See Chapter III for "Words That Smell & Words That Stink." Descriptions of odor are very difficult. We do not really have a vocabulary of odoriferous words. What is "sweet" to me may be "cloying and heavy" for you. I suggest that you read Chapter III with a pen and paper in hand. Get a few bottles of different essential oils. Smell them! Write down your reactions.

Start with the easy oils such as Clove oil, Peppermint oil, Sandalwood oil and a flower oil such as Rose oil or Tuberose oil. Describe the scent with color, with sound, with taste, with as many adjectives as seem to fit. In other words, develop your own odor vocabulary. Write this down and compare with my descriptions. Then as you read along you will more or less know what sort of scent I am describing.

PEO • When you see these initials it means Pure Essential Oil. This is usually identical with EO or Essential Oil.

pH • This is a scale of number from 0 to 14 that is used to measure the alkalinity or acidity of a substance. Neutral is 7.0, and below that is acid such as vinegar or honey. Above 7.0 is alkaline such as soap. Human skin and hair is about 4.0 to 6.0.

Pommade or Pomade • These are pre-pared perfume materials obtained by enfleurage. The fat that is saturated with the essence of the flower after the enfleurage process is termed the pom-made or pomade.

Resin • A hard, brittle substance (Mastic, Amber, Copal) that is transparent or translucent and usually yellow to brown. Formed as a plant secretion and obtained as an exudate (recent or fossilized) or as an extract of plants. Often obtained from Firs and Pines. Resins have antibacterial properties and are used in industry, medicine, incense and cosmetics.

Rosin • Like a resin but usually darker, a bitter, friable resin obtained from the oleoresin or dead wood of Pine trees by the removal of the volatile Turpentine oil, etc. Used in varnish, lacquer, soap and industry.

Salve • A soothing or healing medicinal or cosmetic ointment generally made with healing substances such as herbs infused in oil, strained, and the herbal oil then solidified with wax.

Shellac • A natural resin that is secreted by the Lac insect and deposited on trees. It is collected, purified and used for industrial purposes and for body care or as hair spray. In the '40s and '50s one could always tell who used a hair spray with shellac in it because their hair-dos formed perfect hard shapes unflappable in the wind and sent out little dandruff puffs of flakes throughout the evening. I read that now in the '90s shellac-based hair sprays do not flake (which I sincerely doubt). Also, if your hair does not move in the wind, maybe you are using the wrong spray?

Skin • The stuff that covers all creatures and forms the first line of defense against bacterial, alien, fungal or other substance invasion. Read a good physiology text for a scientific description of skin—ideally you already know the basics: Several layers of cells with glands and follicles that accomplish wondrous healthful benefits. Creams and lotions can soften the external layer, and face-lifts can change your perspective.

Soap • Combine a fat or oil with a base like lye [potassium carbonate (from wood ashes) or calcium hydroxide] and use the appropriate measurements and temperature gradients, and a wondrous chemical change will occur that turns fat and lye into soap. This is call saponification. Generally a well-made soap will be slightly alkaline, which when applied to the skin temporarily changes the pH of the skin—the soap combines with the dirt, strips it off the skin, you rinse with water—dirt gone and the skin quickly reverts to its normal, slightly acid pH.

Spice • A spice is generally described as the dried parts of those very aromatic plants that make their home in the tropics: the hard parts of plants such as berries (Allspice or Black Pepper), flower buds (Cloves), roots or rhizomes (Ginger or Vetivert) or bark (Cinnamon). Spices have their essence in these hard parts of plants, while the herbs have their essence in the soft parts. Herbs usually are at home in the temperate climates and these include leaves (Rosemary), flowers (Rose), stems and leaves (Angelica).

Still • The equipment used in distillation to separate the plant material from its delicate essential or volatile oils usually comprised of (1) a RETORT, which is the chamber that holds the plant material and takes the heat; (2) the HEAD, which collects the steam; (3) the TUBE, which sends the steam to the condensor; and (4) the CONDENSOR, which is where the steam separates into hot water and volatile oils. Aristotle described the use of stills in 350 B.C.

See the drawing on the next page, and *Secrets of the Still* by Grace Firth, EPM Publications, 1983.

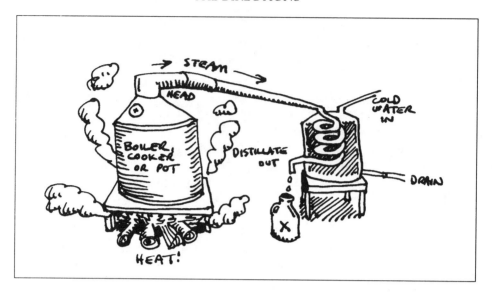

Synergist • A substance that when combined with another increases the effectiveness of both.

Talc • Mostly magnesium silicate, it is a substance that occurs naturally and is used in baby powders, makeup, creams, etc. Unfortunately, most talc occurs in conjunction with arsenic. The best talc comes from Montana and is essentially free of arsenic. Talc is a lung irritant. Use other powders such as Cornstarch or baking soda as your absorbant powder and for your baby. Herbal powders are also very effective and can be made from equal quantities of powders of Orris root, Orange peel, Lemon peel and Sandalwood.

Tea • This means two things: (1) the liquid that is made from the Tea plant, *Camellia sinensis* (contains theophylline and is the best bronchodilator known, and (2) the liquid that is made when you combine water and herbs, strain and drink it. This is another confusing herbal term. A tea is an infusion that is used cosmetically or medicinally—when lots of herb to water is used and infused for a long time it is generally called an *infusion*; when a little bit of herb is steeped in lots of water for 3–5 minutes, the resulting beverage is generally considered a tea. Did I confuse you further?

Terpeneless Oil • Terpeneless essential oils are processed perfume or flavor materials from which all monoterpenes have been removed ($C_{10}H_{16}$). This is usually done to improve the solubility of the essential oil and to concentrate the active aromatic scent and to increase stability. Gattefossé considered terpeneless essential oils to be superior because they were more easily absorbed when used in subcutaneous or intra-muscular injections and were less irritating when used externally. Also the fragrance was more "gentle." He conceived the use of terpeneless Lavender oil for all sorts of deep wounds and sores.

Tincture • An alcoholic solution containing medicinals or aromatics; about 50% alcohol. To make a tincture at home, infuse 1–4 oz of herbs or plant materials directly into 1 cup of 100° alcohol such as vodka or brandy. Shake daily for 10 days, strain and use.

Tisane • Historically a nourishing decoction having a slight medicinal quality. It was originally made from Barley and called a ptisane. We could consider the Chinese herbal soup a modern-day tisane. However, most people would define a tisane as a beverage tea made from flowers and drunk simply for pleasure and taste delight.

Unguent • A preparation made from fat or oil, usually with a medicinal or cosmetic purpose. It liquefies upon application to the body.

Volatile oil • An oil that vaporizes quickly and easily; an oil that easily evaporates. It is also called an essential oil and contains the plant hormones and delicate chemical constituents of the plant. Antonym=Fixed Oil or Fatty Oil.

Example: Peppermint oil is an *essential* or *volatile oil* that is obtained by steam distillation from Peppermint leaf and is easily evaporated, while Olive oil is a *fixed* or *fatty oil* that is obtained by pressing the Olive fruit and does not evaporate.

Water • When this term is used in cosmetics or body care it usually means the waters in which significant amounts of essential oils have been dissolved. This happens during distillation of many essential oils such as Peppermint leaf water, Orange flower water and Rosewater. An herb water can also be a 2% solution (2 ml essential oil steeped in 4 oz distilled water, shake vigorously, shake regularly and use). This can be either a medicinal or cosmetic substance.

Recently when my dog was hit by a car and needed twice-daily disinfectant soaks as well as wet bandaging and then dry bandaging, I used an herb infusion for the soaks, then Tea Tree oil water (2% solution) for the wet dressings. The vet said it was just short of miraculous how quickly the wounds healed and closed up. Cosmetically, Lavender or Orange flower waters are used therapeutically on the skin as well as to "set" makeup.

Water Bath • Also known as a *bain-marie*. A pot containing water in which is placed another pot containing the substance being cooked or heated; used for cooking delicate or sensitive ingredients such as Chocolate foods or fragile cosmetic products.

Wax • An organic compound that melts at low temperature, is solid at room temperature (except for Jojoba), is water-repellent and gives solidity to creams and salves.

I believe in a good glossary and I believe in using the glossary and that is why in most of my books the glossary holds a prominent position, generally Chapter II. How can you possibly discuss a new subject unless you are familiar with the specific words, the terminology of the subject. Please read this chapter over and over again. You will be surprised how easily you will become conversant in the subject of aromatherapy. Test your so-called aromatherapy experts with two simple terms—ask them to define *Fixed oil* versus *Essential oil*. Most will not know the difference, but if you read this chapter—*you* will!

For further definitions of herbal, cosmetic, and culinary terms, read Chapter 2 of

> *Jeanne Rose's Herbs & Things*
> *The Herbal Body Book*
> *The Herbal Guide to Food*

For medicinal herbal terms see the glossary in

> *Jeanne Rose's Modern Herbal*

For some general terminology, see the glossary in

> *Kitchen Cosmetics.*

Chapter III

Descriptions of Some Essential Oils— Words That Smell & Words That Stink

... For the fragrance that came to each was
like a memory of dewy mornings of unshadowed
sun in some land of which the fair world in
Spring is itself but a fleeting memory ...

J. R. R. Tolkien
The Return of the King

All of the oils are marked

because

some oils have been known to cause irritation, allergic reactions or sensitivities on some people. However, all substances have been implicated to some degree in unpleasant reactions on someone ... so it would be wise to try the patch test before using a new essential oil or any other cosmetic substance externally.

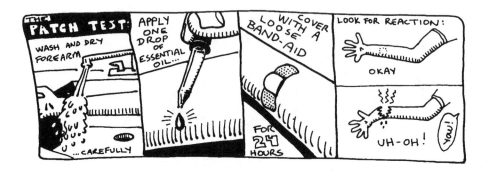

The Patch Test. If you have sensitive skin or a history of allergies, then by all means use a patch test to gauge your relative sensitivity to essential oils. Wash an area on your forearm about the size of a quarter and dry it carefully. Apply a drop of the essential oil. If you are very sensitive in general you may wish to dilute the oil equally with a bland carrier oil such as Olive oil and apply this dilution. Then add a loose Band-Aid and wait twenty-four hours. If there is no reaction—terrific—go ahead and use the oil in your formulas. Keep all essential oils away from the eyes and from moist mucous areas in general.

In addition to the symbol 𝕊 which represents scent wafting into the air, we have used descriptive drops to separate some very particular oils. These little drops mean

🚫 Do not use or to be used only by a certified aromatherapist.

ⓓ Dilute in carrier oil before applying externally, or dilute in alcohol before internal use.

◑ Umm! This oil could cause a problem. Caution is necessary!

◔ Skin irritant! Skin irritant!

◔ . . . No worries . . . user friendly. Okay on children.

⑦ unknown properties

Words That Smell & Words That Stink
Aromatic Words

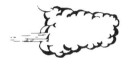

smell

scent

odor

aroma

bouquet

fragrance

stink

stench

reek

malodorous

redolent

fumes

ambrosial

fetid

acrid

putrid

repulsive

fœtor

sweet

Have you ever wondered why there are so few words that actually describe scent? Words that when said actually put a particular scent in your nostrils? Rose—is one of these. And why are these scent words generally eponymous renditions of the name? For example, how else would you describe the scent of Roses but by the word "rose-scented" . . . except possibly when you are describing specific scents of specific Rose types such as "peppery scent of the Cécile Brunner Rose" or the "fruity scent of the apricot Rose."

So I was looking in one of my synonym dictionaries* and came up with the following words for *smell:* "The nouns that describe that which is perceived by the nose" relates to the olfactory sense and *smell* is a general term that we can all relate to. A close synonym might be odor or aroma or fragrance or stink or stench. But *smell* or *odor* can be either positive or negative, pleasant or unpleasant, and even neutral. It takes a good adverb to help the olfactory-unconscious human even begin to decipher what another person means when they say, "Your jacket smells!" or "My hands have picked up an odor." *And* aren't phrases more descriptive when you say "doggy smell" rather than smells like a dog or "outhouse stink" instead of smells like a toilet. The word *odor* has a more neutral connotation, and one begins to understand this when one says "refreshing odor" or "foul odor." How about the Ivory scent of soap or the spicy odor of incense or the burnt woodsy scent of burning fall leaves, or the repellent fetid scent of diseased flesh or how about the unique scent of formaldehyde as it is used to preserve flesh and again the eponymous fragrance of the Violet.

*Choose the Right Word, by S. I. Hayakawa. New York: Harper & Row, 1968.

THE DIRECTIONS

Which brings us to scent. Doesn't that word make you feel that the volatile oils that will get to your nasal mucosa will be pleasant? "The sweet scent of the Wallflowers that remind you of rich wild honey," or "the heavy honey scent of a just-picked Ice Plant blossom," that purple roadside plant that you wouldn't think would have any scent at all?

Fragrance makes you think of sweet things or body powder. Your son might say "I like my mommy's fragrance," or the older daughter says "Mother has a fragrance of talcum." My own daughter always described me as fragrant as Rosemary herb, and while cooking, I was described only as "Garlic"!

And how would you describe the emanations of humans? What do you say when your lover leaves in the morning and you grab and caress the pillow that he slept upon? I remember that one of my husbands' smell could only be described as car grease and diesel. That man is fifty years old now and car grease is still what he smells like, but at the age of fifty with all the other smells he has accumulated over the years, it no longer is very romantic. What this man needs is twenty-seven herb baths in a row, zinc tablets added to his diet, and for the first time in his life some really powerful scent-absorbing deodorant that is in itself unscented. Body odor can be appealing but not when it stinks. It always amazes me when a very young person marries a very old person—how can they tolerate the way each smells?

I love to read phrases in books that truly can give you a scentual picture of fragrance such as "A blissful expression came over her face and her nostrils expanded as if she were inhaling a quite delicious fragrance."*

In my own town of San Francisco and along my own street there is a sweetness to the air before a rain. The air lifts off the earth, carrying up from the branches and boughs, from flower and fence, a fragrance that is pungent and sweet. Down the street lined with trees a scent comes from the tree blossoms noticeable in the autumn and only when the weather changes. Put your nose directly on the blossoms and you actually only smell the dust and car exhaust fumes left there from the passing traffic. But walk a foot or two away and the sweetness of the blossoms is evident. It is a halo that surrounds and grasps the trees. What are these fragrant trees? The city only says that they are "street trees."

And so we proceed to the descriptions of plants and their essential oils, their sexual scent, the sexual exudation or personal bug repellent odors.

How do you describe a scent? Smell these and form your own vocabulary.

---

*Jitterbug Perfume, Tom Robbins. New York: Bantam Books, 1984

AT = Aromatherapy
EO = Essential Oil
PEO = Pure Essential Oil

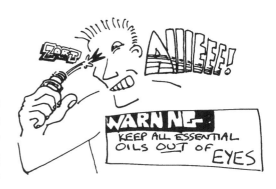

 Ambretta oil or Ambrette oil is steam-distilled from the whole seeds of *Hibiscus abelmoschus* or *H. moscheutes*. It has a strong musky odor and is used in perfumes or potpourris as a fixative. Ambrette seeds and this oil are considered to have a powerful effect on the adrenal glands and could be used in oil mixtures as an aphrodisiac or where the adrenals need to be stimulated to function. It is possible that Ambretta oil could be used as an inhalant or in massage oils when one is detoxifying from steroid drugs.

 Ammi visnaga is a Mediterranean plant of the Carrot family. The seeds of this plant have been used since ancient times as a smooth muscle relaxant and a treatment for colic and asthma. Its use is mentioned in ancient Arabic journals as a diuretic to rid the body of excess fluid. The seeds are small, grayish, egg-shaped and quite aromatic. A common name for the plant, Khellin, also describes the active ingredients and its use has been incorrectly described as a bronchodilator. Actually, when the seeds are taken they can sometimes cause nausea and vomiting. The reconstituted drug came to be called cromolyn sodium or Intal, a trademark of the Fison Company. What Intal does is mask the output of the mast cells that line the respiratory mucosa, thereby blocking allergic reaction in the nasal mucosa and in the bronchial tubes. The essential oil of Ammi is used as an inhalant to do much the same thing. It should be used judiciously, either vaporized in a diffusor or a few drops added to boiling water and the steam inhaled. Use only 1–2 drops at a time. Treatment needs to be continued for some weeks before any effect is felt. It is particularly useful for respiratory problems, for allergic asthma and for bronchial spasms.

Angelica—*Angelica archangelica*, called the Root of the Holy Ghost, is a biennial umbelliferous plant whose root is steam-distilled to produce a powerful musky-sweet, heavy, woody-scented oil. This oil is very much an insect attractant and should not be used by persons who have allergic problems with bugs or bees. The oil can be quite expensive and I have seen it listed in catalogs at prices from $70 to $100 for 5 ml (15 ml = ½ oz). It has great value as a blender oil, especially mixed with Clary Sage, Patchouli or fixative oils such as Oakmoss and Vetiver. This oil is also added with the root to make various liqueurs such as "Cointreau." Specifically, Angelica is best used in the bath (no more than 1–2 drops with other PEO) for its fragrance and to stimulate the circulation to remove toxins. Since the root itself is used as a digestive, the oil can also be used if you have a stomach ache—either bathe in the scented waters or use 1 drop on a sugar cube and suck.

One of my favorite travel and jet-lag remedies is a mixture of essential oils that contains Melissa, Angelica, Peppermint and Ginger. These oils can be mixed together in equal quantities, diluted by half with alcohol, carried on your trips in a small container and when necessary taken. You can also put a drop or two on a compress for a headache or stomachache.

...WILL HEAT YOU UP

The fragrance of Angelica oil is very much a stimulant to the digestive system both to ease pain and encourage appetite, and for alcoholics to cause a distaste for this drug. The root can also be chewed. It is used in massage, bath, facial masks, compresses, lotions, face and body oils and in the diffusor. This essential oil would be very good used in the diffusor just before a dinner party to stimulate appetite. Laplanders believe that chewing on the root prolongs life.

Anise Seed (Aniseed) oil is steam-distilled from *Pimpinella anisum*, a member of the Umbel family. The seeds have much value in various products such as facial steams and hair rinses, and in culinary and medicinal products such as cough formulas. Main constituent of the oil is 80–90% phenol ether called anethole.

Aniseed oil has a spicy, Licorice-like aroma. This essential oil is used as a flavoring in many baked goods and in pipe tobacco as well. Gattefossé mentions it as a cordial, carminative, digestive and lactagogue, but Patricia Davis considers it highly toxic and narcotic and suggests other oils to use for these properties. I have used it extensively in 20 years of aromatherapy demonstrations where the scent has been universally described as reminding people of Christmas cookies and Licorice sticks. Definitely a holiday scent. I consider the scent of Aniseed to be "green" in color, especially useful as an occasional inhalant for harmony and balance, and to soothe a "heartache." Heart palpitations, erratic breathing, vomiting and migraines can be eased with Aniseed oil and can be used in mixtures for baths, massage oils, facial oils, and of course in the diffusor.

It has also been recommended as a fish attractant. Fishermen rub Aniseed oil on their hooks and say the catch of fish is improved.

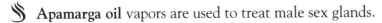 **Apamarga oil** vapors are used to treat male sex glands.

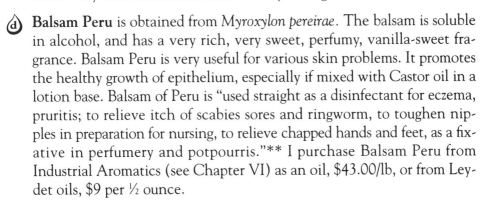 *Artemisia arborescens* oil contains chamazulene. This brilliant blue member of the Artemisia family has anti-inflammative and anti-allergenic properties on account of its high azulene content. It is for the most sensitive of skins and has produced amazing results on actinic keratosis and other skin infections and abnormal growths. It is highly effective on eczema and psoriasis. Combined in a 1% solution with *Aloe vera* gel it works very well on sunburn and severely damaged cellular tissue.*

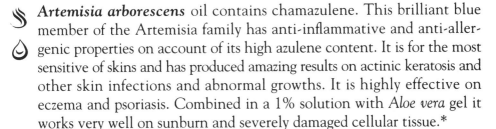 **Balsam Peru** is obtained from *Myroxylon pereirae*. The balsam is soluble in alcohol, and has a very rich, very sweet, perfumy, vanilla-sweet fragrance. Balsam Peru is very useful for various skin problems. It promotes the healthy growth of epithelium, especially if mixed with Castor oil in a lotion base. Balsam of Peru is "used straight as a disinfectant for eczema, pruritis; to relieve itch of scabies sores and ringworm, to toughen nipples in preparation for nursing, to relieve chapped hands and feet, as a fixative in perfumery and potpourris."** I purchase Balsam Peru from Industrial Aromatics (see Chapter VI) as an oil, $43.00/lb, or from Leydet oils, $9 per ½ ounce.

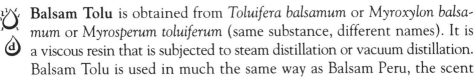 **Balsam Tolu** is obtained from *Toluifera balsamum* or *Myroxylon balsamum* or *Myrosperum toluiferum* (same substance, different names). It is a viscous resin that is subjected to steam distillation or vacuum distillation. Balsam Tolu is used in much the same way as Balsam Peru, the scent

---

*from Victoria Edwards

**from Jeanne Rose's *Herbal Body Book*.

being more Vanilla-like, somewhat richer and sweeter with a bit of Cinnamon scent. Tolu is used in soap making, as a fixative in perfumery and in medicinal preparations. Both Tolu and Peru are pathological products from injuries made to the trunks of trees. The Balsam seeps out, hardens and then is shipped to manufacturers where it is processed for use. Both are soluble in 95° alcohol.

 Basil—There are several types of Basil oil, two of which have the most use in aromatherapy preparations. The true Sweet Basil oil from *Ocimum basilicum* is steam-distilled in several countries including the USA, France, Italy and Spain. Basil oil from the Comoro Islands or the Seychelles is called the Exotic or Réunion type. These two oils can be distinguished by odor. For our purposes of home usage of essential oils, we will concentrate on true Sweet Basil oil. Basil oil has a warm, rich and fiery scent and is used in perfume bases to produce a "green" type of fragrance. It blends well with resinous scents as well as fixatives such as Oakmoss. I have particularly used the Basil oil in preparations to help hair growth, and in massage oils for its warming effect.

Basil oil is especially effective when mixed with Lavender oil and sometimes a sweet type of Rosemary oil called Rosemary Verbenon oil. This mixture is rubbed into the hair roots to stimulate hair growth. To use: take a few drops of the blended oil and with your fingertips rub into the bristles of a soft hairbrush, then use the fingertips to massage the hair at the roots to stimulate blood circulation, and finally the hair is brushed gently but completely with the brush. Do this every day to clean out the hair root follicles and to stimulate growth. If the mixture is too strong it can be diluted by half with Jojoba oil, which has a reputation of dissolving the clogging debris from the hair root follicles allowing oxygen to get in, which further improves hair growth.

Basil oil is very good when used in massage oils and is especially favored in rituals to honor the goddess. It is the oil of kings and queens.

Gattefossé mentions the use of Basil oil as a diuretic, emmenagogue, cleanser for the respiration, good for the heart, good for the digestion, used for the nerves, sinews and tendons, and inhaled to stimulate the mind and intellect. Tisserand found in his library researches that Basil was a stimulant of the adrenal cortex. Cosmetic use is mainly as an external

> **DILUTE ESSENTIAL OILS BEFORE USING**

application to stimulate hair growth and healthy hair, or externally on the skin to stimulate a sluggish complexion.

Very recently Arnould-Taylor in England has been using Basil oil, diluted, for treating herpes and shingles and other debilitating conditions with great success!*

Small amounts of Basil are stimulating and usually tonic, large amounts are too much. Do not overdo.

 Benzoin—A gum resin from *Styrax benzoin*, it is generally used as an extract in alcohol, and as a preservative for cosmetics and lotions. This extract is antibacterial, antiseptic, deodorant and when used internally it is expectorant and diuretic. The gum is used as a sweet fixative scent in incense and potpourris. In the *Herbal Body Book,* many uses and formulas are listed for this gum that was once known as gum benjamin. The gum and tincture of gum Benzoin has a sweet balsamic and Vanilla-like odor. It is very pleasant, and although not strictly speaking an essential oil, it does have much value in aromatherapy because of its antioxidant, antibacterial and preservative qualities. Mr. Gattefossé in his seminal work on *Aromatherapy* in 1937 lists the qualities of the [Benjoin] as "sharp, cutting, penetrating, moderating and softening, to relieve pain, and inhaled for lung ulcers and used externally for gangrene." Tisserand mentions that Benzoin absolute is energizing and is inhaled as an expectorant for mucus and to tone the heart and circulation.

When I had a Great Dane dog that spent most of his time lying down on hard surfaces, he developed (as do many sedentary animals) large sore spots on the "elbows" where the hair became ingrown and the flesh soft and mushy. The treatment was daily applications of gum Benzoin liquified with alcohol. It wasn't strictly the application of tincture of Benzoin but more the resin that killed the bacteria and "hardened" the skin.

---

*from Victoria Edwards

Bergamot oil is the essential oil expressed from the peel of the fruit of the small tree called *Citrus bergamia*. It is a name that comes from another time with many references in literature. This is one of the many citrus scents. It is wonderfully refreshing, uplifting and can also be very relaxing. As with the other citrus scents, it can cause photosensitization and should not be used if you wish to go out into the sun. Bergamot oil when applied in skin and body care is an antiseptic and is used as an application for acne and other skin afflictions. It can be inhaled as a digestive and to relax the nervous system. Gattefossé considers Bergamot to be cordial, cephalic (used for problems of the head) and stomachic (as an antispasmodic and digestive).

Bergamot oil should always be diluted before use and should never be used by those who are allergic or have very sensitive skin. Bergamot is rarely used these days, as it is expensive and can cause skin sensitivities and irritation.

I like to use it in the diffusor or as a blending oil with others in skin preparations. I particularly like Arctander's description of Bergamot oil as "a green or olive green, mobile liquid of extremely rich, sweet-fruity initial odor. . . . The characteristics of this topnote remain perceptible in good oils, and it's followed by a still more characteristic oily-herbaceous and somewhat balsamic body and dryout. The sweetness yields to a tobacco-like and rich note, reminiscent of Clary Sage." Besides cosmetic preparations, Bergamot oil is used to flavor Tobacco and sometimes as a fixative scent. It is a primary component of the ancient remedy called Hungary Water, which was used as a cure for paralysis and to beautify the complexion.

 Birch oil—There are several essential oils and raw perfume materials produced from various species of Birch tree. Birch Bark oil is produced from *Betula lenta*. Birch Bud oil is produced in several northern European countries from the leaf-buds of *Betula alba*. Birch Tar oil, which has an odor described as "Russian leather," is distilled from several Betula spp. such as *pubescens*, *alba* and *pendula*.

Taken separately the essential oil of Birch Bark is produced from the tree that grows wild throughout northern United States and parts of Canada. (A completely non-related species, the Wintergreen, produces a scent and essential oil that is nearly identical with Birch Bark oil.) This is a refreshing oil described as having a Wintergreen scent (think of chewing gum), is native to the New World, and is used in massage oils for muscular aches and pains. It is used in body oils and baths where it can work as a diuretic, for obesity or water retention or edema. It is useful as a refreshing cleanser. Generally speaking, one would never use Birch Bark oil neat, that is, directly on the skin, undiluted.

Once I decided that the fragrance of Birch Bark oil would be useful in a sauna because of the body odors that had accumulated there. I placed a single drop of the oil on my swimsuit. Within moments in the sauna the oil had volatilized and spread throughout the room and all over my body. I developed a serious rash about my waistline and it took a very long, very cold shower and then continuous applications of healing Bruise juice* to heal the rash from the single drop of Birch Bark oil. The other occupants of this very large sauna enjoyed the fragrance very much. Which brings up another point—Birch Bark oil and oil of Wintergreen can cause allergies in sensitive individuals and should be used with caution.

The oil from Birch buds is used in shampoos for scalp treatments and dandruff and externally in lotions for healing skin irritations.

Birch tar (and Pine tar) is a very old, well-known, old-fashioned product that is still of use in healing lotions and ointments for eczema, psoriasis and other skin disease. It has an oily, sweet, charred-wood and smoky fragrance that is well-known to our elders. When mixed with woody scents such as Vetiver, or Patchouli, it becomes a base for many types of men's fragrances.

In herbal use it is often recommended that the leaves be used for women and the bark for men when properly treating skin disease.

KEEP ESSENTIAL OILS OUT OF YOUR EYES

**See Chapter 6, California, *Herbal Body Works*.

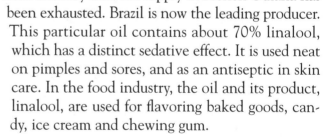 **Black Pepper** oil is a steam-distilled oil from *Piper nigrum* fruits (aka Peppercorns), and is used mainly in essential-oil mixtures as an inhalation for colds, flu and bronchitis. It is an expectorant and blends well with Sandalwood. It is warming and stimulating. See also Pepper, Black, oil.

I personally use a mixture of 1 oz Eucalyptus, ½ oz Basil and ¼ oz each Fennel, Black Pepper and Birch as an inhalant or diffusor mixture for the lungs.

Bois de Rose oil is steam-distilled and water-distilled from *Aniba rosaeodora* and sometimes other species of the genus. It is a tree from the rain forest of Brazil, French Guiana, Surinam and Peru. The synonym is Rosewood (although the word "Rosewood" can mean a variety of species). It is an evergreen tree that grows to 100 feet, and has stiff leathery leaves up to twelve inches long. The leaves are downy yellow on the underside and have woolly-brown terminal flower clusters. In 1875 a

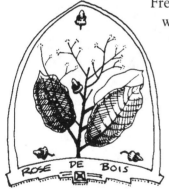

Frenchman first distilled from the bark and chipped wood the fragrant oil that is so esteemed in the perfume industry that the supply in French Guiana has been exhausted. Brazil is now the leading producer. This particular oil contains about 70% linalool, which has a distinct sedative effect. It is used neat on pimples and sores, and as an antiseptic in skin care. In the food industry, the oil and its product, linalool, are used for flavoring baked goods, candy, ice cream and chewing gum.

A relaxing bath mixture would be Rosewood or Bois de Rose 4 drops, Marjoram 2 drops, Lavender 2 drops and 1 drop of Bergamot.

 Cade oil is identical to Juniper Tar oil. It is used externally for psoriasis and many other skin afflictions. Generally, it is used in ointments and salves for all sorts of skin problems. I once applied it externally to my upper

thighs on a reddened patch of skin and nearly drove myself crazy trying to scratch it off. So in the *Herbal Body Book*, I wrote "when applied, it itches like crazy but also anæsthetizes a bad itch. Follow application with a soothing oil or an Aloe rub." Cade oil is often used in soaps as a disinfectant and its fragrance combines well with Thyme oil, Oregano oil or Clove oil.

 Cajeput oil is derived by steam distillation from the fresh leaves and twigs of *Melaleuca minor*, also known as M. *leucadendron* from Indonesia. Since Cajeput oil can be very irritating, its use can be easily replaced by Tea Tree oil or Niaouli oil, both related species of this genus. Like Clove oil, Cajeput oil can be used to dull toothache pain (1 drop in the cavity) until you can get to the dentist. The *Melaleuca* oils all have use as applications for many skin conditions such as fungus, athlete's foot, psoriasis, acne, etc., as a massage on the body for throat and chest infections and as an inhalant to clear the nasal passages. See also Tea Tree oil, Niaouli oil and MQV oil.

 Calamintha nepeta ssp *nepeta* oil is distilled from the tops and leaves from this species of the Lesser Calamint. This is an erect bushy plant that blooms in July and August. Mrs. Grieve, *A Modern Herbal*, states that *Calamintha officinalis*, which is almost identical, contains a camphoraceous, volatile, stimulating oil that is water-distilled but whose superior virtues are better extracted by spirit. The strong odor resembles Pennyroyal and it has a taste like Spearmint only warmer. The herb tea from the leaves makes a pleasant cordial tea taken for weakness of the stomach and flatulent colic. The oil of the Lesser Calamint has a more potent odor, is a lovely amber-pink in color and Kurt Schnaubelt states that "the active principles are monoterpenes, pulegone, menthone and calamenthone. The properties of the oil are hepato-stimulant, hormone-similar (?) and anti-hyperthyroid. The indications are for hyperthyroidism and bronchial mycosis. The contra-indications are for children and pregnancy.*"

 Calendula oil is the infused oil of the Marigold plant, *Calendula officinalis*. This is not an essential oil, but since it is described in many reference works it should also be mentioned here. A quantity of fresh flowers is

---

*Fax received from OSA/PIA, April 3, 1992, courtesy of Kurt Schnaubelt

macerated in warm oil and then gentle heat is applied for several hours after which the golden yellow oil is strained off and used as a carrier oil in aromatherapy products. See also "Carrier Oil" in the formulas section of this book (Chapter VII). The Marigold flowers are very occasionally extracted to produce Marigold absolute, but this has little use outside of the perfume industry. Extractions with water yield an intensely colored liquid that has great value as an herbal hair rinse, or a liquid that can be used in many herbal products, salves and cosmetics. A species of Mexican Marigold, *Tagetes spp.*, can be steam-distilled to produce an essential oil; however, it is not generally available. Again the color and content are more intense when extracted with water. This is used as a reddish tint to rinse hair. It is also called Periçon in Mexico and drunk as tea.

Regarding the Calendula oil used as a carrier oil: this is one of the easiest and simplest basic ingredients that can be homemade. It is generally grossly overpriced, often costing $9.00 to $18.00 for 50 ml (under 2 ounces). You can make it at home for approximately 50 cents for 50 ml. This is a wonderful carrier oil containing quantities of carotene and is used for dry skin or for a healing and relaxing massage. See also Tagetes oil.

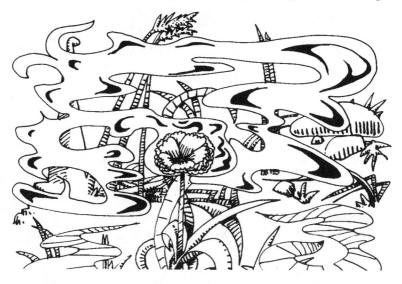

Calophyllum inophyllum oil is an oily-looking, viscous dark-green oil steam-distilled from the bark and seeds. These oily seeds are dispersed by bats and the sea. The EO is used on the scalp for healthy hair and mixed with *Helichrysum* for burns and wounds.

⬦ **Camomile** (or Chamomile*) is that wonderful yellow daisy-like flower that is used for everything: cosmetics, fragrance, oil, herbal baths, soothing tea. The root is used for toothache and the entire plant in herbal therapeutics. The whole plant is used from root to flower. The essence is obtained by steam distillation of the flowers. Camomile smells sweet, resembling fresh golden apples, and this fruity scent has given it the name of Manzanilla in Spanish-speaking countries.

Externally, an infusion of the flower heads is used as a facial steam to cleanse the pores, and as a wash and poultice to reduce facial puffiness. The infusion and poultice can be used as a rinse for the hair. The lighter your hair is, the more golden will be the effect of the floral poultice on it. On dark hair a thick decoction of Camomile flowers will supply bright highlights.

The Egyptians had a great reverence for Camomile and used it in massage oils to remove aches and pains. Sports-minded people will like using the flowers in a bath for relaxation and to ease aching muscles. This plant was one of the favored strewing herbs of the Middle Ages, to sweeten the air of a room and create a relaxing atmosphere.

Camomile oil is produced in several countries: France, Morocco, Spain, Egypt and others. The distillate from the *Anthemis nobilis*, the Roman Chamomile, is golden yellow while the oil of *Matricaria recutita* or *chamomilla*, the German or Hungarian Chamomile, is a lovely deep blue, due to the presence of azulene.

⬦ Chamomile is much used in aromatherapy. It has a pronounced effect on the mind and nervous system. The scent is rejuvenative and especially helpful to those of a sensitive nature. Inhaling the herby, aromatic, slightly bitter but always refreshing scent of the golden Chamomile blossoms will ease your depression, soothe your irritable nature, lull you into a restful sleep and calm you. Use the oil straight or use it in combinations to relax and soothe a busy household after a trying day. A busy woman might like dabbing a drop or two of Chamomile oil on the forearm, to inhale occasionally during the day, for relaxation and to allay temper. Remember that oil of Chamomile is recommended for use in

---

*Throughout this work and all other references as well, you will note the variant spellings of this daisy-like flower. Usually, Camomile is a common name and Chamomile is a scientific name. But inconsistency is the rule and both spellings are acceptable.

Various Chamomiles, Camomiles

Chamomiles—The plants called Chamomile have been in use for herbal products and body care for thousands of years. There are two main plants in use: one is an annual and the other is a low-growing mat-like perennial. Unfortunately, the Latin binomials have become a confusing array of various names. Scientists have changed the names to suit themselves and their particular form of taxonomy.

	1973 *The Herbal Body Book*	1991 *The Aromatherapy Book*
German Chamomile annual Chamomile Hungarian Camomile contains chamazulene for severe skin problems use externally anti-inflammatory anti-allergenic	*Matricaria chamomilla*	*Matricaria recutita*
Roman Chamomile mat-like Chamomile perennial Camomile English Camomile azulene inhalation oral use anti-inflammatory anti-allergenic	*Anthemis nobilis*	*Chamæmelum nobile*
blue Chamomile Moroccan Chamomile contains chamazulene mixta Chamomile Moroccan Chamomile	*probably the same plant used as an adulterant*	*Ormensis multicolis* *Oremis multicolis* *Anthemis mixta*

the diffusor, in a child's room, for the æsthetic, for the calm that will come, for sweet sleep.

The herbal uses of Chamomiles have been documented in many sources including my own *Herbal Body Book*, where dozens of formulas and recipes are given for the external uses of these wonderful plants. These plants have been used for centuries as medicine for both external application and internal use. Primarily this medicinal use is due to the azulene content, although the two plants are quite different in their essential oil and chemical composition.

Roman Chamomile oil is steam-distilled from the flower heads of *Chamæmelum nobile*. This oil is almost insoluble in glycerin but quite soluble in mineral oil and some other oils. It has one of the highest contents of esters of any known essential oil, 250–310. The chamazulene is formed during distillation and the quantity decreases with time during storage. The oil contains a lower concentration of azulenes than the German Chamomile and does not stimulate liver regeneration after subcutaneous application. Taken orally, it is an effective therapeutic agent. Occasionally, contact dermatitis has occurred with this oil and it should probably not be used by those who are allergic to the Ragweed family. This Chamomile as with the German Chamomile has almost no incidence of allergic reaction itself, but since herbal samples are sometimes contaminated with other types of Chamomiles, notably *Anthemis cotula*, it is best to collect or grow your own flowers for water infusions and internal and external use. Roman Chamomile oil is used in perfumes and all sorts of cosmetic preparations.

German Chamomile oil is collected from flower heads of *Matricaria recutita* by either solvent extraction or steam distillation. Some components of the oil are only available by using large quantities of water, so the product is often redistilled. The deep blue color of German Chamomile oil is due to the content of azulene (chamazulene). Acid value of the German oil is higher than the Roman and so more azulene forms. Certain chemotypes* of this oil produce more or less amounts of alpha-bisabolol, chamazulene and farnesene, and these various amounts determine what the specific chemotype will be used for. For example, when Chamomile is

---

*Chemotype-certain particular varieties are grown to produce essential oils that predominate in one chemical constituent or another. Generally depends on the plants' growing environment.

collected in the morning, the essential oil retrieved will be high in far-nesene and bisabolol, but these chemical compounds change and alter during the day and only traces are found in the oil when the plants are collected in the evening and distilled. The azulene of the German Chamomile is known to stimulate liver regeneration, and subcutaneous treatments will initiate formation of new tissue. There is much bisabolol and here it acts as an antimycotic, anti-inflammatory and ulcer-protective. The anti-inflammatory effects of German Chamomile extracts predominate externally while the smooth-muscle relaxing effects predominate internally. Extracts are useful for persons who have infections of the skin or mucosa.

Using Chamomile oil—Generally speaking, use Roman Chamomile oil by inhalation and orally; use German Chamomile oil by external application and massage. Both are anti-inflammatory and antiallergenic. When used by inhalation the oils are immunostimulant, calming and relaxing. Menstrual pains are soothed from any source. The oils ease headaches and insomnia and are used as a rub for arthritic joints. They are also antispasmodic. One of the five most important essential oils (Chamomile, Eucalyptus, Lavender, Myrrh, Rose).*

§ **Cananga oil** is water-distilled from *Cananga odorata*; see also Ylang-Ylang oil. It is said to stimulate the adrenal glands.

§ **Caraway oil** is steam-distilled from the ripe, dried and crushed fruits (seed) of *Carum carvi*. This small herb is native to Asia, Europe and United States where it grows wild, and is cultivated in many countries including those of Eastern Europe, Spain and India. Caraway herb or oil can be used in facial steam mixtures to stimulate the complexion. It is best used by pale-complected persons to give their skin color and "life."

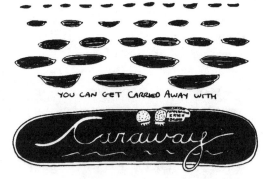

YOU CAN GET CARRIED AWAY WITH
Caraway

---

*For further information see *The Chemistry, Pharmacology, and Commercial Formulations of Chamomile* by Mann and Staba; Dept. Med. Chem, Coll. of Pharmacology, University of Minneapolis, Minneapolis, Minnesota 55455.

A poultice of the seeds with Chamomile is helpful to reduce inflammation and bruises. The essential oil is used *internally* to stimulate the circulation, as a flavoring agent in foods, to kill intestinal parasites, as a digestive stimulant and carminative and to stimulate the lymphatic system. This oil is used *externally* to help cure mange in dogs, to kill scabies, as an all-over body stimulant. It is inhaled to refresh the conscious mind, as a stimulant and to enhance alertness. The oil can also be rubbed around an aching tooth to reduce pain. The main constituents of Caraway oil are carvone and limonene but the percentages change depending on how long the fruits are on the still or how old the oil is.

I have a dog with a propensity to skin irritation, and hot spots. The mixture of oils I use to keep this chronic problem under control is 20 drops each of Caraway oil, Tea Tree oil, Lavender oil and Carrot Seed oil, in 4 oz of water. This is a 4% solution. Use in a spray bottle. Shake and spray on problem areas twice a day.

 Carrot Seed oil is steam-distilled from the dried seed of the common Carrot, *Daucus carota*. Carrot Seed oil contains quantities of carotene that just might provide Vitamin A to the skin. The pores of the skin do not just work one way; toxins go out and herbal nutrients *can go in*. So start with clean skin before applying Carrot Seed oil or any aromatherapy quality essential oil.

This oil is only used by application and not by inhalation. It can be used in massage, facials, lotions, potions, masks and with carrier oils in full-body massage. This is an excellent all-purpose oil that is used as a tonic for the skin and relieves any sort of skin irritation or rash, helps to deter and to reduce wrinkles, and is used with such oils as Parsley or Celery or Birch to reduce edema in the tissues. It is definitely a stimulant to the reproductive system and should not be used internally unless abortion is desired. In massage oils, Carrot Seed oil is useful for menstrual troubles and as an emmenagogue. It is a stimulant for all the glands and a stimulating oil in general. Might have some use to create appetite in the anorexic in full body or abdominal massage. Carrot Seed oil has a very earthy, very rooty, very heavy odor. When inhaling this scent, salivation is apt to occur. Price ranges from $10 to $35 (!) per 5 ml although I have seen it advertised at $10.50/oz (29 ml). This oil has one of the greatest price ranges I have seen.

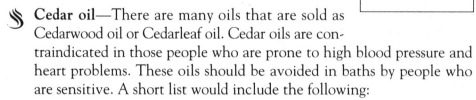

DILUTE
ESSENTIAL
OILS
BEFORE
USING

 Cassia oil is used to stimulate the pancreas.

 Cedar oil—There are many oils that are sold as Cedarwood oil or Cedarleaf oil. Cedar oils are con-traindicated in those people who are prone to high blood pressure and heart problems. These oils should be avoided in baths by people who are sensitive. A short list would include the following:

 1. Cedarleaf oil or Thuja oil from *Thuja occidentalis*, which primarily contains thujone, a skin irritant that is somewhat poisonous. Generally this oil is used only as a disinfectant; a few drops mixed with water would be a handy way to wash down counter tops and wooden tables. A drop can be applied directly to a wart (verruca).

2. Cedarwood "Atlas" oil from *Cedrus atlantica*. The oil is primarily of use in aromatherapy as an application or inhalation for the respiratory system. It is antiseptic, fungicidal and reduces oily secretions. It can be added to shampoos or facial washes. Inhaled it has great uses in the respiratory system and is excreted via lungs and urine. A drop of oil in ½ cup water is used as a gargle for sore throat. A few drops with Eucalyptus in a steaming bowl of water is a wonderful measure to reduce nasal and lung congestion.

For bronchitis and asthma keep a small bottle of this oil mixed about half and half with Eucalyptus and Chamomile (2 oz water + 10 drops Cedar + 10 drops Eucalyptus + 2 drops Camomile), and inhale whenever necessary. You can also use it on a hanky that you can inhale discreetly whenever necessary to reduce asthmatic symptoms.

Atlas Cedarwood oil is a fine addition to any massage oil, especially when respiration improvement is the target of the massage. In the perfume trade Atlas Cedar oil is used for its tremendous fixative effect. *Cedrus atlantica* is a Pine not a Cypress. This is the tree that is believed to have originated from the Lebanon Cedars of Bible fame.

3. Cedarwood oil from East Africa is steam-distilled from a type of Juniper called *Juniperus procera* and is used primarily to scent and fragrance soaps or in perfumery.

4. Himalaya Cedarwood oil is steam-distilled from *Cedrus deodara*. This tree is very closely related to the Atlas Cedarwood and it is possible that the oil could be substituted for it in various formulas.

5. There is also a variety of oils that are produced from Japanese Cedarwood and go under several names such as Sugi, Hiba or Hinoki oils.

6. The famous tree, *Cedrus libani* or Lebanon Cedar, is possibly the oldest perfume material known. The trees are protected on Cyprus and in Lebanon and the essential oil is no longer used. Distillation of this oil probably began over 5500 years ago.

7. Port Orford Cedarwood from *Chamæcyparis lawsoniana* has a delicately fragrant needle that is used in potpourri. The steam-distilled oil is wonderfully fragrant but has as yet no particular use in aromatherapy. However, I have occasionally used it as an inhalation for congested respiratory passages.*

8. Texas Cedarwood is steam-distilled from *Juniperus mexicana* and is used as a disinfectant and in perfumery.

Champaca oil or Champa oil is obtained by extracting *Michelia champaca*, a lovely flower that is very deep yellow in color. Champaca is native to Indonesia and the Philippines and has been grown in similar areas. An infused oil is made from the flowers and used in massage and as a hair dressing. The absolute is obtained by extraction and this expensive product is sometimes cut with Ylang-Ylang, which is somewhat cheaper in price. Champaca oil has a warm, luscious odor and mixes well with Sandalwood. The oil diluted with Calendula-infused oil can be used in massage or when mixed with essential oils used as a perfume.

---

* Regarding Port Orford Cedar; it no longer grows to reproductive maturity as a result of an unknown pathogen. This is a great pity as the scent is wonderful. It is a very rare wood and if you contact Mark Wheeler at Pacific Botanicals, it is possible that he may be able to have some gathered for you.

Chilé (Red) Pepper oil is the oleo-resin obtained from *Capsicum annuum*. This is a powerful, extremely concentrated substance. I recommend it*— for only one use—and that is to deter animals from eating your plants and dogs from defecating on your sidewalk. I am not sure where or when I received the gallon of viscous reddish-black substance, *Capsicum* oleo-resin, that resides in my basement but for years I could not conceive how to use it. However, I do live in the city and my one poor tree in a hole in the sidewalk kept dying and being replaced mainly because the loose dogs in the neighborhood used the tree for their own private bathroom. Well, one day I added a scoop of this oil to some Crisco and stirred it up really good and with a narrow paintbrush painted the sidewalk around the tree with this mixture. Then I stood near the window overlooking the sidewalk and waited. Sure enough, along came the neighbors' squeaky little dog. It got a good whiff of the mixture, lifted his leg, put it down and ran squeaking out of view. The next dog walked over the line to take her dump, smelled her paws; licked them and "goodbye" dog. So now I paint the sidewalk at regular intervals and have not had to clean up dog doodoo since.

This mixture works as well in the garden. Paint a rock and drop one down each gopher hole. Paint your fences and keep cats out. For deer make a double fence, 2 feet between and surrounding your yard, and

---

Cellulite and Lymph Congestion

mix
        1 drop to 1 oz carrier oil or

1 drop Chilé Pepper oil
3 drops Cypress oil } mix with 4 oz carrier oil
1 drop Cumin oil

After a bath (see Chapter IX) rub into the areas of cellulite.

—*Victoria Edwards*

---

*Victoria Edwards uses Chilé Pepper oil and says it is good in massage oil mixtures for poor circulation, and as a rub for cellulite and lymphatic congestion.

paint the outer fence only. This can be painted directly on trees but must not be used on tender plants. For snails, put a flat barrier like rocks or bricks around the area that you wish to protect and paint the barrier.

Please don't get this mixture in your eyes—if you do you will end up jumping around screaming and howling, while you splash water in your eyes. The burning sensation goes away in 4 hours.

> KEEP
> ESSENTIAL
> OILS OUT
> OF YOUR
> EYES

 Cilantro oil—see Coriander oil.

Cinnamon oil is steam-distilled from *Cinnamomum zeylanicum*. Both the bark and the leaf are distilled to create two products. Generally we are familiar with the bark oil that has a distinct germicidal effect, even stronger than Clove oil. Cinnamon oil is very strong and usually not recommended for the aromatherapy beginner to use. In the hands of a competent aromatherapist, Cinnamon bark oil is used as a stimulant for the circulation, as an antiseptic, as an occasional aphrodisiac especially as an inhalant, and by direct application to kill head lice and scabies. Once a friend of mine who was visiting from Big Sur tried Cinnamon oil on his pubic lice— his screams could be heard around the block. Cold compresses and then the application of Bruise Juice* eased the skin irritation and the pubic lice turned up dead. Cinnamon oil is especially wonderful when sprinkled on rolled Cinnamon sticks and then placed in potpourri. Cinnamon oil should only be used highly diluted. Inhaled it is used as a sudorific (makes you sweat) and in ritual incense against malice or spite. The aroma of Cinnamon is said to increase your ability to tap into your psychic mind and to increase financial prosperity.

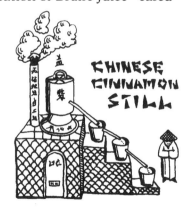
CHINESE CINNAMON STILL

*See Chapter VI, California: *Herbal BodyWorks*

Cistus oil—See Labdanum.

 Citron oil—See Lemon oil.

 Citronella oil—The oil is steam-distilled from a variety of Managrass or Lemon Balm grass, *Cymbopogon nardus*. Who does not remember smelling this intense scent on nights filled with bugs and mosquitoes? The oil is mainly used in bug repellents or applied as a mosquito repellent. It can also be used in lotions and soaps to repel insects and deodorize. Mixed equally with Virginia Cedarwood oil it is used as an application to repel bugs. Inhaled, the scent has an effect on the heart, often speeding up the beat. This is definitely not recommended in aromatherapy demonstrations where there are people present with heart problems. In dilution anyone can use this oil externally.

Citronella oil is generally very cheap and can be used as an antiseptic to sanitize and deodorize surfaces where food is cooked or chopped or handled. Mix 5 drops of essential oil in 1 ounce of fixed oil such as Olive oil and rub into a chopping block after you have cleaned it. Or mix 5 drops of essential oil in 1 ounce white vinegar as a wash for any surfaces used for serving or cooking. The scent of this oil is repugnant to cats and so can be used as an application to plant tubs or table legs or fences to repel these felines. The herb itself is used for oily skin or hair in shampoo, washes or vinegar rinses.

Citrus Scents include:

Citrus aurantium, see Neroli and Petitgrain;
Citrus bergamia, see Bergamot;
Citrus bigaradia, see Neroli;
Citrus limonum peel, see Lemon;
Citrus medica is the fruit Citron;
Citrus medica var. acida, see Lime;
Citrus nobilis, see Tangerine or Mandarin;
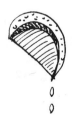
Citrus paradisi, see Grapefruit;
Citrus reticulata peel, see Mandarin and Tangerine;
Citrus sinensis peel, see Orange;
Citrus vulgaris, see Neroli.

Clary Sage oil is distilled from the flowering tops and leaves of *Salvia sclarea*. This is a perennial plant that became as tall as me when I grew it in my urban yard. The tops were sticky and the smell was herby and sort of bitter—I sometimes described it as smelling like a cat. This oil is much used in perfumery, as it contains a large quantity of linalool (linalol)* which is easily synthesized and often adulterated. True Clary Sage oil that is genuine and natural will cost approximately $10–$14 for 5 ml (about ⅙ oz).

This oil is used in aromatherapy as an application for people over 50, for aging skin, to regenerate skin, reduce wrinkles, with Sandalwood oil for menstrual irregularities, and inhaled to reduce tension or as an antidepressant, and for "grounding." Clary Sage oil mixed with Jojoba is a fine application to hair roots to stimulate growth (4 drops/1 oz). As with many oils that can be considered to be a Mediterranean type, the best comes from soil that is not too rich, not too moist and on the alkaline side. The herb is easily grown and is used in bath herb mixtures as an aromatic astringent. For relaxation and quiet sleep, take a 20-minute herb bath of Clary Sage and Lemon Verbena, and while you are in the tub drink a cup of warm Lemon Verbena tea, rub 1–2 drops of Clary Sage oil on your bath towel, pat yourself dry with it, jump into your silk jammies and pop into bed for a delicious night's sleep. Clary Sage EO can be used in home diffusors set on 20-minute bursts of operation for hot flashes, menopause symptoms, adrenal problems and heat waves for people who use steroids, and for the elderly who often suffer from waves of heat and other disorders.

 Cloves, *Eugenia caryophyllata*, have been in cultivation for at least 2000 years. The immature flower buds or Clove buds are water-or steam-distilled to produce the oil. Historically, the flowers, buds, leaves and twigs were used for scent. A famous scent of the 16th century was Rondoletia, which is synergy of Cloves and Lavender. The original scent included musk and ambergris and could probably not be duplicated today. See *The Magic of Herbs* by C. F. Leyel, page 196, for the formula. In older days it was thought that you could not walk near Clove trees while wearing a hat because the tree would become frightened and would no longer bear fruit. Septimas Piesse determined that fragrance could be correlated to

---

* Linalol—Kills bacteria, relieves discomfort.

sound and color: Cloves were one of the seven primary odors. The Clove scent was considered to vibrate in the key of B and in the color of violet.

Medicinally, Clove oil is antiseptic, stimulating, pain-killing, a carminative, parasiticide and sometimes aphrodisiacal. It is generally applied externally, greatly diluted, as an application for rheumatism, arthritis, for muscular aches and pains. It is inhaled to stimulate the mind, to overcome exhaustion, to stimulate memory, to stimulate the respiratory system and as an antiseptic for various infectious diseases. If too much is inhaled it can act as a soporific; it can cause a good sleep generally culminating in stimulating dreams. This was one of the first oils to be directly applied in therapy — in aching teeth to anesthetize them or on warts to remove them. However, it is considered strongly allergenic — take care.

Clove bark oil is steam-distilled from *Dicypellium caryophyllatum*, commonly called Brazil Clove, Clove Bark or Cayenne Rosewood. It is a native of the central Amazon region of Brazil to French Guiana. This is a small tree and all parts smell and taste like Clove buds. The flower buds are used in Brazilian cookery. The distilled oil is now in little demand.

Coriander oil is steam-distilled from the fully ripened but dried fruit of *Coriandrum sativum*. This is a smallish plant and the seeds (fruit) are crushed just prior to distillation. Coriander oil is mainly used in the food industry as well as in aromatherapy. The oil is warming, smells sweet and woody, is a spicy aromatic and a nice addition to mixtures to be used in perfume.

Aromatherapy uses are: *Internally* as a medicine; a carminative to ease flatulence; an antispasmodic for digestion problems; and a stimulant to the entire body. It is used *externally* in rubs or massage oil mixtures as a warming pain-easer for arthritis or rheumatic complaints; rubbed on the temples to ease pain of a migraine headache; as a revivifying stimulant to be used during convalescence from long-term illness; an application for oily skin, blackheads and skin impurities.

It blends well with such oils as Anise, Cardamom, Sage, Bergamot and Clary Sage. Mixed with other members of the *Umbelliferae* family such as Dill, Anise, Fennel and Caraway, it is used as a stimulating digestive.

Coriander oil should be diluted 1:5 with carrier oil before application on external skin problems.

Coriander is an herb, considered a spice, and has been in use for thousands of years to flavor food and especially the true curries of India, where it was introduced by the Arabs. Coriander was found in the tomb of Tutankhamun and later Pliny mentions Egyptian Coriander as a remedy for the bite of the two-headed serpent.

Cilantro oil is distilled from the leaves of the Coriander plant. It has a very fresh powerful scent.

Croton oil is very toxic but has historical use as a stimulant for the pineal gland. I do not know how it is used.

Cubeb oil (*Piper cubeba*) is occasionally used as a stimulant for the parathyroid glands and is considered a substitute for *Litsea cubeba*. See also *Litsea cubeba*.

Cumin oil is distilled from the dried, ripe fruits of *Cuminum cyminum*. This oil is used mainly in the food industry. It has medicinal value as a digestive stimulant, is used for flatulence, and could probably be a wonderful cure as an inhalant for constipation. And here is where I have my experience from Cumin oil. In 1972 I was researching for the *Herbal Body Book* and making numerous formulations using essential oils. By 1973 I was married and pregnant and had finally gotten to the writing part of the *Aromatherapy* chapters. My son Bryan was born in November and he had a very pleasant disposition except for the odd but normal habit of only having a poop about every 5–7 days. This was wonderful if we wanted to go out with him because there was never a need to change a stinky diaper. However, it wasn't so wonderful towards the end of those 5 or 7 days if we expected to go out, because the thought of changing those enormous overflowing diapers was frightening. One evening while breastfeeding Bryan and smelling various essential oils, I opened the Cumin oil. It smelled rich and delicious like a really good curry. I let Baby Bryan have a whiff and he immediately rewarded me with a very full and yeasty diaper. I thought this was very interesting. The next time we had to go out, we let Baby Bryan smell the Cumin oil and again he had his weekly poop (after only 3 days). So this became our standard treatment to encourage Bryan to have a BM prior to any event or any family dinner and it worked 100% of the time.

> ### DILUTE ESSENTIAL OILS BEFORE USING

I would say that there is little use for Cumin oil externally, but inhaled it has a fragrance of good food and would be stimulating to the appetite if a bit were vaporized in an aromatic lamp prior to a dinner party. You might also let your baby inhale it if you wish to encourage a bowel movement. A very novel way to use aromatherapy!

Victoria Edwards recommends using Cumin oil for lymphatic congestion and poor circulation. She says a few drops in a massage oil blend work wonders.

Cyclamen oil—I have seen this oil listed on labels of various products but can find no reference for it nor can I determine a source.

Cypress oil is steam-distilled from the needles, twigs and cones of *Cupressus sempervirens*, an evergreen tree that no doubt originated in the Mediterranean area. This rather reasonably priced oil has great use, primarily for the respiratory and circulatory systems. It is warming and stimulating and uplifting. And it can also be soothing and relaxing when inhaled just before bedtime. This is a very good oil to be added to mixtures for oily hair, oily skin, or sweaty palms and feet. It is astringent and helps to reduce overactive sweat and oil glands. It is useful in mixtures to reduce fluid retention and cellulite. Use in baths or massage oils for aching muscles, abdominal cramps or menstrual cramps. Mix it in with your alcohol rubs for arthritis pain. Inhaled through a vaporizer or AromaLamp this oil is particularly beneficial for those who suffer from respiratory problems, congestion or asthma. It is antispasmodic and antiseptic; a drop in ½ glass water can be gargled for sore throat, coughing or laryngitis. Mrs. C. F. Leyel in *Cinquefoil* mentions "the balsamic resin of the Cypress, if inhaled, heals diseased lungs, and when it is burnt has a beneficial effect on the mucous lining of the nose." Price ranges from $8 to $18 for 15 ml (½ oz). Cypress is excellent for smoothing transitions, particularly the loss of friends and loved ones or the endings of relationships. Inhale the fragrance for strength and comfort.

An ancient Cypress tree, the Sahara Cypress (*Cupressus dupreziana*), also called "tarout" by the Tuareg tribespeople, has been in use for at least 2500 years for utensils and light construction. It is possible that this ancient tree was used centuries ago for its aromatic resinous wood as an inhalant and medicine when the Sahara was green and rain was more abundant. Now the few trees that are left (only 160) are numbered and protected against vandals and wood choppers. See *Natural History*, September 1991, for an interesting story of this tree.

Daru Haridra oil vapors are used to treat female sex glands.

Dill Seed oil is steam-distilled from the ripe, dried and crushed fruits (seed) of *Anethum graveolens*. This small herb is cultivated in the United States, Germany, England and some other countries. The oil is almost identical with Caraway oil and can be used much in the same way and even substituted for Caraway in most formulations.

Dill Weed oil is steam-distilled from the entire plant and to date has found little use in aromatherapy.

Elemi oil from *Canarium commune*, a plant native to the Philippines, is used to treat the thymus gland.

Eucalyptus oil is steam-distilled from a number of different types of the tree *Eucalyptus spp*. Leydet oils has the greatest number of these diverse types of Eucalyptus as follows: *E. globulus*, *E. australiana*, *E. radiata*, *E.* chemotype from *E. globulus*, *Eucalyptus* chemotype A from *E. australiana*, *E. citriodora* and *E.* chemotype SP from *E. globulus*. Each of these oils and chemotype oils are from one specified chemical race, rather like Zinfandel wine is of one variety but each vineyard produces a Zinfandel of a particular quality and taste.

In general, Eucalyptus oil is used as a specific for the respiratory system. It is an antiseptic stimulant with a very specific balsamic odor that can only be eponymously described as smelling like Eucalyptus. This oil has great value in a vaporizer to stimulate and loosen bronchial secretions so that they can be coughed up, and is used primarily for coughs, colds, bronchial infections and asthma. Eucalyptus oil is very effective in killing bacteria and for clearing the system when used in a vaporizer. It is antiviral and cooling. I like Eucalyptus oil mixed equally with Peppermint oil and white vinegar added as a cooling spritz for a fever. This is also used in an application for the skin as an effective treatment for acne or boils. Naturally, the cooling spritz is also cleansing to the body. Used singly or with other oils such as Citronella it is a very good insect repellent. I find that Eucalyptus oil can be used singly but the strong camphoraceous odor is wonderfully adaptable to a number of other oils that both enhance the effects but soften and soothe the scent. Besides those mentioned, mix Eucalyptus oil with Tea Tree oil for external fungus infections such as athlete's foot; with Rosemary oil as an anti-inflammatory for aching muscles or arthritis; with Ammi visnaga as an inhalant for allergic asthma; or with Sandalwood or Black Pepper in the vaporizer for bronchitis.

 Fennel oil is steam-distilled from the ripe fruits of the Fennel seeds (*Fœniculum vulgare*). There is bitter Fennel oil and sweet Fennel oil. In my uses of essential oils I have had very little use for Fennel except in scenting spicy potpourri. Fennel seed oil is very reasonably priced and could be used as a digestive or a tasty addition to certain types of food. But why bother? The Fennel seeds themselves are just as aromatic and tasty.

Fennel seeds and the oil can go into mixtures of herbs to steam-clean the skin or in baths when weight loss is desired. Fennel seed oil and Dill seed oil, 1 drop of each, can be used as an inhalant to soothe the stomach, and can be used as well in a vaporizer. I have used this mixture for those days just after the holidays when every day I felt as if I had overeaten.

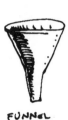 Inhaling a bit of Fennel oil is certainly nicer than taking Maalox or drinking some strong medicinal herbal tea. The fragrance of Fennel lends itself to scenting the house for any holiday. A dab of Fennel oil and a dab of Fir oil on your Christmas tree is just the thing to keep your house fragrant for Christmas.

FUNNEL   FENNEL

The properties of Fennel are mildly antiseptic, strongly antispasmodic and carminative, slightly diuretic and expectorant. It is used for flatulence, nausea, obesity and vomiting. Mix it with Orange oil, Almond meal (ground Almonds) and Cornmeal and use it after your bath to scrub away dead skin cells and cellulite. See the formulas for a more complete recipe. Fennel seed tea or a drop of Fennel oil in a glass of water are used to encourage milk production in first-time mothers.

Fennel oil is antibacterial, antispasmodic, aperitif, carminative, digestive stimulant, weak diuretic. It is also a slight emmenagogue, galactagogue, influences estrogen production and is a vermifuge. It is eaten as an herb or the oil used externally and internally as an aid to weight reduction.

There is a nice long monograph on Fennel in *Aromatherapy World*, Issue 1, January 1991, published by ISPA in England.

Fir Needle oil is steam-distilled from various species and types of the leaves and twigs of *Abies, Larix, Picea* and *Pinus*. Most companies that retail oils seem to prefer the Siberian Fir, *Abies sibirica*, or the Balsam Fir Needle oil, from *Abies balsamea*. These are extremely low-priced oils that are just wonderful used during the winter or holiday seasons to scent the house, the decorations or the holiday tree. The scent is wonderfully refreshing bringing to mind the crisp heady scent of a forest just after a rain. This scent can elevate your emotions and "ground" you or make you feel comfortable and at home.

Fir Needle has several uses, primarily on the antiseptic side. Both oils are "warm" and refreshing scents and are used in the nebulizer or vaporizer for all sorts of respiratory problems and as a gentle tonic to the nervous system. To refresh your home and to bring the clean scent of the outdoors inside, use a spritzer to spray the air and to spray over the carpets, then vacuum—it will smell great. My feeling is that the scent of the Firs and Pines are a gentle sedative and can be used to stimulate the thinking while the body rests and relaxes. I primarily use this oil to scent potpourris and bath herbs, and especially in a product that I call Deep Forest Bath. See the formula section for the recipe.

Frankincense oil is steam-distilled from the *Boswellia carteri*. A resin exudes in drops when the tree bark is damaged, and this resin is collected and used in religious service as an incense. From the burning incense a fragrance issues that floats on an invisible thread to heaven to attract god's attention. Frankincense is one of the very first products used in ritual. During Roman times, when cremation was widely practiced, it was also customary to burn it in the funeral pyre. This may have been to propitiate the god, but Pliny the Elder suggests that it was intended to disguise the unpleasant odor of burning flesh.

After the resin is collected and some used for incense or sold as "tears," it is then steam-distilled and an essential oil produced. This oil is powerfully antiseptic and astringent and tonic. It is used for external skin afflictions such as boils and pimples, and as an inhalant for bronchitis, colds, coughs and excess mucus production. Generally speaking the essential oil is inhaled for the respiratory system as well as used externally for skin care. Physically when you inhale the scent of the oil or the incense it seems to slow you down, to deepen the way you breathe, to cause introspection that helps with meditation and prayer. This is one of the finest ritual oils.

Soaps made with Frankincense and Myrrh are used as a ritual cleansing for the body prior to serious meditation or special rituals. The soap and the oils are of particular use for aging or wrinkled skin but should be mixed with a carrier oil for best effect.

For mental problems, for depression, for those who cannot get on with their lives, there is no equal to Frankincense, although for best results it should be mixed with other oils to enhance the effects. Frankincense works on the 6th chakra and can be mixed with Myrrh and Balsam Tolu as well as Lavender.

The ancient Egyptians used Frankincense not only as scent and fragrance but also as a fumigant, incense or in medical prescriptions. In their hieroglyphs it is described as "being from the land of Punt," which is present-day Somalia. Pliny tells us further that an entire year's production of Arabian Frankincense was burned in the funeral pyre of Poppaea, the wife of Emperor Nero. What he doesn't tell us is that Nero kicked his pregnant wife to death and tried to propitiate the gods and cleanse his guilt by burning this enormous amount of Frankincense.

In November 1991, it was reported that the ancient fabled center of the Frankincense trade, the lost city of Ubar, was found using ancient maps and modern survey cameras from space. Ubar is in Oman near the Arabian sea. Ubar was in use as far back as 2000 B.C. and its destruction by collapsing into the limestone cavern upon which it was built is chronicled in the *Arabian Nights*.

See also Myrrh.

Galanga oil is steam-distilled from the finely chopped and pulverized rhizome of *Alpinia officinarum*, which is related to both Ginger and Cardamom. It is native to China but is now grown elsewhere. This rhizome is used in Asian cooking sometimes as a substitute for Ginger but it has its own very particular uses in food. The essential oil is woody and spicy and smells like a combination of Ginger and Cardamom. It tastes warm but has a cooling aftertaste sort of like Peppermint oil. A drop can be added to store-bought Ginger Ale to improve and intensify the flavor. It is used as a disinfectant and an antiseptic and sometimes to treat the pancreas. Do not confuse Galangal, Galanga or False-Ginger oil with *Kæmferia galanga* which is also known as False Galanga oil.

Galbanum is a natural fatty gummy resin obtained from *Ferul galbanifera*. The oil is steam-distilled from this resin. It has a very strong odor and is a useful fixative in perfumery and incense. Another name is *Peucedanum galbaniflora* or Sulphur wort. This was considered a "green" incense by the ancient Egyptians and is mentioned in their earliest texts as having been imported from Persia. Theophrastus mentions it as being used in an ointment to warm. It soothes aching hands and feet and joints. In Coptic medicine it was used to expel little beasts and bugs from the home. Galbanum has a very strong Green Pepper or fresh Green Pea smell and is very harmonizing and balancing for the psyche.

Victoria Edwards says that M. Maury suggests great benefits for revitalizing aging skin when Galbanum is mixed with Violet leaf oil and Rose oil in a facial blend. She warns that Galbanum should not be used on young skin. It is sometimes used to treat the pineal gland.

 Garlic oil, *Allium sativum,* is the oil made when you infuse large amounts of Garlic in a vegetable oil such as Olive oil. There is no such thing as an essential oil of Garlic. But if you do make a Garlic (Garlicked) oil, by all means keep it refrigerated at all times, as there is danger of botulism germs growing in the product that would certainly do your health no good at all when you went to eat it or use it on something. I use the infused oil of Garlic carefully strained as ear drops to relieve middle ear pain, brushed onto French bread to make a delicious appetizer, or for croutons.

Garlic oil has other uses, mostly in the area of cooking. But if you have a child that suffers chronic ear infections, nothing is quite so effective as well-made ear drops of Olive oil in which Garlic has been allowed to macerate for a few days and is then strained out.

Garlic mashed in water and then strained through very fine silk cloth makes a great nose drop to cure sinus infections. This, however, must be *freshly made* each time you wish to use the drops. Ten drops of the liquid are snorted three times per day for three days. This is just about 100% guaranteed to cure even the most obstinate sinus infection. See *Herbs & Things* page 210, for more information.

Geranium oil, or Rose Geranium oil, is also called African or Algerian Geranium oil, and is steam-distilled from *Pelargonium graveolens*. It is also steam-distilled from *Pelargonium asperum*, according to Victoria Edwards, who retails it for about $9/5 ml. It has a lovely greenish color with a very distinctive flavor and scent that can only be described eponymously as "geranium-scented." There are many different fragrances in this fragrant-leaved plant called Geranium, *Pelargonium spp.*; and these scents range from "apple" to "apricot" to "lemon," "lime," "rose," etc. But for our purposes here we will only discuss the essential oil that is steam-distilled from the Bourbon type Geranium.

The oil comes from both the flowers and flowering tops and produces an herby-scented flower oil. This oil is of most use in applications for aged, wrinkling or older skin, as well as for healing balms and salves after facial or plastic surgery. When *inhaled* the scent is antidepressant, uplifting, averts tension and is stimulating to the psyche. It can be mixed with Rosemary oil and inhaled to aid the memory. As an *external* application this oil can be used slightly diluted with a carrier oil and then simply applied directly, but it has much more value when added to any sort of lotion, hand cream, shampoo, etc. In this context it is healing and antiseptic as well as a cellular regenerative. It has value in body and facial preparations where it acts to balance the function of the oil glands, and so it can be used for both dry skin and oily skin.

Geranium oil seems to be an adrenal cortex stimulant and so it mixes well with Camomile and Myrrh. It seems that it would have value as an inhalant for those with adrenal function problems, such as persons with asthma or even male or female menopause. I use this particular mixture in the vaporizer as a stimulant to the adrenal glands so it will act as an anti-inflammatory to my lungs and as a stimulant to the thyroid. Simultaneously, another vaporizer is used with Clary Sage to reduce the hot flashes of menopause. These two vaporized oil blends are perfect to keep asthma and menopause symptoms totally at bay.

Rose Geranium has many facial, body and therapeutic uses.

Ginger oil is steam-distilled from the rhizomes and roots of *Zingiber officinale*. It has a strong odor that gives you a warm feeling and is used as such in the perfume trade to introduce "warmth" to the final product. The taste is very strong and spicy. The scent of Ginger oil will often make one's mouth water, and so it can be used to aid in the treatment of anorexic persons. Ginger oil is somewhat greenish-yellow and it gets darker with age. It is used as an aperitif (1 drop in Ginger Ale or carbonated water), for the stomach, to ease gas pains or for flatulence. It is a stimulant to the system, and compresses can be used to reduce fever and pain.

> **KEEP ESSENTIAL OILS OUT OF YOUR EYES.**

Internally, Ginger oil is taken for diarrhea, stomachache, or over-eating that results in painful digestion. It is especially good taken as a tonic drink (either the root boiled in water or a drop of oil in a glass of water) after a big meal or as a treatment for jet lag (here it is mixed with Rosemary oil as a stimulant to wake up). It is wonderful used in foods to perk up the taste.

Externally, Ginger oil is used in compresses for arthritis or rheumatism or chest pains from cold or flu, sore throat or swollen glands.

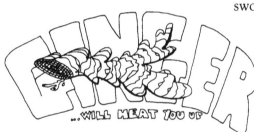

Inhaled, the scent is stimulating, eases confusion of the mind and is a warming scent to "warm the heart."

I find Ginger especially useful as an herb steeped in water for stomachache or flatulence or as a treatment for the common cold or flu. Take the infusion with honey. A drop of Ginger oil is wonderful in commercial Ginger Ale to spark the taste and remind you of the delicious Ginger Ale that seems only to be available in Singapore (definitely a memoristic taste and fragrance). The inhaled scent is soothing and warming especially if you are lonely or when traveling.

A good first-aid oil for the traveler.

Paul Duraffourd in *En Forme Tous Les Jours* mentions the use of Ginger oil in a formula to treat aches and pains:

Mix together 10 ml each of Ginger oil, Cypress oil and Rosemary oil with 5 ml of Oregano oil and 500 ml of Eau de vie. Use this as a friction rub twice a day, morning and night for aching joints. Use the treatment for at least 15 days.

Grapefruit oil is steam-distilled from *Citrus paradisi*. It acts on the gall bladder and can be taken *internally* for this organ as well as the entire digestive system. *Externally* it is astringent and is used as a facial toner, to stimulate dead-looking or lifeless skin, and applied neat to treat herpes.

Inhaled, Grapefruit oil is an anti-depressant, relieves anxiety and is used to treat menstrual problems such as PMS and menopause "hot flashes." It also makes a very good air refresher and eliminates cooking odors in the kitchen.

Grapefruit Seed oil is used as a preservative in fine cosmetics and can also be applied to Candida and other fungus infections as a fungicide. It works well with Rosemary Verbenon. There are several sources of Grapefruit seed oil. Most are prepared with glycerin and can be used directly in any product. Grapefruit seed extract is also available in pill form and taken for Candida, bacterial and parasitic diseases as well as intestinal diseases that result in diarrhea, abdominal pain and fatigue. It is considered a natural alternative to pharmaceutical antibiotics.

Helichrysum italicum **oil** (subspecies *italicum*)—This plant is a subspecies of the commonly known plant Everlast or Immortelle. The essential oil distilled from it has a distinct fragrance and a unique chemical composition. According to J. Paltz, it is useful for phlebitis, whooping cough, liver fatigue and spasms. The oil is said to have anti-viral activities. According to Dr. Penoel, it is outstandingly effective in stimulating production and protection of new cells, even in the case of deep, bleeding wounds. This regenerative effect is also apparent in minimizing and smoothing scar tissue when mixed with *Rosa rubiginosa* (wild Rosehip seed oil). These oils are perfectly suited for external application. Helichrysum oil is very valuable for skin-care preparations to regenerate the skin and at the same time it is totally non-irritating. Applied neat to bruises as soon as possible, the bruise will usually not form and the oil will prevent swelling and discoloration. It combines very well with Roman Chamomile and azulene-containing essences, such as *Artemisia arborescens* and many *Achillea* species (Yarrow). Helichrysum mixed with

Rose Geranium is healing for burns.

"The main constituent is neryl acetate and according to J. Paltz in *Le Fascinant Pouvoir des Huiles Essentielles*, 1984, this aromatic is useful for phlebitis, coronary complaints and liver fatigue. Helichrysum is used for detoxifying people from drugs including smoking (nicotine). The affinity with skin care is observable. Treating acne tissue with Helichrysum in dilution has proven more effective than the use of any other essential oil. The French Helichrysum is green and honey sweet. The Yugoslavian oil is orange and not as refined in its scent quality. The sweetness is so rich there is also a fruity-tea undertone. The fresh plant has a Maple sugar scent."

—*Victoria Edwards*

Heliotrope—This wonderful vanilla sweet scented plant called Heliotrope, *Heliotropium peruvianum*, has purple or white blossoms and is commonly called Cherry-Pie. The scent is a delicious combination of Cherry and Vanilla. Unfortunately at this time it is not grown commercially for its oil and steam distillation seems to be unsuccessful. I have tried over and over to extract this delicious nerve-soothing scent from plants grown in my own garden to no avail. I have tried enfleurage as well as a home-still. I suggest that you buy the plants and inhale their delicious sweetness to soothe your nerves and relax your body. You can make a pretty colored tincture of the blossoms and use this as a compress for a headache or as a gargle for a sore throat.

In the *Herbal Body Book*, I reported on the use of a cold infusion of the flowers as a rinse for the hair or body, and I have also made a cold-oil infusion of the flowers and used this as a massage oil. The fragrance is partially made up of heliotropin, and this is used as an inhalant for relaxation when a patient intends to undergo Magnetic Resonance Imaging (MRI). It would seem more appropriate

> ### DILUTE ESSENTIAL OILS BEFORE USING

for physicians to simply use Heliotrope plants in their offices to reduce stress and to control anxiety rather than give their patients synthetic molecules to inhale. Physicians are actually beginning to see the benefits of using particular fragrances to make certain unpleasant treatments easier for patients to undergo.

The Heliotrope is indigenous to the Americas and was used by the original inhabitants of Peru in their medicine.

In folklore, the Heliotrope is the symbolic flower of August. This is a group of plants that always turn towards the sun. In folkloric history, Apollo was attracted to a water nymph named Clytie but, as with most narcissistic self-loving persons, Apollo eventually grew tired of Clytie. The nymph was madly in love with Apollo and pined away for the love she felt for him. She languished for nine days and nights while she watched his chariot move across the sky from dawn to dusk. She took no food or drink during the time that she watched Apollo. The other gods took pity on poor Clytie and turned her into the beautiful, sweet-smelling Heliotrope. (Helios=sun and tropos=to turn to.) The Heliotrope thus means in the language of flowers devotion and faithfulness. To dream of a Heliotrope means that you are lost in love for someone who is ignoring you. In ritual use, if the flowers are picked in August and used for good, the good will return to the ritual user up to ten-fold, and if the flowers are used for evil, the evil will turn upon the evil-doer ten-fold. My suggestion is that you perform a healing, cleansing ritual in the month of August using the Heliotrope flowers and think only good thoughts.

 Honeysuckle oil—This lovely white when youthful and yellow when mature flower is easily grown in the home garden. An absolute is professionally produced from the flowers of the genus, particularly *Lonicera caprifolium*, and other species. It produces an intensely sweet odor that can be almost nauseating. The absolute is only available to perfume houses. Steam distillation has been attempted and an oil produced that costs about $15/ml. This was the first scent that I produced in my home still and by oil infusion when I was making massage oils in the late '60s. My method has been outlined fully in previous material, but briefly here is how to extract Honeysuckle fragrance from the flowers:

Fill a clean quart-size mason jar with young flowers, then add Olive oil until the jar is full and just to the point where the flowers are submerged. Keep in a warm place (but not in the sun). Strain out the oil every 24–36 hours and add new flowers to the oil until it takes on the scent of the flowers. Do not squeeze the flowers. Bottle in small containers and refrigerate.

Here are some points to remember: (1) as you add the oil to the jar, it weighs down the flowers so that a full jar of flowers becomes only about ½ jar of flowers; (2) use a lightweight Olive oil or Jojoba oil; do not use Almond oil or any other so-called aromatherapy carrier oil because they go rancid too quickly; (3) pick the flowers in the early morning hours before the sun is up and dries them out, as Honeysuckle produces its essential oil in the early A.M. and after that the EO retreats back along the vine; (4) most fragrant flowers when picked continue to produce essential oil up to 36 hours after being picked, and after that they begin to fade and fail, so it is important to remove the dead flowers the moment they begin to fail; (5) the spent flowers may be used immediately as a healing, soothing poultice for sunburn or irritated skin, or they may be frozen for use at some later time; and (6) to the bottles of infused Honeysuckle oil you may add a teaspoon of Vitamin E or tincture of Benzoin or even a small pinch of the Benzoin resin itself to act as a preservative.

Honeysuckle-infused oil is perfect for massage therapy. It is soothing and relaxing and can be used as well in any sort of dessert where oil is needed but will not necessarily be cooked. The fragrance of Honeysuckle is notable because it is relaxing, soothing and uplifting.

 Hops oil is an essential oil steam-distilled from *Humulus lupulus*. This vine is grown throughout the world not for the beauty of the flowers but in particular for the very fragrant resin that occurs in the tiny yellow glands under the flower petals. This resin is of particular use in the brewing industry.* There is a large processing center in the United States in Willamette Valley near Portland, Oregon, and near there is a very small privately owned still to extract the essential oil.

---

* For information regarding the harvest of Hops see Natural History magazine, January 1992, publication of the American Museum of Natural History.

This oil is used in perfumery but it also has importance in aromatic medicine to aid the insomniac. Three drops of Hops in a diffusor is enough to ease those who have difficulty sleeping. This essential oil should be more intensely studied by the medical profession as an aid for those in pain who need to sleep but who may be harmed by more potent medications. A Hops pillow is an old but valued sleep remedy for adults who have difficulty going to sleep. Simply take 4 ounces of freshly dried Hops (moisture about 10%) plus 2 ounces of Rose leaves (*Rosa eglanteria*). Stuff into a fabric casing and sleep on this. Hops flowers are also drunk as a tea for restlessness and used by alcoholics to ease the fantasy of DT's. Mixed with other herbs it can aid in the reduction of fever and pain. It can also improve the appetite in those who are anorexic or recovering from wasting diseases. Hops and Hop pillows and extracts of Hops have been in use since at least the 8th century.

Hyssop oil is the steam-distilled oil from *Hyssopus officinalis*. "Hyssopus" is an old name originally used for another plant, and "officinalis" means a plant used medicinally. Hyssop is used as an antiseptic, digestive and fluid extractor (diuretic or emmenagogue, expectorant), fever reducer, nerve soother and sleep helper. It is used for such problems as asthma, bronchitis and other respiratory difficulties including cough and dyspnœa (difficulty in breathing), for various skin problems such as eczema, for emotional stressors, and medicinally for wounds and sores. Hyssop is somewhat toxic because of its high ketone content, and it should be kept in mind that Hyssop should be moderated with other essential oils. It makes mucus more fluid and helps one to spit out this mucus thereby relieving bronchial distress and spasms. Of the three main organ systems that Hyssop treats—skin, digestive and respiratory—its most important use is for the respiratory system. Hyssop is considered a "sacred" herb and has value in ritual use, cleansing of sacred spaces and as a strewing herb.

Immortelle oil—See *Helichrysum*.

Inula oil is steam-distilled from *Inula graveolens*. It is also known as Elecampane or Sweet Inula. It contains bornyl acetate and lactones. This oil is very effective when inhaled for persistent or hardened sinus mucus, bronchial problems and breathing problems. Drink teas containing Elecampane and other herbs for the respiratory system while inhaling this scent. It is also used externally for heart complaints, skin rashes, herpes and skin eruptions, as it reduces itching and promotes healing. See also J. Paltz, *Le Fascinant Pouvoir des Huiles Essentielles*, 1984.

Essential Oil Mixture for the Respiratory System

1 ml (20 drops) each of Basil, Hyssop, Inula, Lavender, Myrrh, *Ammi visnaga* and Chamomile oils

¼ ml (5 drops) of Peppermint oil

2 ml (40 drops) of Eucalyptus oil

Use in a diffusor and inhale the scent 20 minutes three times per day.

Inula odorata, an oil from another species, is also called Sweet Inula. It is a very unusual emerald-green essence of the same botanical genus known as Elecampane in the Compositae family. It has mucolytic and expectorant properties, as well as being a potent anti-inflammatory. It is hypothermic, sedative, cardio-regulative, diuretic and depurative. It can be applied in cases of bronchitis, asthma and sinus mucous-membrane infections.

Note: These may actually be the same oil but grown under two slightly different names and conditions.

Iris is an incredibly fragrant plant. It grows well in Boulder, Colorado, and is harvested there for its flowers. It is considered a late spring plant, which it is in regions like the Rockies, but it is more an early spring plant in the Mediterranean-like weather of San Francisco Bay Area. It comes in the most outrageously brilliant hues and colors of purple, true indigo, sky blue, salmon and "knock your socks off" yellow . . . And the fragrance is unbelievably warm, soft, sexy and so voluptuously sweet.

The Iris is the sacred flower of the goddess of the rainbow, *Iris*, who takes the message of love from heaven to earth (ergo the Rainbow). Iris means "eye of heaven" and is the name given to the goddess, this flower, and the center of your own eye, meaning that each of us carries a bit of heaven with us. The Iris is considered the symbol of communication and messages. The root of the Florentine Iris is called Orris root and is one of the most expensive perfumes available. Unfortunately, the lovely scent of the Iris is not captured by enfleurage or steam distillation. So if you want to experience the joyful feeling of uplift and an end to anxiety and lethargy, plant some of the fragrant Iris and inhale the scent directly from the flower.

See Orris root for more information.

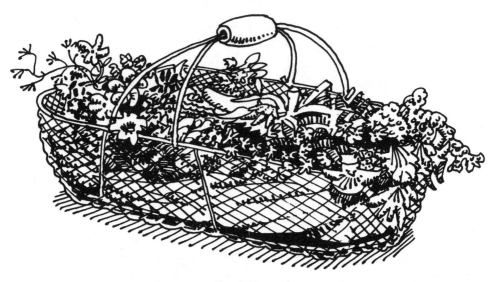

NOTHING QUITE SO FINE,
AS A BASKET OF FLOWERS
IN THE SUMMERTIME

Jasmine flower oil is obtained by several methods including enfleurage to obtain an absolute from the châssis, concrète and pommade (for definitions see Chapter II). These products are obtained from the nighttime picking of the flowers of *Jasminum officinale* and *Jasminum grandiflorum*. Jasmine is a night-blooming plant and the essential oil is produced during the dark hours rather than during the day. The scent is heavy, musky, romantic, somewhat reminiscent of Orange flowers with a touch of honey, beeswax and green herbs thrown in. But only if you have walked out into a warm southern night, whether in Louisiana or France, and been enveloped with the dusky scent of the Jasmine can you ever really know it. It is a remembered pleasure.

As with many thick-petaled flowers the essential oil is produced for up to 36 hours after picking. This makes it an ideal flower for the home

usually solvent extracted otherwise

maker of scents to practice the art of enfleurage. In the *Herbal Body Book* and *Herbs & Things* I describe detailed ways of using the enfleurage method at home: see also Chapter V of this book.

Jasmine oil is used as an aphrodisiac through inhalation or as an application to treat various problems of the reproductive tract. I have used it directly to massage the abdomen for menstrual cramps and uterine pain. A drop rubbed on the temples will clear up a headache within moments. It is a powerful treatment for men with prostate problems and impotence, and for frigidity in men and women. This oil when rubbed on the body makes you feel warm and good inside. The therapeutic effects are both emotional and physical. It is warming but not reddening. In skin care, Jasmine has value for the treatment of dry skin, sensitive skin, in formulations for wrinkles and to rejuvenate aging or mature skin.

Inhaled, it is powerfully relaxing but not a soporific. It is calming and useful for many mental stresses. It is uplifting and soothing.

Jasmine Enfleurage . . . Simply put a layer of Olive oil-or Jojoba oil-soaked cotton wool in a flat white enamel pan. Flowers are handpicked in the evening and placed on the cotton and left there for several days. Flowers are removed and replaced with new flowers several times. The cotton is then wrung out and the oil collected in a container. At this point the oil can be used directly or you can then mix it with pure alcohol, letting it stand for several weeks, shaking the container daily. Then the alcohol and oil are separated by pouring off the Jasmine-colored and scented alcohol (and the otto or perfume is filtered off). Where do you buy this alcohol? Look in your Yellow Pages. Various chemical companies sell 190° and 200° alcohol for small-business use in tincture or perfume. It costs about $8/gallon plus about $26 to the government as a tax, or $34.

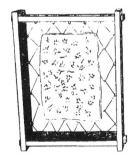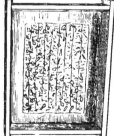

Use this oil in compresses, directly on the skin for headaches or pain in the abdomen and in moisturizers. It is a waste to use Jasmine oil in soaps or facial steams. Use it in massage oils. If you make your own Jasmine oil, you can use the spent flowers to make a flowery tonic water that can be sprayed on the skin or used in scenting fine desserts. Also you can make your own cologne and toilet waters with the spent parts of the flowers and alcohol. The oil is very expensive: 1 ml costs $50, but little is needed as its scenting power is intense.

Juniper Berry oil is steam-distilled from the crushed, dried or partially dried fruit (berry) of *Juniperus communis*. Juniper Berry is what makes gin gin. The essential oil is used as an antiseptic. It is used externally as a cleanser, to help the body release fluids and in all sorts of products such as massage oils, compresses and cosmetics. It can be taken internally in very small amounts to act as a diuretic for cystitis and to detoxify the body. I would encourage the use of Juniper Berry tea instead, especially mixed with Fennel Seed and Rosemary herb. A very good mixture of oils to be used in an alcohol rub or a compress for cellulite or arthritis would be Rosemary, Juniper Berry and Lemon. Juniper Berry oil is used for problems of obesity, urinary infections, problem skin, arthritis or gout.

Sitz baths are in order for urinary problems, genital warts, itchy vulva or jock itch. Just a few drops in a bowl of warm water will help. Use the sitz bath several times per day.

For obesity and cellulite, make a formula using alcohol or vinegar with 2% Juniper Berry essential oil instead of the usual Olive oil or other vegetable oil. People who are obese can even absorb fatty oils through their skin. A vigorous skin brushing with loofah or brush, a vigorous massage, and then the application of 5 drops of Juniper Berry oil in 1 ounce of white vinegar is in order. For arthritis or gout, make a massage oil with 5 drops of Juniper Berry to 1 ounce of Olive oil and massage several times daily.

For poor memory, inhale the scents of Rosemary and Juniper Berry in a diffusor or AromaLamp.

Victoria Edwards says that Alpine Juniper oil is used for those with sensitive kidneys, as it is softer and milder than other Juniper Berry oils.

See also Cypress and Cedar for related oils.

Kanchamara oil—The vapors are used to treat female sex glands.

Kewda oil is also called Attar of Kewda or Keawa or Keora oil. The oil is obtained by maceration or through steam distillation from these unusually large fragrant flowers of the *Pandanus odoratissimus*. A well-developed Pandanus plant may only have 25 flowers (each up to 165 grams in weight or 5–6 ounces) and the yield can be several kilos of oil.

> **KEEP ESSENTIAL OILS OUT OF YOUR EYES**

Attar of Kewda is obtained when Pandanus flowers are steam-distilled with Sandalwood oil. In Ayurvedic medicine it is used for the spleen. Victoria Edwards describes the scent as a strange combination of Horse-radish and Gardenia.

Labdanum is a natural exudation from the plant *Cistus ladanifer*. It is not to be confused with "laudanum," which is the name for a number of opium preparations originally obtained from alchemists. Labdanum is a small shrub called Rock Rose. The resin is obtained by boiling or steaming this plant. This resin is extensively used in soapmaking and as a fixative in perfumery as well as a blender in various herbal preparations. The fragrance of Labdanum oil is fiery and sweet. The uses of this plant are mainly to treat skin disease. A decoction is made of the more delicate top parts of the plant with the flowers. This decoction is used as a wash several times a day for acne, psoriasis, and sore, burning or irritated skin. The essential oil is used in much the same way, as a fixative in perfumery or as an application for skin disease. Use Jojoba oil as a carrier oil.

The odor of Labdanum is probably the only one in the vegetable kingdom that closely approximates that of ambergris.

Cistus oil is steam-distilled from crude Labdanum or from the absolute from concrète of Labdanum, not from the plant itself. Cistus oil is used in urinary infections as a diuretic, and on wounds or boils for its drying effect. Cistus oil is inhaled and this is stimulating to the senses (sense of touch, feeling, sight and sound). It is inhaled for its effects on the upper part of the brain. It is useful in ritual work and magic. It can also be inhaled as a quieting tonic for the nerves, for the insomniac and to elevate the emotions in meditation.

 Lavender is like a soothing breath of fresh air. The scent—whether as a freshly plucked plant scenting the garden, or the dried flower tops woven into a spear and then placed among your linens, or the oil fragrancing the air in the diffusor—refreshes and cleanses the air. Lavender, sometimes spelled Lavander, is the most versatile of the essential oils and is steam-distilled from *Lavandula vera*, aka *L. officinalis*. Lavandin oil is from a hybrid of true Lavender and Spike Lavender, called *L. hybrid grosso*. And a Lavender oil is also distilled from *L. latifolia*. Each of these oils has particular uses and each varies depending on the place and altitude grown. Plants grown at high altitudes are distilled there, and the lower-temperature boiling results in a higher ester content of Lavender oil.

Lavender vibrates in the musical key of A and affects the 6th chakra, that is, the pineal gland or the third eye, and it vibrates in the color of indigo. These are useful bits of information for those who are interested in harmonizing healing rituals or meditations.

Stately Lavender's fragrance has been recorded in history's fondness for scent. Francis Bacon said in one of his essays, "And because the breath of flowers is far sweeter in the air (where it comes and goes like the warbling lilt of music) than in the hand, therefore nothing is more fit for that delight than to know what be the flowers and plants that will do best to perfume the air . . . set whole alleys of them [Lavender], to have the pleasure when you walk. . . ."

As spring approaches, the scents and aromas of flower buds waft through the air, tantalizing your nose with memories of times past. These "aromemories" are brought to the surface of your mind by evocative scents. When you inhale an odor directly, the scent affects the mind in a psychological way, although direct physiological effects can also occur, such as inhaling Eucalyptus oil from a steam bath or vaporizer to thin mucus secretions, as it acts as an expectorant for clogged respiratory passages.

Much has been invented about Gattefossé's learning of the wonderful therapeutic uses of Lavender oil. The event is related in his book, *Aromatherapie* (1937), as follows:

". . . External application of small quantities of essential oils rapidly stops the spread of gangrenous sores. In my personal experience, after a laboratory explosion covered me with burning substances which I extinguished by rolling on a grassy lawn, my hands were covered with a rapidly changing gas gangrene. Just one rinse with Lavender oil stopped the gasification of the tissues. This treatment was followed by profuse sweating and healing began the next day. (July 1910) . . ."

Gattefossé had 50 years' experience with essential oils before he wrote the seminal aromatherapy book. He was particularly influenced by Lavender oil's especial virtues. He used it for everything including open wounds and where all tissue had been excised and the bones revealed.

On the day that I wrote this article regarding Lavender oil, my dogs were accidentally released from our property and Sumo-dog hit by a car. He was dragged along the pavement on his right side, losing hair on his haunch and a piece of skin about the size of a salad plate. The most serious of his injuries was to his right rear leg, where the ligaments and tendons were severed and partially excised to his toes, and the skin and muscles torn off in a 180° rotation around the hock joint, leaving the bones exposed. The vets had him washed and cleaned up in no time but the exposed tissue and bone were really going to be a problem. The vet recommended amputation but I refused to have the procedure done, preferring aromatherapy treatments instead.

The leg was soaked two times a day with a cleansing solution, and dirt and pebbles removed with a Water Pik. Then we soaked gauze in a 2% Tea Tree and Lavender solution (1 ml each of Tea Tree and Lavender oil and 4 ounces of water). This was wrapped about the ankle and then the leg bandaged. Victoria Edwards was visiting for the day and she suggested Ylang/water solutions (1:1) sprayed on the area for pain. I also used a diffusor with Lavender oil in the daytime and Ylang oil in the evening to calm Wolfie-dog, who seemed to be traumatized and agitated. This calmed her down and soothed her. I noticed that she would stay near the diffusor for about 20 minutes and then would leave the area to rest elsewhere but she was calmed and relaxed. At this writing, our Sumo-dog is doing well with the Tea Tree/Lavender wraps, the edges of the wound are pink and healing, and scar tissue is forming to cover the joint. I hope to have more positive results to discuss later, using aromatherapy on our dog.

Note: Within two months the large wound was totally filled in with granular tissue and covered with scar tissue. Although the muscles and ligaments cannot regenerate and the loss of a chunk of bone weakens the leg, Sumo-dog now has the use of his leg, it was not amputated, and he need only walk with an occasional limp.

English Lavender oil has a high linalool content, which makes it ideal as an anti-bacterial and to relieve discomfort. Lavender oil can also be produced that is terpeneless (see Chapter II) and this would be best used on open wounds. Lavender oil properties are stimulating, antispasmodic, decongesting to the respiratory system and sinus, antiseptic and healing for all external skin conditions including deep wounds and burns, and for weakness and swelling of the limbs. Inhaled the oil is calming but stimulating, antidepressive and anticonvulsive.

This is definitely one of the oils that should be on your number one list—and particularly of use in a first aid kit and for children and pets. It is good for camping because it repels fleas and flying creatures like mosquitos.

Lavandula vera oil—This essential oil highlights the universal qualities of Lavender. Some of its many uses are for small wounds, cuts and burns. Whenever the skin is inflamed or disintegrated, Lavender is the oil that can be applied instantaneously. The other main uses of Lavender oil include in massage oil for cramps and cramp-related headaches. This oil can also be applied inside the ear.

—Victoria Edwards

Lemon oil is expressed from the peel of the Lemon *Citrus limon*. To make 1 pound of oil you need to express (squeeze to break the oil glands) the peels of about 1500 Lemons. The scent that we call Lemon (Citron) comes primarily from the chemical compound limonene, which makes up approximately 90% of the Lemon's essential oil. It is modified somewhat by citral. According to *Encyclopædia Britannica* the Lemon was known to the ancient Greeks and Romans and was introduced to Spain about 1000 A.D. At about this time it was distributed through Europe by the Crusaders after they found Lemon trees growing in Palestine. About 1494 the fruit was cultivated in the Azores and most of the crop shipped to England. The tree is rare both in China and India. It grows well in the Mediterranean and United States. The scent of Lemon is distributed throughout the plant world: most notable of these plants are Lemon Balm, Lemon Basil, Lemon Catnip, Lemongrass, Lemon Thyme and Lemon Verbena.

DILUTE ESSENTIAL OILS BEFORE USING

According to Valnet: *internal* uses include bactericide, antiseptic, to activate the white corpuscles in defense of the organism, fever reducer, tonic, diuretic, to repel internal parasites, vitamin C and to calm; *external* uses include antiseptic, cleansing, astringent, skin care and insect repellent. Internal indications are for infections or infective states, fever, loss of appetite, worms and parasites, urinary disturbance, dyspepsia, flatulence and burping, for reducing fat in the obese and for respiratory problems such as asthma, flu, pneumonia. *Externally* indications are for gargling for sore throat, tonsillitis, nosebleed, mouth inflammations, skin sores and acne, infected wounds, first-aid remedy for insect bites, insect repellent for such as ants and moths, and added to drinking water to purify.

There are many ways to use Lemon oil and the juice of Lemon. An old grandmother cure for colds and flu is to squeeze the juice of Lemon into a glass, add water and a shot of brandy, add a piece of the Lemon peel and 1 drop of Lemon oil, and drink this hot or cold when you have a fever or flu. My Irish "grandmother" used Irish whiskey and my Italian "mother" used Sambuca as a substitute in this remedy that seems world renowned.

Another use for Lemon juice is to extract calcium from an egg shell. Use a shot glass. Put a whole unbroken egg in the shot glass, add the juice of a Lemon. Let sit overnight. Drink the Lemon/calcium in the morning and prepare the egg for your breakfast. The acid of the Lemon leaches the calcium out of the egg shell without harming the flavor of the egg. The Lemon peel from the squeezed lemon is then cut into strips and dried and can be used in potpourris, drinks and making medicine.

Lemon oil is also very good to disinfect chopping blocks. Make a mixture of 3 drops Lemon oil to 3 ounces of water, shake, and use this to wipe wooden furniture or children's toys. A whole Lemon peel can be rubbed on these wooden items which will express some of the oil and then they can be cleansed with the solution.

Lemon oil is one of the most useful of the essential oils and should have a place on everyone's shelf.

Lemongrass oil is steam-distilled from *Cymbopogon citratus*, which means Cymbo=cup or cup-like, pogon=bearded racemes, citratus=smells like citrus. The scent is very strongly citrus, lemony with an herbal tone.

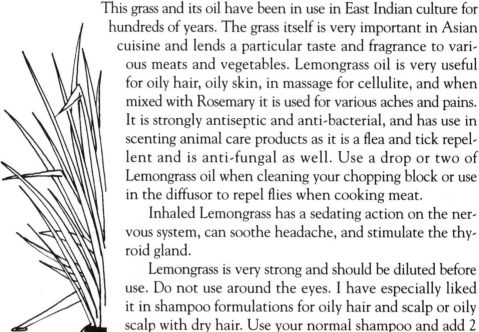

This grass and its oil have been in use in East Indian culture for hundreds of years. The grass itself is very important in Asian cuisine and lends a particular taste and fragrance to various meats and vegetables. Lemongrass oil is very useful for oily hair, oily skin, in massage for cellulite, and when mixed with Rosemary it is used for various aches and pains. It is strongly antiseptic and anti-bacterial, and has use in scenting animal care products as it is a flea and tick repellent and is anti-fungal as well. Use a drop or two of Lemongrass oil when cleaning your chopping block or use in the diffusor to repel flies when cooking meat.

Inhaled Lemongrass has a sedating action on the nervous system, can soothe headache, and stimulate the thyroid gland.

Lemongrass is very strong and should be diluted before use. Do not use around the eyes. I have especially liked it in shampoo formulations for oily hair and scalp or oily scalp with dry hair. Use your normal shampoo and add 2 drops to every ounce for lathering.

Treatment for Oily Hair or Scalp

One ounce good quality dry castile soap, shaved and diluted with 8 ounces of water or 8 ounces of herbal tea water. Heat gently until the soap dissolves. Add 4–8 drops of Lemongrass oil that has been mixed with ½ oz of tincture of Benzoin or alcohol to dissolve the oil. Shake gently and put away for use. This makes 4–8 shampoos.

Hints: Use plain castile soap available from Indiana Botanic* or Barbara Bobo Castile Soap for Shampoo in Ohio.* Also, a mixture of Lemongrass and Lemon peel herbs, 1 ounce mixed herbs/8 ounces of water, simmered and strained, makes an excellent herbal base for your aromatherapy shampoo.

---

*See Source List, Chapter VI

Lemon Petitgrain oil is steam-distilled from the leaves and twigs and undeveloped fruits of the Lemon tree. It contains up to about 50% citral. At this point I have seen it listed on only one price sheet of those who sell aromatherapy products.

Lemon Verbena—See Verbena oil.

Lime oil is expressed from Lime peels or steam-distilled from the peels of *Citrus medica var. acida*. It can be used in much the same way as Lemon oil and blends well with Lemon oil. Inhaled, the oil may stimulate the muscles around the eye. How this is accomplished I do not know.

Litsea cubeba **oil** is steam-distilled from the small pepper-like fruits of a plant commonly called May Chang. It is a shrub or tree of the Laurel family with fragrant flowers, fruits and deciduous leaves up to four inches long. It grows wild and is cultivated from northeastern India to South Vietnam. All parts possess a pleasant lemon scent. The delightfully fragrant flowers are used for flavoring tea and they also yield an essential oil prized in perfume blending. The young fruits are also fragrant and peppery-tasting. They resemble and are used as a substitute for Cubeb Pepper (*Piper cubeba* of the Pepper family). May Chang fruit is especially employed as a seasoning to overcome the strong odor and taste of old goat's meat and not-so-fresh fish. A small amount of the alkaloid laurotetanine in the bark, leaves and fruit renders them slightly toxic. The taste is pleasant and it is used with Lemon and other scents as a room freshener.

MADAME

MAY-
CHANG

also known as......

Litsea Cubeba

Lovage herb produces an essential oil both from the herb or celery-like top part of the plant as well as from the root. It has a very powerful fragrance of Celery. Lovage herb oil is steam-distilled from the freshly harvested above-ground parts of the Lovage plant when it is fully mature. I have used this oil to flavor foods when I really want a strong Celery flavor, and in aromatherapy demonstrations—reactions to this scent range from "smells green and like it would taste good" to "too strong, too grassy-scented." Lovage root oil is steam-distilled from the roots of *Levisticum officinale*. This is a very large and tall plant. The scent of Lovage root oil is very strong. I think it would make a wonderful fragrance for the entrance of a restaurant, as the scent is warm and smells like good cooking.

Mandarin oil is expressed from the peel of the true mandarin, sometimes called "European type," *Citrus reticulata*. Other varieties of C. reticulata, particularly those found in the United States, are called Tangerine. The fragrance of Mandarin oil is very sweet and typical of the true fruit. It is generally indicated in problems of the digestive system, especially for the young or the elderly, as it is very gentle. The oil is used externally in massage oils and inhaled for calming and soothing. For pregnancy use, make a massage oil of 5–10 drops of Mandarin oil with 1 ounce of Olive oil and use this daily to massage the abdomen. Substitute Jasmine oil in the evening as a calming, soothing evening massage. These two oils will help prevent stretch marks. They are also useful for young girls when their breasts and hips are beginning to grow as an A.M. and P.M. massage oil to prevent stretch marks.

See also Tangerine.

Marjoram oil is steam-distilled from flowering tops of *Origanum marjorana* and is valued for its antifungal and antibacterial abilities. This species of plant is well known as Sweet Marjoram and is grown all over the world as a seasoning herb. The properties that make it valuable for *internal* use are: antispasmodic, if *inhaled* causes drowsiness, expectorant and digestive stimulant. For *external* use it is tonic and soothes pain.

It is prescribed for anxiety, sighing or grief (inhaled), digestive spasms or flatulence (1 drop sucked on a sugar cube), respiratory distress (inhaled), insomnia or migraine headaches (inhaled), irritability (inhaled), overactive sex drive (inhaled or massage oil) and for any weakness or during recovery from illness (in baths or massage). This is a very effective oil used in massage products for athletes after heavy physical workouts, as it increases circulation by dilating arteries.

This is one essential oil that is really useful when used with the herb. Make infusions of Marjoram and use the strained liquid in baths or as a tea to drink. To every 8 ounces of strained infusion add 1 drop of Marjoram oil. This is also useful to drink or gargle with if you are a singer, as it can improve and strengthen your voice.

See also *Flavour and Fragrance Journal*, Volume 5, pp. 187–190 (1990) for more information.

Sweet Marjoram oil is also steam-distilled from *Majorana* hortensis*, and Wild Marjoram oil from *Thymus mastichina*.

 Mastic is a resin that comes from an evergreen shrub, *Pistacia lentiscus*. The bark is cut and the odorous transparent resin oozes out. It is cultivated on Chios, a mountainous island in the Aegean Sea. Mastic is used in perfumery as well as the paint industry and in dentistry. The Mastic shrubs have been used for thousands of years, to purify the blood and to treat rheumatism. *National Geographic* (January 1992) mentions that Columbus, sent by Genoese traders to cash in on the money-making crop, visited Chios at least once.

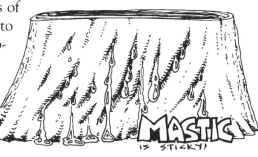

MQV, *Melaleuca quinquenervia viridiflora*, or True Niaouli, is steam-distilled from one of two trees that are physiological forms of the same botanical species. The other form produces the essential oil called Niaouli. MQV has a fine balsamic odor. Victoria Edwards says, "It is used inhaled for the respiratory tract and allergies, and applied directly for infections and hemorrhoids, and has been shown to increase the levels of immune globulines. Together with Ravensara it is probably the oil with the highest overall value to counter infections. However, it also has other important qualities, as it is recommended for respiratory allergies (often producing tremendous relief). As this oil has not shown any toxicity, it can be used as liberally and universally as Lavender. The applications are similar to Tea Tree but some people find the scent more delicate and sweet than that of Tea Tree."

My dogs really dislike the scent of Tea Tree when I open up the bottle but run away less quickly from the scent of MQV.

See also Niaouli and Tea Tree.

***Majorana** Miller = *Origanum*

Melilot herb and Melilot infused in oil, from *Melilo-tus officinalis*, is used for the eyes, brain and head. The herb is used in baths to take away melancholy; it is the fragrance that is effective. Melilot tea is drunk to strengthen memory. The fragrance is inhaled to give mental comfort, ease pain in the head, and to help people "who have lost their senses." It may also be drunk as a cordial for these latter effects.

> **KEEP ESSENTIAL OILS OUT OF YOUR EYES**

In folklore this plant sprung from the blood of the lion that the Emperor Adrian slew.

Melilot has a wonderful fragrance variously described as honey or Carnations.

Melissa oil is steam-distilled from the tops of *Melissa officinalis*, a lemon-scented herb called Balm or Lemon Balm. This is a lovely plant grown in many gardens. The herb itself is used as a calming tisane; it induces a mild perspiration and eases the pain of fever and headache. There is little scientific evidence concerning the effects of Melissa. Most of the published work has been done in Germany. Melissa essential oil has been shown to be sedating, probably due to its constituent citronellal. Robert Tisserand wrote a profile of Melissa in *The International Journal of Aromatherapy*, Winter '88/Spring '89, in which he discusses some known Melissa therapeutic effects: antimicrobial against *Streptococcus hæmolytica* and thus useful in throat infections, for erysipelas, combined with Rose oil effective in the management of herpes zoster and herpes simplex by external application, useful for children because they like the scent and therefore they can be treated without too much squirming. For cold-sore blisters, three applications of undiluted Melissa oil are made directly on the blisters during the day. The oil must only be applied to the blisters, so a preliminary application of glycerine to the surrounding area is in order.

 Mint oil is steam-distilled from *Mentha arvensis*. It is also called Cornmint oil. It contains such large quantities of menthol that it is solid at room temperature. Mint oil is used as a substitute for Peppermint oil when the menthol effect is desired, although the fragrance of Mint oil is much less sweet than that of Peppermint oil.

Muguet oil is the created version of Lily-of-the-Valley, which is only rarely available as a natural oil.

Mugwort oil is steam-distilled from *Artemisia herba alba* or *A. vulgare*. It is called Armoise in French and often referred to as Armoise oil. This oil is considered an emmenagogue and so can be used to stimulate the menses; it is also a vermifuge and indicated when one has internal parasites. The herb tea as well as the oil are used in this case. Mugwort has been sprinkled on pillows for wild dreams, but care should be taken because the thujone content may cause nightmares and sickness if used to excess. This herb in a "dream pillow" has been used through the ages to induce "dreams of the future," and with a drop or two of oil added to this mixture you have a very powerful tool to investigate the psyche.

Myrrh oil is steam-distilled from the resin of *Commiphora molmol* or *C. myrrha*. Among the ancient high cultures of the East, none is so little known as the one that flourished in Southern Arabia, the "Arabia Felix" of classical times in the 1000 years before the birth of Christ. Several herbs are mentioned in the ancient papyrus and two of these are Frankincense and Myrrh. These were luxury commodities, both are gum resins exuded by trees. Frankincense comes from two species of the genus *Boswellia* and Myrrh comes from *Balsamodendron myrrha* (the old name). The trees are found only in southern Arabia. It is probable that their restricted range is determined by some unique combination of soil, elevation, temperature and rainfall.

In antiquity the two resins had many uses. Myrrh was used primarily in cosmetics and perfumes. The 18th Dynasty Egyptian Queen Hatshepsut, for example, is reported to have rubbed Myrrh on her legs to make them fragrant. Theophrastus and Pliny inform us that Myrrh was one of the chief ingredients in three famous cosmetic preparations of classical times: Egyptian perfume, Mendesian ointment and another substance named Mageleion.

Both these resins were among the classical materia medica (medical treatments) and were prescribed to promote menstruation and for such ailments as paralysis of the limbs, "broken head" and dropsy. Because of the many uses for the resins in ancient times, the rising demand could not be met by the limited supply. As a result the price was driven up, and in Biblical times these resins were ranked alongside gold as a suitable gift for the Christ child. Pliny states that in Alexandria where Frankincense was processed, workmen were required to strip for inspection before being allowed to leave the factory. Thus the same motive that drives men to seek their fortune in gold or oil may have caused the northern Semites to move to Southern Arabia.

In 1000 B.C. Solomon's fleet carried the resins to various markets by sea. The fame and fortune of the cultures of Southern Arabia rose and fell with the use and then disuse of Frankincense and Myrrh. One of the reasons for the declining use of Frankincense was that the Christians replaced cremation with a simple burial.

There is still a small market for Myrrh and Frankincense as a church incense and a medicinal substance, but the quantity required for this is minuscule compared with the amount required in former days.

Myrrh oil is useful in skin-care products for revitalizing aging and wrinkled skin. It is *inhaled* for the following indications: to cool the air or emotions, to regulate all secretions of the body, used at the time the thyroid gland begins to function in the morning (6 A.M.) to stimulate and regulate function (useful for those who are dieting), as an astringent and antiseptic for the lungs and medicinally as an application for thrush and other fungus infections. Inhale the oil to stimulate the 6th and 7th chakra. Myrrh vibrates in the color blue to indigo and is useful for problems of the throat region.

Neroli oil is the name of the essential oil derived from the sweet-scented flowers of *Citrus aurantium*, *C. vulgaris* or *C. bigaradia*. This powerfully sweet oil has extensive use in skin-care products, particularly for dry or sensitive skin. The Orange flower water or hydrosol produced during the steam distillation can be used in desserts and sweets as well as skin care. I particularly like using Orange flower water to moderate the stimulating effects of Coffee: a few drops in a cup of Coffee is very nice. Orange flower water is also a perfect addition to all sorts of Chocolate foods and drinks.

Orange flower oil or Neroli oil vibrates in the 2nd to 4th chakra, and is of considerable use inhaled for all states of grief and depression. It is quietly soothing, calming and sedating. A drop of Neroli oil in a teaspoon of honey and added to a cup of Marjoram tea is good to drink in the evening if you have trouble sleeping. Keep this tea beside your bed and you can also sip it if you wake up in the night. Valnet lists the properties of Neroli as diminishing cardiac contractions, dulls the nerves and lightly hypnotic. It is indicated for cardiac spasm, chronic diarrhea and insomnia.

A drop of Neroli oil mixed with honey in a cup of warm water is a good drink for cranky children. The scent can also be inhaled through a diffusor used in a child's room.

Oil for Skin Rejuvenation
10 drops each of Neroli, Frankincense, Fennel and Carrot. Add this to Calendula-infused oil, about 2 ounces. Squeeze in the contents of 4 vitamin E capsules. Use nightly on face and neck after you have cleansed your skin with a gentle soap.

 Niaouli oil is steam-distilled from *Melaleuca viridiflora*, a tree that grows in Australia and is one of two physiological forms of the same botanical species that produces true Niaouli oil or MQV. Niaouli oil is used like Cajeput oil. It has antiseptic properties, is stimulating and encourages the organism to defend against disease. It is used for all sorts of inflammations and infections, for the respiratory system, both internally and externally. Inhale 2 drops mixed with Eucalyptus oil for respiratory problems. Use this same formula with 5 droppers of carrier oil (100 drops) as a friction massage on the throat and chest.

Niaouli and Tea Tree oil cost about $5 for 5 ml, while MQV costs about $7 for 5 ml. They are used in the same fashion, with MQV having the more sweet and refined scent and Tea Tree and Niaouli oils being stronger in both scent and action.

See also MQV and Tea Tree.

 Nutmeg oil is produced by steam distillation of the fresh, finely ground, dried Nutmegs, *Myristica fragrans*. The oil is employed in friction rubs for rheumatism and neuralgia, as it is analgesic. A drop of oil can be used on an aching tooth. Ground Nutmeg is used in foods to combat intestinal infections, for chronic diarrhea, and to aid digestion and ease flatulence. The inhaled scent is stimulating and combats mental fatigue. This is one of the most potent oils, and high doses are considered to be stupefying and a circulatory sedative.

Oakmoss oil is produced from a simple plant, the lichen *Evernia prunastri*. The scent is lovely, full of the forest, the salty scent of seashore plants, barks, woods and green things. Oakmoss grows on Oak tree trunks and branches. It is pale gray or greenish gray. It has been used in perfumery as early as the 16th century and seems then to have been forgotten. The *Encyclopædia Britannica* states, "Baskets filled with it have been found in the ancient royal tombs of Egypt, but whether intended for perfume or, as some suggest, for making bread, is not known." Oakmoss oil is mainly used in perfumery to supply a masculine scent and as a fixative. I use it in a special blend of citrus scents to add a masculine note.

"Massage therapist Ann Sibbet reports that using a small amount of diluted Oakmoss oil over the forehead and sinus area brings great relief to people congested in this area."

—*Victoria Edwards*

Olibanum oil is steam-distilled from *Boswellia carteri*.
See also Frankincense and Myrrh.

Opopanax oil is steam-distilled from *Commiphora erythraea*. The root and stem of this plant exude a liquid that hardens into lumps. These lumps are steam-distilled and used as a fixative in perfumes. An inferior quality of Myrrh is also known as Opopanax. The word means "all-healing vegetable juice." See *Herbs & Things* and *The Herbal Body Book*. Arctander describes the scent of Opopanax: "the vegetable-soup-like, slightly animal-sweet odor of Opopanax oil is entirely different from the medicinal-sharp freshness of Myrrh oil."
See also Myrrh.

Orange Flower oil—See Neroli.

Orange Peel oil from Bitter Oranges produces the main ingredient in liqueurs such as Triple Sec and Curaçao.

Orange Peel oil from Sweet Oranges is produced by expression of the peels and then steam distillation of the expressed product of *Citrus sinensis* or *C. aurentium dulcis*. It can have a very sweet typical orange or Sweet Valencia orange scent. Orange oil is wonderful in blends with other citrus scents using Oakmoss oil as a fixative. This makes a very delicate scent, Orange/Oakmoss masculine aroma.

Orange Peel oil is a digestive and helps the digestive processes including the kidney and gall bladder (1 drop on a sugar cube), inhaled as an antidepressant and nerve sedative, applied locally to disinfect surfaces, diluted and applied locally as a skin-care product, to scent black tea, and used with lemon juice as a tanning agent.

Orange Peel oil is for the 2nd chakra and encourages energy, gives courage and counters the emotion of worry.

This is a good oil for your children's first-aid kit, and for your kitchen to refresh the air and dissipate bad odors. There are several products on the market using Orange oil in their blends that are said to safely eliminate allergy-causing pollen, smoke and other odors.

 Oregano oil is steam-distilled from the tops of *Origanum vulgare*, while some say it is *Thymus capitatus*. This is a strong, spicy, herby-scented oil and is a powerful antiseptic, bacteria killer and virucide as well. It is used internally (1 drop in a spoon of honey) immediately upon feeling the flu or for treating all sorts of internal infections, digestive problems, flatulence (although Peppermint oil is safer) and amenorrhea. It is used externally on parasites such as scabies and diluted for head lice. It may be mixed with other oils for the external treatment of cellulite and obesity (mix with Lemon and Juniper), and inhaled it is used for respiratory problems, asthma, bronchitis, and viral and bacterial pneumonia.

In the *International Journal of Aromatherapy*, Winter 1988, page 12, there is an interesting article listing the potential application of essential oils in the treatment of viral diseases. Oregano oil is among those discussed.

 Orris oil is obtained from the rhizomes of the *Iris florentina* or *Iris pallida*. This is not strictly an aromatherapy oil, although if you could obtain it you would find some powerful uses for the inhaled scent. Orris is the most expensive of all the natural perfume materials. First the plant is grown and then when the rhizomes are harvested they must be aged for three years before an absolute or concrète is obtained. Bugs love the plant so there is damage from insect invasion before the rhizomes get to the factory. The fabulous scent is violet and fruity.

See also Iris.

 Palmarosa oil is steam-or water-distilled from wild, fresh or dried grass, *Cymbopogon martini*, from the Philippines. (For other members of the genus, see Citronella and Lemongrass.) This oil is considered a cellular regenerative and so is used *externally* for skin problems, acne, dry skin, and old and wrinkled skin. It is antiseptic, stimulating and soothing. *Inhaled* it is considered to have a normalizing effect on the thyroid gland. Arctander states that Palmarosa oil is the best natural source of geraniol of all essential oils. Other therapeutic uses would be related to the content of farnesol and geraniol (see Rose Geranium).

 Parsley oil is produced by steam distillation of the top of the flowering Parsley plants, *Petroselinum sativum*, the common domesticated culinary herb. This plant has been known and used as food for thousands of years. The herb itself is used as part of an abortive process and this effect (emmenagogue) can be intensified with use of the Parsley oil taken internally (1 drop three times per day).

 Parsley Seed oil is produced by steam distillation of the ripe fruits/seeds. It is toxic and if used at all should be treated with great care. Parsley Seed oil can be used in teeny tiny amounts to flavor what otherwise might be bland foods and meats.

 Patchouli oil is produced by steam distillation of the dried leaves of *Pogostemon patchouli*. The scent is evocative of the "hippies" of the Haight-Ashbury days. Since those days of the late '60s and early '70s I have come to truly dislike this ubiquitous scent. In aromatherapy demonstrations, many persons describe the scent of Patchouli as "dirty, musky, sweaty human bodies all packed together in a noisy room." This is a direct quote from a class that I gave in San Francisco in 1975. I can't say why these people of the late '60s liked Patchouli as much as they did, but they certainly did give this formerly lovely, earthy scent a very bad name. It is the new Hippie revivalists' oil of choice.

Inhaled, the scent of Patchouli (for those who like it) is a nerve sedative and antidepressant, for some it is an aphrodisiac (it may remind people of their younger, more sexually free days), it affects the pituitary gland, and 7th to 1st chakra ☉.

Externally it can be used in skin-care products to treat dry, old or wrinkled skin, to rejuvenate, invigorate and restore. It blends well with Oakmoss, Geranium, Lavender, Rose, Orange flower and Myrrh, and can be used in creams and lotions for tissue regeneration. It is considered antiseptic and anti-inflammatory.

I like Tisserand's statement that "it sharpens the wits." We can all certainly use more wit sharpening.

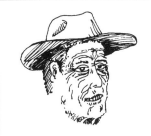

Old Man Wrinkle Cream
Mix together 10 drops each of Patchouli, Myrrh and Rose Geranium. Add to 2 ounces unscented cream or carrier oil. Apply daily. This smells good and if used regularly in time will diminish wrinkles.

Pennyroyal oil, American, is steam-distilled from the freshly harvested slightly dried tops of *Hedeoma pulegioides*.

Pennyroyal oil, European, is steam-distilled from the freshly harvested, slightly dried tops of *Mentha pulegium*. Both can be used in insect-repellent sprays and lotions. Both these oils can be used as emmenagogues but are considered dangerous and toxic. The herb tea is the recommended way of using the herbs, and the oil is saved only for repelling insects.

Pepper oil or Black Pepper oil is produced by steam-distilling the dried and crushed but not quite ripe fruits of *Piper nigrum*, a vine native to India. The flavor of the oil is not pungent like the spice because the flavor principles cannot be distilled. Black Pepper oil when taken *internally* is used to stimulate the digestive system, and to stimulate the reproductive system as an aphrodisiac. It is considered useful to soothe stomach pains and as a preventative against food poisoning. It is used *externally* (always dilute for external use) in rubs and lotions. It acts as a pain killer and stimulates blood circulation and is best used in blends. *Inhaled* the scent is stimulating and comforting and considered to be good for the 1st chakra.

Black Pepper oil is good mixed with Fennel or Anise for flatulence and belching and with Cumin to treat constipation. Mixed with Juniper and Lavender it is used in baths to warm you up in winter or cold months or when you have a cold and the main symptoms are the chills.

Manniche says in her book *Egyptian Herbal* that "Black Pepper was used in the mummification of Ramses II" along with the usual balsams and gums such as Myrrh, Frankincense and Cinnamon. The Black Pepper was found in the nostrils and abdomen of Ramses II.

See also Black Pepper oil.

Pepper oil or **California Pepper Tree oil** is steam-distilled from the red fruits of *Schinus molle*, a tree native to the northern parts of South America. When I was growing up, we had one of these lovely trees growing in the backyard, and as a kid I would pick off the ripe fruits and chew them. My mom would pick the small berries (fruits), dry them and use them in cooking as a substitute for whole Black Pepper. Arctander says that an intoxicating beverage can be produced from these ripe berries but I am unfamiliar with this particular usage.

California Pepper is often called "false Pepper." This essential oil rarely if ever appears on the market but if you have a California Pepper tree in your yard, you may collect the ripe berries and use them, as follows: *Culinary*, whole or ground as a fragrant red substitute for Black Pepper; *Externally*, infused in oil or simmered in water and used to massage aching sore muscles or joints (it is a stimulant); *Internally* only as a food spice.

 Peppermint oil is one of the most important and most used of the essential oils. It is steam-distilled from the partially dried plants of *Mentha piperita* when they are fully mature and in full bloom. Peppermint odor and flavor is extremely well-known in all sorts of culinary items, chewing gum, tea, toothpaste, medicine, candy, baked goods and what-have-you. If you chew on a Peppermint leaf and then suck in air, a distinct cooling effect will be felt in your mouth. This cooling effect is from the presence of menthol, which is useful in making cosmetics and body-care products. This coolness of menthol is useful in dandruff shampoos that are also made with Chilé Pepper oil for that prickly effect—people think that if it is cool and prickly, it is working on their scaly scalp! Is it?

Peppermint oil is extremely useful when you are hot either from a hot fever, hot flashes or hot weather. Inhaled it cools a fever, decongests the sinuses, calms the mind, soothes a headache, acts as an antidepressant, stimulates the nervous system and mind, also calms the tendency for your mind to race along, acts on the 7th chakra and can be used to increase spirituality and possibly clairvoyance during meditative states.

Externally, Peppermint oil is used as an antiseptic to wounds and sores (use diluted), as a chest rub for respiratory diseases (use in a blend of oils or fats), as a skin cleanser (hydrosol or water spray) and in rubs for aching muscles and limbs.

Internally, Peppermint oil has a proven reputation to cure nausea and vomiting (1 drop on a sugar cube is slowly sucked, or 2 drops in 8 ounces of water is sipped), to help clear up the effects of jet lag (mixed with Rosemary and Lemongrass and sipped and inhaled), and the herb tea is taken for fever and colds that are "hot." Always use Peppermint oil diluted, as it can burn and irritate when used neat. Peppermint oil in a lotion has an interesting feature in that it cools while it warms. The menthol increases blood flow wherever it is applied, soothes while it gives a cooling feeling. Try it as a muscle rub or for tired feet.

My favorite Peppermint tales are two: Once I had a Great Dane dog who as he aged would let loose with the most incredible, nauseating, smelly farts. I would then give him 1 drop of Peppermint oil in a teaspoon of water. Soon the smells would become Peppermint tainted and shortly thereafter there would be no smell at all.

Tale 2. Shortly after I met my newest set of in-law parents I was told that one of the boys had just changed from a carnivorous to a vegetable diet. His bowels had not caught up with the change, however, and the air was filled with sulphurous emanations. I suggested the Peppermint oil in water remedy and sure enough, the cure had its expected effect but the Peppermint odor lingered in the house for days. What I found out much later was that he had used 1 teaspoon Peppermint oil in 1 glass of water and had sipped it over a two-hour period. Certainly this was an unnecessarily large amount of Peppermint oil. One drop in ½ glass of water is adequate.

"Peppermint is a typical first-aid essence as its effects usually set in very fast. Nausea, sore throat and travel sickness are symptoms that are traditionally countered with Peppermint. Published research documents its value for 'Irritable Colon'."

—Victoria Edwards

 Petitgrain oil is steam-distilled from the leaves and twigs of *Citrus aurantium amara*. The scent is sharp and biting with a real hint of Citrus. It has a pleasant, floral, slightly woody odor. It is used in soaps and perfumes and in blends, often to soften the heavily sweet scent of Neroli. Petitgrain has therapeutic qualities that are similar but less strong than Neroli. This is a wonderful oil to use in oil blends to harmonize the aspects of stimulation and sedation. Petitgrain is used internally in tiny amounts as a digestive stimulant, where it acts to increase digestion and decrease spasms and flatulence. It is used externally in many body-care products more often as a blending ingredient rather than for its tonic or cleansing ability. It is very refreshing used 2% with distilled water as an after-shave spritz. Inhaled, Petitgrain is used to refresh the senses, clear confusion, reduce mental fatigue, reduce depression and as a tonic scent, as it is uplifting and refreshing.

An interesting fragrance blend for men might be:

    10 drops each of Orange and Bergamot
    6 drops each of Rose Geranium and Grapefruit
    5 drops each of Lemon Peel and Petitgrain
    3 drops each of Sandalwood, Myrrh and Marjoram

Mix this with 4–6 ounces of unscented cream as a hand lotion, or with 6 ounces distilled water for after shave or for exhaustion, or use directly in your diffusor for a wonderful, sweet, refreshing, citrus scent for the home.

As with other citrus oils, Petitgrain can cause photosensitivity and so should not be used in tanning lotions or before going out in the sun.

Pine oil is produced by steam distillation of various *Pinus* species. When the Pine wood is distilled it is called Turpentine, and when the needles are used it is called Pine Needle oil. *Pinus sylvestris* is the species most used for Pine Needle oil. This is a powerful antiseptic whether used externally or internally. Valnet mentions that it can be used internally to stimulate the adrenal cortex.

Internally, Pine oil is used for all sorts of infections including respiratory, urinary and intestinal, although the Pine Needle infusion rather than the oil is to be recommended. *Externally*, Pine oil is very good to stimulate blood circulation for arthritic pain or muscular aches and pain in general. *Inhaled*, Pine Needle oil is good as an antiseptic for the respiratory tract, and to soothe mental stress and relieve anxiety.

Other *external* uses are to repel bugs and skin parasites and to refresh the air in homes and act as a tonic in the sauna. Mixed with Eucalyptus oil and Peppermint oil and solidified with Cocoa butter or beeswax you have an excellent application to rub on the chest to relieve sinus or bronchial congestion. A drop of the oil can be snuffed for nasal catarrh (a bit of a rough remedy in my opinion).

For the Japanese, Pine is a comforting scent that they use in their cleansing rituals. For people of the United States Pine has most definitely been overused in cleaning solutions. Often when you give an aromatherapy demonstration the participant will only say it "smells like housework" or "smells like cleaning solutions."

DILUTE ESSENTIAL OILS BEFORE USING.

In general Pine oil is antiseptic, kills germs, is anti-inflammatory, refreshing, deodorizing and stimulating. A good oil to have in your first-aid kit.

A useful way to take Pine Needle oil is mix a drop with a teaspoon of honey, add ½ cup hot water, stir and sip. Dose: 6 times per day.

Ravensara aromatica is a tree up to 40 feet in height belonging to the Laurel family and indigenous to Madagascar. The essential oil is steam-distilled from the leathery clove-scented leaves and sometimes the equally aromatic fruit and bark. This oil contains a high proportion of terpene alcohol and cineole, and this is used to treat flu caused by *Myxovirus influenza*. Other oils in this group are *Laurel nobilis*, *Eucalyptus radiata* and MQV.

Ravensara is used to treat flu symptoms and bronchitis. It is particularly useful to counter virus infections and to rid the body of toxins produced during such illnesses. It has also produced astounding amelioration, even in bad cases, of zona (shingles) especially when used in combination with the extract of *Calophyllum ino-phyllum*. The scent is a mixture of Clove and Eucalyptus and the taste is that of Clove and Nutmeg. See also Dr. D. Penoel, *Phytomedicine*, 1981.

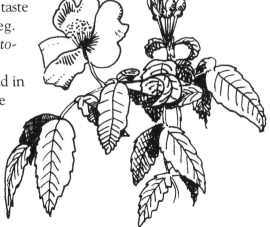

Ravensara is also cultivated in Sri Lanka. The seed kernels are popular as spice in Madagascar and have been exported to France. Leaves and bark are also used for seasoning. The bark is employed in native rum.

The Rose distils a healing balm
The beating pulse of pain to calm.
—*Anacrean, 500* B.C.

Rose essential oils are distilled from the following:

Rosa centifolia, the Rose de Mai, Cabbage Rose, Moroccan Rose or Indian Rose, pink flowers;

Rosa damascena, the Bulgarian, Turkish or Moroccan Rose, red flowers;

Rosa damascena bifera, Castilian Rose, Rose of Castille, pink flowers;

Rosa eglanteria, Rosehip Seed oil, Apple Rose, Eglantine or Brier Rose, pink flowers;

Rosa gallica officinalis, the Apothecary Rose or Rose of Provence, red wide-open flowers with crisp yellow centers;

Rosa rubiginosa, Rosehip Seed oil.

Rosa centifolia, the thousand-petaled Rose, grows to six feet, has one annual flowering and is used for fragrance, potpourri, Rosewater and perfume. Redouté, the famed Rose portrait painter, immortalized the Roses at Malmaison, the favored home of Josephine and Napoleon.

when solvent extracted

Rosa damascena bifera, the lovely, heavenly, fragrant pink Castilian Rose, grows to four feet. This is called autumn damask rose and it flowers repeatedly. This is the Rose that has been praised by Virgil and Ovid and was grown by Roman florists. The beautiful blossoms are dried and used for potpourris and fragrance.

Rosa damascena trigentipetala grows to four feet, has one annual flowering and is cultivated in Bulgaria in the Kazanlik Valley. This is the Rose used for Attar of Rose, Rose oil and Rosewater. Over one million blooms are used to make one kilo of essence. It has semi-double rose-red blossoms and the oil is used for rejuvenating and regularizing the menstrual cycle. The Damask Rose is used in the manufacture of triple Rosewater. Also used for Attar of Rose is *Rosa alba semi-plena* and *Rosa rubra.*

Rosa eglanteria has apple-scented leaves, grows to twelve feet and generally has one annual flowering. This is a wonderful plant whose thorn-edged canes grow quickly and can be used as a barrier to keep animals out of your property (hence the legend of Sleeping Beauty). The leaves are used for their green-apple scent in potpourris, the small, fragrant, pink whole buds and petals can be used for fragrance, and the Rose hips or mature fruit are used for vitamin C, cough syrup, pancake syrup and medicinal preparations.

> **KEEP ESSENTIAL OILS OUT OF YOUR EYES**

Rosa gallica officinalis is a very sweet, deep-red Rose, grows to five feet, has one annual flowering, and is used in high-quality potpourris and for the extraction of Rose oil that is used for fragrance and medicine, hence the common name, Apothecary Rose. This Rose became very popular in the 13th century and is also known as the Provence Rose.

The Rose scent is easily one of the most used, most prized and most costly of plant materials. Prices range from $10/ml for Moroccan Rose to $50/ml for Indian Rose, depending on the quality and perfection of the Rose scent. The Rose plant, petals and oil are very important in cosmetics, body-care products and home pharmaceuticals. Rosewater was distilled by Arabs and Berbers of Morocco around 700 A.D. Rose herb is considered to be a cellular regenerative, as is Comfrey herb, and both can be used externally in any body-care product for dry skin, wrinkled skin and sensitive skin. Rose lotion is a wonderful moisturizer for young and old alike. Rose oil can be taken internally but tea of petals is more often recommended for the reproductive system, as it is considered to aid those who have menstrual problems, or frigidity and impotence in women and men. The Rose petal juice and tea are mildly astringent when used either externally or internally. Rose oil inhaled or applied to the forehead relieves headache. It is an antidepressant, makes you feel better (stimulating), and soothes emotions such as shock or grief.

THE ALCHEMIST ROSE

A Good Rose Deodorant
Mix together equal quantities of baking soda and Orris root powder. Scent 1 cup of the mixture with 10 drops of the Rose oil, 10 drops of Sandalwood and 5 drops of Vetiver or Oakmoss. Shake together, sift and let age for at least several weeks so that the fragrance and powders can meld together. Use as an underarm or foot deodorant. Apply with a powder puff. This wonderful mixture will help prevent the bacterial degradation of perspiration.

Physically Rose scent works on the 1st chakra and is symbolic of strength and vitality; it can overcome fear. In meditation, Rose scent works on the heart or 4th chakra and is used for harmony and balance. Many put a dab of Rose oil or Rose pommade on the forehead to center themselves before beginning ritual or meditation.

Rose oil contains farnesol, which is a very important cosmetic ingredient. Farnesol is bacteriostatic, is attracted to the skin (dermatophile) and is good for mucous membranes. So Rose oil can be used in deodorant products for both underarm and sexual parts. Farnesol appears in other essential oils such as Jasmine, Citronella, Neroli, Sandalwood and Tuberose.

I personally use as an underarm deodorant a spritz that is a mixture of equal parts of Rose oil and water.

Of all flowers
Methinks a Rose is best . . .
. . . Shakespeare—*The Two Noble Kinsmen*

Rosehip Seed oil (Rosehip oil) is obtained from several Rose species, most notably *R. rubiginosa*. This Rose is also called *R. mosqueta*. Pliny was the first to note the fragrance of the leaves, which is somewhat green-apple and cinnamon (also called Eglantine Rose). The Rosehip oil is obtained by solvent extraction and smells like fish liver oil. It is a drying oil in that when refrigerated a solid substance will "come down." The claim is that Rosehip oil can be used as a carrier oil with essential oils. It can be applied in the following ways: reduces scarring, when rubbed daily on the face will reduce facial lines, heals burns, softens scars and allows more mobility for the tissue, retards premature aging. Since this is a dry-ing oil the recommendations are that it should not be used on acne.

My experience with Rosehip oil is that it seems to go bad rather quickly, so my recommendation is that you only buy small amounts at any one time from a reputable source that has high turnover. Then you will always be assured a fresh supply of the oil.

Rosemary oil is steam-distilled from the tops, leaves and smaller twigs of *Rosmarinus officinalis*. Several chemotypes are defined, depending upon where the plant is grown and what the local conditions are:

☿ *R. officinalis*	CT I*	Camphor	France
◐ *R. officinalis*	CT II	Cineol	North America
◑ *R. officinalis*	CT III	Verbenon	France

Rosemary plant is one of the most useful of the cosmetic and medicinal plants along with Rose and Mint. It has a long and fascinating history with ritual and meditative applications as well.

The herb tea is taken *internally* for all physical and men-tal problems, for impotence, as an antiseptic to all the organ systems, to stimulate the adrenal cortex and restore its func-tion (with Licorice), to soothe stomach pain, for arthritis, gout, neuralgia, to stimulate menstrual blood flow (possibly abortive), as a diuretic and sweat producer (sudorific), for all problems of the respiratory system including asthma and bron-chitis, for headache or headpain, and in strengthening baths for children as well as adults. With all these applications, the essential oil of Rosemary can be added to the herb tea but no more than 3 drops are taken daily. *Rosemary oil in undue quan-tities when inhaled or taken is considered to induce epilepsy* in peo-ple and create fear and timidity in animals.

Externally, the strained herb tea with essential oil added can be used to clean wounds and sores, added to a carrier oil is a useful massage product for all forms of joint or muscular pains, and directly applied kills lice and scabies (but burns if applied directly to the pubic region).

---

*CT=chemotype

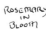

ROSEMARY
IN
BLOOM

Inhaled, Rosemary oil stimulates the 6th chakra, is used to encourage intuition, to increase sensitivity to situations, and helps increase the power of the third eye. It is said to cure forgetfulness and encourage remembrance. The scent is pleasing and offsets brooding. It is is used to strengthen the pineal gland. It vibrates in the color of indigo and purifies sacred places.

Rosemary is a powerful ingredient in all sorts of body-care products and has a reputation to stimulate hair growth. A formula to use for the hair is to mix Rosemary oil and Jojoba oil equally together; to every ounce of this mixture add 5 drops of Basil oil. Use a few drops on your hairbrush every night before going to bed and brush your hair from the scalp to the ends in long sweeping strokes. Remember to apply the mixture primarily to the scalp. The Jojoba unplugs the hair-growing cells and the Rosemary oil stimulates their function to encourage hair growth.

Queen of Hungary Water is an ancient formula of Rosemary herb, Lemon Verbena leaves and Peppermint tops which is distilled with triple Rosewater, triple Orange flower water, and 90% alcohol added, then allowed to age six months. The liquid is then carefully filtered and used to massage and rub on the body. The result is rejuvenative and will give you the beauty of a young woman!

 Rosemary Verbenon is a chemotype of Rosemary that is used therapeutically for treatment of acute middle-ear infections or otitis. An ointment is made with equal parts of MQV and Rosemary Verbenon and rubbed around the ear and the throat where the glands are located. Lavender oil or *Thymus vulgaris* CT linalool is applied inside the ear, 3 drops three times a day. Then a poultice of minced Onion is applied over the ear for two hours. Do this until the infection is cleared. Also, take an herbal cleansing or antibiotic formula internally to clear the blood.

Rosemary Verbenon is used for liver and gall bladder support, cramps, and skin-care for dry skin. It is strongly regenerating and has low-or non-irritant properties.

"In my personal experience Rosemary Verbenon has proven to be very effective for hepatitis. An internal dose can be made with 2 to 4 drops in 4 ounces of water hot or cold with a teaspoon of honey. Also it can be applied directly over the liver area for relieving pain and swelling in a dilution of 5 drops to ½ ounce of Olive oil. One of the interesting side effects of using Rosemary Verbenon internally is improved digestion and relief of arthritis symptoms. As a body oil or facial oil for chronic dry skin combines well with Lavender, Roman Chamomile, Carrot Seed oil and Neroli. Used in a base oil of 10 drops to one ounce of a base oil, e.g., Almond, Apricot, Avocado, Grapeseed, Olive or Sesame."

—*Victoria Edwards*

See Dr. D. Penoel, *Phytomedicine 1/2*, p. 23 ff, 1981;
J. Paltz, *Le Fascinant Pouvoir des Huiles Essentielles*, 1984.

Rosemary Borneol (*Rosmarinus officinalis borneol*) is a Rosemary chemotype that is used for fatigue, infections, cramps and as a heart tonic.

Rosemary Cineol (*Rosmarinus officinalis cineol*) is a Rosemary chemotype that is used for pulmonary congestion, slow elimination and for chronic fatigue.

Rose Geranium oil—See Geranium oil.

Rosewood oil—See Bois de Rose.

Sage, Clary, oil—See Clary Sage oil.

Sage oil is sometimes known as Dalmatian Sage and is steam-distilled from the dried leaves of *Salvia officinalis*.

Sage is from the family of plants called the *Labiatae* (the flowers have lips) and it is a common garden plant, grown throughout the world. It is widely used as a popular remedy and is one of the best-known medicinal plants whose main use is to reduce secretions throughout the entire body. In general the steam-distilled oil is used in perfuming soaps, as a blender fragrance in herbal colognes, in industrial perfumes to mask strong odious commercial odors, and at home to make blends of massage oils, facial oils and hair conditioners. Sage oil mixes well with Lavender, Rosemary and Basil oils. Drops of Sage oil can be mixed with powdered dentifrices and there it will act as a bactericide. It makes a great mouth cleanser.

Since Sage herb dries up secretions from the body, the herb is recommended to be smoked for asthma (a dubious recommendation in my opinion). The oil can be burned over a lightbulb to disinfect rooms. Sage oil and herb tea can be used in many skin care products where excess secretions are a problem, for oily skin, and oily hair. Black Sage tea can be used to darken hair.

The herb tea is used *internally* as a tonic, as a general stimulant to the nervous system and adrenal cortex, as a calmative, it is antiseptic, stops sweating and lactation, encourages menses, has a restorative effect on the body, is used to reduce night sweats, can be taken during menopause and is indicated for all kinds of illness. The essential oil and large quantities of herb tea are not recommended to be taken internally due the presence of thujone (see Table 8). Thujone also occurs in Wormwood and Thuja and is the principal ingredient in the generally banned drink Absinthe. Valnet mentions that Sage essence can be taken 2–4 drops/day in an alcoholic solution or honey water.

Externally, Sage oil and herb is astringent, healing and antiseptic and can be used as a mouth rinse, vaginal rinse or anal rinse. The oil can be directly applied to insect bites and stings and can be mixed with alcohol as a disinfectant for household or sickroom surfaces.

Inhaled the oil is antidepressant (although too strong for many), sometimes uplifting (depressing for some), and useful for mental strain, too much bookwork and mental exhaustion. When any oil is *inhaled* through the diffusor or via a pot of boiling water, it enters the mucous membrane of the nasal mucosa, is absorbed into the blood circulation and affects the entire body and mind.

Physically, Sage tea and the inhaled oil are excellent to activate the nervous system and the adrenal cortex, making them useful both for asthma and to regulate the hot flashes of menopause (with Clary Sage). Hot flashes are those rivulets of heat that flow over the body of so many women (even some men) during their middle years and are caused by a surge of hormones from the adrenal glands.

Too much inhalation of Sage oil can sometimes cause vertigo but in small doses it reduces giddiness and intoxication. As with many oils it is toxic in high doses. When you use Sage oil, inhale it no more than 10 minutes every 4–6 hours. Sage oil acts on the psyche and the emotions to soothe and act as a nervous tonic.

Sage oil is a fragrant disinfectant and the leaves are especially nice when they are burned and the smoke is used to cleanse the air of a home or the room where a sick person sleeps. This is wonderful cleansing odor. Try it!

Don't forget to use a few drops in the bath of your teenagers to refresh them, especially after sports. A drop between the toes will stop athlete's foot before it starts.

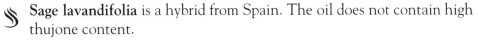 **Sage lavandifolia** is a hybrid from Spain. The oil does not contain high thujone content.

St. John's Wort oil is obtained from *Hypericum perforatum*. This oil has only recently been available. Both the infused oil and the essential oil in a carrier oil make a very good massage oil for sore muscles. It is astringent and aromatic and in shampoo formulas is an excellent cleanser for dandruff, oily hair and scalp. It can be externally applied for pimples and pus'y sores.* This oil is traditionally used for neck and back injuries and spinal trauma. Some use it in treating AIDS patients. In ritual use St. John's Wort oil balances all the chakras.

Sandalwood oil is steam-distilled from the coarsely powdered wood and roots of *Santalum album*. Sandalwood is one of the oldest known materials, and its history of use is more than 4000 years old (2000 B.C.). It has a warm woody aroma and blends well with Rose scent, Lavender, Tuberose, Clove and Cinnamon. Rose potpourris generally have Sandalwood in them as a fixative. The tea and oil taken *internally* are antiseptic, tonic, aphrodisiac (with Rose) and astringent (especially for the urinary system). Sandalwood is indicated wherever there is a problem in the respiratory or urinary systems. It has often been used to treat impotence and cystitis. Valnet recommends 5 drops of oil in a capsule once to four times per day. If you do take the oil this way you will feel a heat in your stomach and sometimes nausea. It is better to take Sandalwood oil one drop at a time mixed with honey or oil in the capsule, up to ten times per day, depending on body weight.

Sandalwood can be purchased as decorative small boxes, beautifully carved furniture or elegant fans. If you purchase a fan, spray it with water or Sandalwood water and then fan yourself in the heat of the day for a pleasantly scented and cooling breeze.

Inhaled Sandalwood is used for bronchitis, to scent rooms and during meditation to open the third eye. It vibrates between the 7th and 1st chakra ᘒ—and so is stimulating as well as grounding. It affects the pituitary gland. Sandalwood incense is traditional for meditation and ritual work.

---

*[Author's note: I could have said a pussy sore but that does not really convey *pus*.]

Externally, Sandalwood oil is good in baths, mixed with other anti-acne oils and in salves for chapped lips and skin. It is slightly healing, moisturizing and soothing when used in lotions, bath and massage products.

Sandalwood oil has a masculine scent.

In my daughter's baby book there is an entry dated August 1964: "In the hospital I used Sandalwood scent, and at home it was in all your clothes in sachet form. I wonder if you will remember this smell and love it when you are older or if you will forget it. It is my favorite scent and I use it constantly." Amber later told me the scent of Sandalwood was very soothing and comforting. It always helps her if she is under stress or doesn't feel well.

Sassafras oil* is steam-distilled from the roots or root bark of *Sassafras albidum.* This is an indigenous North American tree native to the eastern and southeastern USA. It grows wild and has been known to non-native Americans since they stepped upon our Continent. To Native Americans, Sassafras tea was a stimulating diaphoretic aromatic used for all sorts of skin eruptions. Now we use the tea mixed with Rosewater to clear the eyes and mixed with lanolin as a salve for every sort of skin disease. The essential oil is used in a sauna or native steam bath to treat general weakness, to treat mental problems of all sorts, as an anti-inflammatory and to stimulate the body to increase menstrual flow. Sassafras oil is used in all sorts of body-care products including massage oil (for mental balance), and in skin conditioners to treat skin inflammations and infections.

Inhale the oil for mental balance and thought-provoking mental changes.

May be a skin irritant if used neat.

Savory oil is steam-distilled from various plant species, notably *Satureia hortense* and *S. montana. Hortense* is a cultivated species in France while *Montana* is a wild species. If you smell Savory oil it will remind you of Sage and Thyme and maybe a bit of pickles and Indian curry sauce. The oil is used to flavor many commercial foodstuffs. The oil may be used *internally* to aid digestion, make the stomach feel good, relieve digestive spasms, relieve flatulence (although Peppermint oil is a third the price and works more effectively) and expel intestinal parasites.

---

*Used to make MDA.

Externally, Savory oil relieves the itch of insect bites and can be used in the treatment of wounds.

Mix Savory oil with a carrier oil and use for any problem that requires an analgesic or external stimulant.

See also Lavender oil and Tea Tree oil. Don't you have them yet?

 Spearmint oil is produced by steam distillation of the flowering tops of the plant *Mentha viridas*. The herb tea is a popular and well-known tonic drink almost everywhere in the world and especially in Egypt where this sweet, fragrant herb tea is poured after every meal. It is especially delicious if sugar is added. The oil is used in all sorts of pharmaceutical products especially dentifrice, tooth powders and all sorts of toothpaste flavors.

Spearmint tea and oil are used *externally* in body-care products. The herb is a mild antiseptic. The oil can be used directly on acne and skin irritations (it might work more effectively mixed with Tea Tree).

The oil or tea can be externally applied for headache or applied to the stomach as a compress for any sort of digestive disturbance. Chilled Spearmint tea with a dash of Spearmint oil can be applied to the body to reduce fever. Tea and oil can be taken *internally* for digestive aliments. It is a mild stimulant and mild antispasmodic. It can be used for headache, nausea and vomiting.

Inhaled, Spearmint oil is truly a memoristic anti-depressant (who can be depressed when you think of your carefree childhood, chewing gum and throwing spitballs?). It relieves mental strain and fatigue, cheers you up and tonifies your entire system.

Therapeutically, I believe that there are certainly more effective essential oils that will work better in any category, but for remembrance of childhood and a feeling of freedom and lightness, Spearmint oil is the best.

 Spikenard oil or Nard oil is derived from the roots of *Nardostachys jatamansi*, also known as False Valerian Root. The plant is cultivated in India and grows wild in various Southeast Asian countries. The steam distillation comes from the dried, tiny, minced pieces of the root. Tisserand calls Spikenard "one of the most fascinating and obscure essential oils . . . difficult to obtain."

The oil is tonic, cooling, laxative and fever-reducing but whether these effects are from internal use or inhalation, research is not clear.

Spikenard was one of the most precious and costly substances 2000 years ago. It was brought to the Middle East in tiny, beautiful boxes from the Himalayas via India and only opened in the presence of the person to whom it was presented. In the days of Christ a small box of Spikenard ointment would have cost over $400 in today's money. Mary of Bethany* washed and anointed Christ's feet with it and of this event Judas Iscariot says, "Why was not this ointment sold for three hundred pence and given to the poor?" Spikenard is mentioned several times in the Old Testament, Cant. (Song of Songs) 1:12; 4:13,14; and New Testament Mark 14:3-5; John 12:3,5.

Dietrich Gumbel mentions Nard oil as regulating heart beat, harmonizing the blood circulation and externally ". . . as uniting the functions of the skin layers into a harmonious, balanced skin picture, with an initial regeneration of all its functions. It is a soothing oil for the skin and is excellent when used against all kinds of skin irritations and allergies." He considers it of most value for the mature skin that is in fairly good balance. Hair and teeth are skin formations and Nard oil is the best treatment ". . . because it transmits balancing, soothing and harmonizing, characteristics via the mucous membrane of the mouth . . . via circulation into the whole organism."**

Victoria Edwards recommends Spikenard for staph infections, scleroderma and wounds that will not heal.

(d) **Spruce oil** is steam-distilled from the needles and small twigs of several species:

Picea marina, Black Spruce;
Picea alba, White Spruce;
Tsuga heterophylla

Most aromatherapy oil price lists use the Black Spruce. It is used in soap, in baths for arthritis and aching joints, in air refreshers as a cleaner and bactericide and in household cleaners to lend a fresh scent and act as a disinfectant.

---

*Mary of Bethany was not considered to be Mary Magdalene (Saint) until the time of Gregory the Great.

**Gumbel, Dietrich. *Principles of Holistic Skin Therapy with Herbal Essences.* Heidelberg, Germany: Karl F. Haug Publ., 1986. pp. 206–209.

Inhaled the oil is used to stimulate healthy function of the respiratory system as well as a stimulant and healthy expectorant for "wet" asthma and bronchitis. It is said to stimulate the adrenal glands and as such would be a useful inhalant for asthmatics. This oil has a wonderful pleasing scent, reminding one of the outdoors and moist fragrant forests. It is used as an incense and burned in rituals and meditations for "grounding." The fragrance also relieves anxiety and stress.

 Star Anise oil is steam-distilled from the fresh or partly dried fruits of *Illicium verum*. It has a sweet anise/licorice fragrance and is used to flavor foods and candies.

 Styrax oil is obtained by steam distillation of the crude styrax resin of *Liquidamber orientalis* or *L. styraciflua*. The best resin and oil has a luscious lemony, vanilla fragrance. The worst smells like a petroleum product. It is used in perfumery and has medicinal applications somewhat like Benzoin. I personally use Benzoin and keep Styrax oil around just to stimulate memory. Love this fragrance!

Styrax oil is used to make "Amber resin" by mixing with Labdanum gum resin.

 Tagetes oil, see also Calendula. Tagetes flowers do yield a quantity of oil, but this is more often used to color food. This oil is used in England for fungus infections on the feet.

 Tangerine oil is expressed* from the peel of the American variety of Mandarin, *Citrus reticulata* (also called *C. nobilis*). It is used, as is Mandarin Orange, *internally* as a digestive stimulant and for all sorts of digestive problems. It is antispasmodic and helps to control flatulence and belching. With Fennel it can be used to help one secrete excess fluid and so has value in obesity. Fennel oil plus Tangerine oil can be added to a tea of the same herbs. *Externally*, Tangerine is used in various carrier oils as a massage oil to break down cellulite and pockets of fat, as it helps to stimulate draining of the lymphatic system.

As an *inhaled* oil, the aroma is clearly Tangerine-scented, very citrus, and used to soothe the psyche. It is calming, sedating, eases nervous

---

*to release the oil by crushing or breaking open the oil glands in the peel.

tension and with Marjoram soothes emotions such as grief, anger and shock. This is one of the oils that I used on my Wolfie-dog during a time of shock and trauma. When my dogs got loose, Sumo-dog was hit by a car and Wolfie-dog, a beautiful Siberian Husky, came home traumatized and whimpering. We mixed Marjoram, Tangerine and a bit of Ylang-Ylang and put it in the diffusor. She would stay near the diffusor for twenty minutes at a time, would move and then come back to it. It seemed to be very effective in calming her down.

See also Citrus.

 Tarragon oil is steam-distilled from *Artemisia dracunculus*. Tiny amounts can be used to flavor foods. However, it is not recommended for other internal use. The herb itself and the oil have been used as a vermifuge (removes parasitical worms). *Inhaled* the oil has a strong, herby, celery scent and is used to ease digestion, relieve intestinal spasms, for hiccups, belching and farting. A very strong oil—there are others easier to use and just as effective. Cost is about $2/ml.

The herb has no use in skin-care products. The herb *infused* in oil with a bit of the essential oil is very effective as a massage oil on the abdomen for all sorts of abdominal pains and spasms or to massage sore muscles.

Valnet mentions that Tarragon oil can be taken *internally*; it is considered to be an abortive, stimulate menstrual flow, and he further recommends it for aerophogy and for malignant conditions (?). It is considered to be anti-cancer, 2–3 drops in honey water, 3 to 4 times per day.

 Tea Tree oil or Ti Tree is steam-distilled from a particular type of Australian tree, *Melaleuca alternifolia*. Tea Tree oil has been used in Australia by its native people, who introduced it to the Western world via Captain Cook in 1770. Tea Tree oil has been much in use and demand recently, but it is only in the last few years that its use has burgeoned. This is one oil that most definitely will get lots of use in your medicine chest and should positively be part of the home first-aid kit.

It is used *externally* on deep wounds, road burns to dislodge dirt and bacteria, cuts, scratches, abrasions, sunburn, insect bites, any sort of pruritis (generalized itching of the sensory nerve endings) whether anal or vaginal, burns and scalds, herpes lesions, ringworm, lice and tick bites, sores from eczema and psoriasis, thrush, candidiasis, head and pubic lice, athlete's foot, fungal infections, treatment of staph sores, boils, pimples, acne, halitosis, stinky feet, sinus congestion, etc.

Very sensitive skin may need the oil diluted but generally this is used "neat." My only complaint is that even though it cures "hot spots" on pets due to skin disease and fungus, the pets hate the scent and will run the moment the bottle is opened. The scent is strong, clean and powerful—maybe too powerful. If you are a teenager, apply Tea Tree oil to your zits in the evening and in the morning apply Niaouli oil or MQV oil.

Tea Tree oil is 4–5 times stronger than household antiseptic. Its bacterial action is increased where blood or pus is present. Externally used on deep wounds and cuts it will remove necrotic tissue and leave a healthy surface.

There are many many publications available that go into great detail regarding the use of Tea Tree oil. I suggest that if you care to get your medical doctor using this most miraculous of oils, you contact Thursday Plantation (see Source List, California or Australia) and request their certification information.

Tea Tree is a powerful killer of all sorts of bacteria. It is non-caustic to the skin, non-toxic to the body, it produces no negative side effects, it is a natural solvent (may dissolve some plastics), it has strong cleaning capabilities, it has a well-balanced pH level, it is mildly anesthetic and very aromatic.

The oil is best used applied externally but can be taken internally. *Inhaled*, it cleanses the air and purifies the respiratory system and so is useful for disease of the respiratory system.

Use on yourself, your pets, and your children.

See also Niaouli and MQV.

 Terebinth oil is essence of Turpentine. Turpentine is a natural oleo-resin formed as a physiological product in the trunks of Pine trees, *Pinus spp*. The rosin is removed, leaving the Turpentine or Terebinth oil. This is used in many household products and once was a very important part of the home pharmacy.

It can be used as a douche for vaginal problems, taken *internally* for all sorts of hemorrhage, to kill tapeworm, with Opium to treat cystitis, and as a syrup with Balsam Tolu to treat chronic bronchitis.

It is very antiseptic and cleansing, and is *inhaled* for all sorts of problems of the respiratory system.

> DILUTE
> ESSENTIAL
> OILS
> BEFORE
> USING

It is used *externally* to clean sores and wounds, in foot baths for fetid foot odor, to clean gangrenous sores and boils, as a friction rub for aching limbs, in liniments as a pain reliever, and to get rid of fleas and body lice.

 Thuja oil is produced by the *Arbor vitae* tree, *Thuja plicata* or *T. occidentalis*. The leaves and bark are water- or steam-distilled. This contains thujone, and although some aromatherapists occasionally recommend internal use, this is to be discouraged. *Externally*, the oil will kill the virus wart— apply a ring of glycerine around the wart, plantar wart or verruca, and apply the oil only to the wart itself.

The leaves and bark can be *infused* for baths. The scent is refreshing and stimulating, and the infusion itself will clean the skin of the oils of Poison Oak and Ivy.

Thuja oil is considered a convulsant poison.

The delicious-smelling Cedar tree that grows on Waldron Island, Washington State, is also a *T. plicata*.

See also Cedar.

 Thyme oils are made from several species of plants:
> *Thymus vulgaris*, Thymus oil;
> *T. hiemalis*, Lemon Thyme oil;
> *T. vulgaris* **linalol**, Sweet Thyme oil;
> *T. vulgaris* **or** *T. zygis*, Red Thyme oil;
> *T. capitatus*, Oregano oil—See Marjoram and Oregano;
> *O. vulgare*, Oregano oil—See Marjoram and Oregano;
> *Origanum majorana*, Marjoram—See Marjoram and Oregano;
> *Thymus mastichina*, Wild Marjoram oil—See Marjoram and Oregano;
> *Majorana hortensis*, Sweet Marjoram oil—See Marjoram and Oregano.

For herb care see *Jeanne Rose's Herbal Body Book*.

Thyme herb is one of the most useful medicinal herbs for body care, both internal and external, and Thyme oil intensifies all aspects of care. Thyme oil is aromatic, antiseptic, diaphoretic, stimulant and disinfectant. It is used internally, externally and by inhalation.

Thyme oil is used *externally* as an antiseptic and antibiotic. It can be used anywhere on the body or face, and even to cleanse sickroom surfaces (always use diluted). Thyme oil is used in lotions and massage oils to stimulate circulation and clean wounds and burns (Tea Tree is more often recommended). It is recommended to be used externally to kill parasites, for hair loss, in baths and in a solution of honey or diluted alcohol as a mouthwash.

Do not use neat on the skin—always dilute before use.

Inhaled, Thyme oil is uplifting and relieves depression, stimulates the respiratory system and relieves the spasm of asthma, is an antiseptic for all sorts of mucoid conditions, kills bacteria in the air, and is used for bronchitis or pneumonia. Thyme oil is also mildly sedating and can be used for insomnia.

Internal dose is 3–5 drops in honey water 3 times per day.

Thyme Linalol is especially recommended to kill bacteria and relieve discomfort. It is non-irritating and gentle, and especially recommended for treating children and the elderly or infirm.

Thyme oil, Type IV with high thujanol, is considered the best antiviral oil, *Thymus vulgaris* (Chemotype Thuyanol). This essence is quite new. It captures much of the overall strength and stimulating properties of the "regular" essence of Thyme as well as its anti-infectious properties. The difference lies in the much higher content of highly desirable terpene alcohols (non-toxic) and the much lower content of irritant and slightly toxic phenols. This oil is strongly germicidal (yet non-irritant) and a very good liver stimulant. Recent conversations with French researchers point to its efficacy against Chlamydia. As the Thyme is non-irritant it can be used vaginally and on mucous membranes.—Victoria Edwards

Tuberose oil is produced by "washing" the pommade or absolute of Tuberose with alcohol. The flowers of *Polyanthes tuberosa* are picked before the petals open. This is a beautiful, stately plant with a central spike of flowers. Since the flowers produce oil up to 36 hours after they are picked, the enfleurage method is usually used to extract this long-lasting scent. I have grown Tuberose for 20 years in my greenhouse so that I may enjoy this fabulous, flowery-sweet scent during the short flowering season (short in San Francisco). I have especially enjoyed Tuberose flower in champagne (1 per glass) as an aphrodisiac.

Inhaled the oil is an aphrodisiac, it centers the emotions, and for those who like it, strengthens the emotions as well.

> KEEP
> ESSENTIAL
> OILS OUT
> OF YOUR
> EYES

Underarm Odor is a natural product formed by the interaction of cutaneous microflora and the secretions of axillary apocrine glands. The underarm scent can regulate a woman's menstrual cycle and create a regular menstrual cycle. Women who have sex at least once a week are generally more regular than those who have sex less often. Male underarm odor may be the key to these regular cycles. In a study reported at the Meeting of the Society of Cosmetic Chemists in 1985, seven women with irregular menstrual cycles had an extract of male underarm odor placed on their upper lips, three times a week for three months. They were not to wash the area around their nose for at least six hours afterward. Nine other women were given a placebo extract. Dr. George Preti, an organic chemist, and co-workers at the Monell Chemical Sense Center, Philadelphia, found that four of the seven women, better than 50%, had regularized their menstrual cycles by the end of the study. Only one woman in the control group had regularized. According to Dr. Preti, "It appears that you need consistent intimate contact for the odor effect to work; simply living under the same roof won't do it."*

Is this why we women always like to sleep under the arm of our male companion?

There is a possibility of future products such as scent-based drugs, scented tampons or just scented nose patches that act as birth control systems.

I recently read of a company in London, Bodywise Company, which discovered and patented a substance based on androstenone, a pheromone found in the sweat men produce in their armpits. This substance is used to treat bills that are sent to customers; 17% more people pay up when their bills are treated with androstenone than when it just smells like paper. One whiff of a bill treated with male underarm odor sends most recalcitrant debtors directly to their checkbooks to pay it off.

Another study reported by Britain's University of Warrick (about 1990) showed that a tincture made from a steroid extracted from human

---

*From a personal facsimile from Dr. Preti, January 29, 1992.

sweat produced a significant tranquilizing effect when sniffed.

Rather an interesting application of aromatherapy, don't you think?

 Vanilla planifolia is an orchid, a large climbing vine indigenous to Central America. The flower is pollinated by a particular insect that can get inside the orchid, or the flower can also be hand-pollinated. As the pod or fruit develops it elongates, and just prior to complete maturity this sexual part, the pod (the outer capsule), is harvested. The pods are now dried and cured, a chemical fermentation process that releases enzymes and during which the pod gets brown and flavor and aroma begin to develop. As the fruit dries, crystals appear on the outside, the vanillin. Sometimes this may take up to a year, sometimes the fruits are dried by infra-red light.

See also Tonka and Vanilla in *Herbs & Things* by Jeanne Rose.

The pods are then processed in various ways to give us Vanilla oil and Vanilla extract. Although it is true that most of the Vanilla used in flavor work is a manufactured product, there is also definitely a natural Vanilla available. My suggestion is to buy whole Vanilla pods and to make your own alcohol extract using 151-proof rum.

Vanilla is more than just a particular scent. It is a recognizable flavor that revolutionized the taste buds of the peoples of the Olde Worlde. Vanilla, a native of Central America, was used by the indigenous peoples, including the Aztecs, along with Chilé Pepper and Chocolate to make a very tasty drink that only the god/kings were allowed to partake of. This drink and these foods were exported to Spain about 1575 along with most of the Aztec gold.

Vanilla oil can be used in body-care products but why bother? It is the fragrance itself along with the taste that is the true aphrodisiac. It mixes well with Orange and Chocolate tastes.

Vanilla pods, chopped and *infused* in oil make a dynamic massage oil for the impotent, frigid or sterile person—it is warming, soothing and an aphrodisiac. Mixed with a bit of Olive oil, a Vanilla massage oil preparation can be used to lubricate the outside of the vaginal area. Sex will be delicious, nutritious and sweet-smelling as well.

Inhaling the scent of Vanilla will almost always remind you of mother, home cooking and sweet baked goods, and it will be calming, soothing and stimulating to the feelings of the 1st chakra. Prolonged exposure to Vanilla scent can have a deleterious effect on the nervous system.

Vanilla Tincture

125 grams chopped or ground Vanilla pods are macerated in 1000 grams of 95% ethyl alcohol for 2 weeks and then carefully filtered. This can be used directly in cooking or mixed with Olive oil to make a massage oil. One teaspoon Vanilla pod tincture to 8 ounces, more or less, of oil.

See the monograph on Vanilla in *Food* by Waverly Root, published in 1980, by Simon & Schuster, NY, for more Vanilla information.

Natural Vanilla is expensive: extracted from the bean it costs about $1,200 a pound. By contrast, flavoring made from synthetic vanilla costs only $7 a pound.

Using a relatively new technology called cell culturing, however, a small California company has patented what it says is a way to produce natural Vanilla at less than $200 a pound. "You have a much fuller-bodied, rounded flavor, rather than the sharp chemical aroma," said Raymond J. Moshy, president of Escagenetics Corporation in San Carlos, California. The cell-culture process can cut the cost of flavoring to less than $200 a pound, which makes it economical for use in premium ice creams, baked goods and other foods.

TRUE **Verbena oil** or **Lemon Verbena oil** is produced by steam distillation of the freshly harvested leaves of *Lippia citriodora*. This oil has a wonderful fresh, herby-smelling lemon scent. This plant is considered an herb, although in my backyard in San Francisco it is a tree kept about 20 feet high, annually clipped and topped of about 3 feet of new growth. The leaves are used in body-care products and in facial steam mixtures to stimulate the pores. It is cleansing and tonifying. In shampoos it helps degrease the scalp and gives shine to the hair.

Externally, the oil can be used in bedtime bath mixtures, 1 drop Lemon Verbena to 2 drops Rosemary or Lavender for sleeping. In lotions,

Lemon Verbena is used to degrease the skin, for acne or blemishes.

The tea can be drunk. It is calming, soothing, non-addicting and can be used regularly by the insomniac.

The essential oil is taken *internally* in small amounts (1 drop). It acts as a digestive stimulant to soothe the stomach and relieve digestive disturbance. Lemon Verbena tea with a drop of the essential oil is a wonderful aperitif or after-dinner cordial for those who are prone to overeating.

Inhaled the oil of Lemon Verbena is relaxing and soothing, calms excess nervousness and improves concentration.

Vetiver oil is steam-distilled from the small cleaned, washed roots of *Andropogon zizanioides (muricatus)*. This is a tall perennial grass whose rootlets are cut and dried and then soaked in water before the distillation process. The scent of both the roots and the oil is clean, refreshing and slightly woody. Also called Vetivert or Khus-Khus.

Externally, Vetiver oil is used in perfumery and potpourris as a fixative. It is used in lotions to stimulate the circulation for aching joints or arthritis, and for dry, irritated, mature or aging skin. As it is moisturizing, it is a humectant for dry skin. It blends well with other oils that are used for mature skin such as Frankincense, Myrrh, Rose, Patchouli and Sandalwood.

There is no real use for Vetiver taken *internally*.

Inhaled, the scent is calming and sedating, used for comforting and for people who feel "uprooted" or without stability. It affects the parathyroid glands.

Duraffourd recommends "drops placed on a handkerchief and placed among the underwear."

The roots are also used to make fragrant fans and screens. When these are dampened during a rainstorm or when water is sprinkled on them, breezes blow through, the scented water evaporates, and a clean and refreshing scent is left.

Violet Flower and Leaf—A concrète is made of the flowers or leaves of *Viola odorata* and this is washed to obtain the fragrance material. However, since the flower absolute is astronomically expensive, possibly $100,000/kilo, often the more obtainable item is a Violet Leaf Absolute. I have had bits of Violet flower absolute and treasured it, but more often I have had a deep green-coloured, green-smelling, sweet-green scented Violet leaf. Neither is used much in aromatherapy—it is just too expensive—but if you have a Violet patch in your garden you can easily obtain the scent for personal use. If you can't grow it or don't wish to trouble yourself with the extraction process, call Leydet oils. The owner, Victoria Edwards, sells Violet Leaf, 1 ml/$40.00, or try Herbal Endeavors, $27/ml. The former is therapeutic and the latter is PEO from Tisserand.

Externally, Violet flower and leaf are used to treat anything near the throat or 5th chakra. Violet leaf has a historical reputation for treating throat cancer. To learn the uses of the herb and flower, please refer to the *Herbal Body Book* by Jeanne Rose. Briefly stated, Violet treats all problems of the skin. The essence or essential oil in products is used for all forms of skin inflammation. Use the herb or flower as tea or compress.

Taken *internally* the tea (the essential oil is tooooo expensive) is used to treat nervousness, stomach cramps, headaches and stress and is gargled for sore throat.

Inhaled the scent of Violet is sweetly soothing for annoyed or cranky children, and for restless or overexcited pets or humans. It subdues acute inflammation, encourages sleep, comforts the heart, soothes anger, cures dizziness and relieves headache.

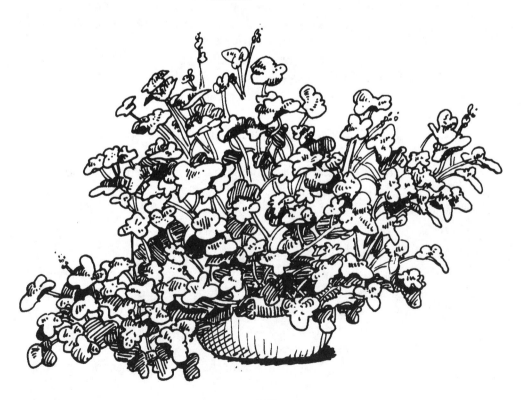

Wintergreen oil is an oil of American origin, water-distilled from the leaves of *Gaultheria procumbens*. It has a wonderful bright fragrance typical of the Wintergreen gum and candy of youth. During the distillation process, methyl salicylate is formed by enzymatic action. Some people are very allergic to methyl salicylate. Wintergreen oil is very useful in various skin preparations for problem skin, but if you are allergic to it then its use will often cause skin problems. Always use the patch test before trying Wintergreen oil.

The herb is used as an astringent aromatic in lotions, creams and salves. Infused in oil, it is used as a rub for arthritis and sciatica.

The oil should not be taken internally.

Externally, if you are not allergic you may use 1–4 drops of oil per ounce of carrier oil or lotion for external application to eczema, acne, blemishes or external skin problems.

Inhaled, the fragrance is memoristic of youthful pleasures.

 Yarrow oil is steam-distilled from *Achillea ligusticum* and *A. millefolium* in Belgium, Bulgaria and California. It is quite expensive, about $10/ml. It can be used wherever azulene as an anti-inflammatory has use. Victoria Edwards says, "Yarrow has been under experimental research as an antidote for radiation exposure, as an anticancer as well as anti-tumor agent, as an aid to detoxification from drugs and alcohol. It is useful in severe skin rashes and for wounds that will not heal."

 Ylang-Ylang or Ilang-Ilang fragrance is delicious, delightful and heavenly sensual. The oil is obtained by water and steam distillation of *Cananga odorata*. The large, sexy, drooping yellow-green flowers of the tree are distilled within a few hours of the early morning picking.

The top note, the first impression of the scent as it is applied to the skin, is rather fleeting and ephemeral but richly sweet and powerful. The middle and bottom notes are most lasting, fading out slowly over the course of a day. The flowers can be infused directly into oil, making a delightful aphrodisiacal massage oil. This oil as it is being applied also has a distinct antidepressant effect. I have used it after a warm bath when my day has been unusually difficult, as it relaxes me and soothes jangled nerves.

Ylang-Ylang (ee-long, ee-long)—even the name has an exotic sound —means "flower of flowers." The flowers themselves if they are available can be wrapped in the hair to scent it.

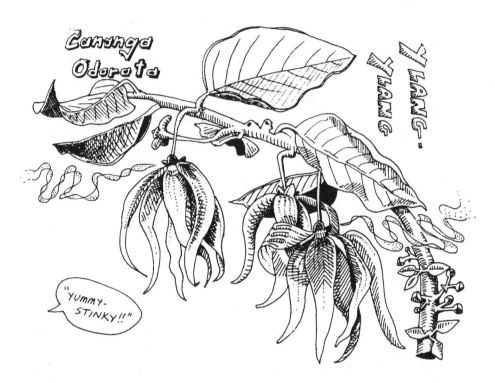

This tree grows in several places in Madagascar and the Philippines. Ylang-Ylang occurs wild from Burma to Queensland, Australia, and is cultivated commercially in the Comoro Islands, northwestern Madagascar, and to a lesser extent on islands in the Pacific and the West Indies. The tree (60–80 or even 120 ft.) is esteemed in all warm regions as an ornamental. It has drooping branches, evergreen leaves (5–8 inches long), richly scented flowers, and inedible fruits. Essential oil distilled from the flowers (usually picked at night when they are most fragrant) is regarded as the "Queen of Perfumes." It is extensively used in fine scents, face powder and various other cosmetics. It has a little-known role in commercial fruit flavors (especially peach and apricot) for candy, icings and baked goods, and also enters into soft drinks and chewing gum.

Externally, the essential oil can be diluted with a bit of carrier oil or scent-free alcohol to make a lasting scent or perfume. The essential oil in a small amount of carrier oil can be mixed and used for massage or a scalp treatment (to soothe or to treat dry scalp). It can also be used in all sorts of cosmetics lotions or soaps to treat dry, aged or mature skin. You can

150

scent cotton balls with Ylang-Ylang and place among your fine lingerie for a delicious scent.

Inhaled, the scent stimulates the adrenal glands. In *The Aromathera-py Demonstration*, some participants found that the oil made their heart race, although it is indicated in cases of tachycardia. We always recommend that it be inhaled in a diluted state or through a diffusor as it can cause headache. In the diffusor, Ylang-Ylang is anti-depressant, soothing, antiseptic and an aphrodisiac, useful for insomnia, nervous depression, states of pain, to treat anger, anxiety and, some say, rage and low self-esteem.

Ylang-Ylang is used in medication to treat the thymus gland (as a stimulant to the immune system).

Valnet mentions it can be taken internally, 2–5 drops, 3 times per day in honey water, for intestinal infections, purulent secretions, impotence or frigidity.

The Fairchild Tropical Gardens in Miami, Florida, has a tree blooming most of the time.

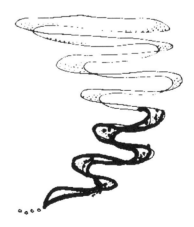

Chapter IV

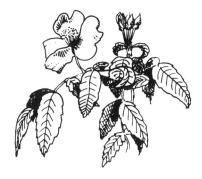

Special Tables & Lists

Autumn Morning to the Five Senses
I hear the finches twittering near their feeder
And see the soft sunlight glowing on the yellow Nasturtiums
*   that live high up on my neighbor's hedge*
Smelling the sweet wild fragrance of the white Jasmine . . .
I taste the tart sweetness of the bright red rosehips
*   the mature fruit of the Apple-scented Rosa Eglanteria*
And feel the prickly Rosemary leaves as I brush by them
*   they release their camphoraceous odor*
*   It fills the air.*
I bent and touch the velvety green softness of the
*   Peppermint-fragrant Peppermint Geranium, AND KNOW*
ALL IS WELL this Monday.
                            —Jeanne Rose, October 14, 1991, 10 A.M.

Table 3
Weights & Measures

Grain	Solid	Fluid
15 grains	= ¼ teaspoon	= 15 drops
20 grains		= 20 drops = 1 milliliter
40 grains		= 40 drops = 2 milliliters
60 grains	= 1 teaspoon	= 60 drops

Essential oils are delicate, highly concentrated essences of plants and only a tiny bit of oil is ever used in a product. If you wish to measure in milliliters only, go to the pharmacy and buy a measured pharmaceutical eye dropper. They only cost a few cents and are a valuable investment in order to duplicate the recipes that you will find in this and other books.

When you double and triple the size of recipes used solely for scenting, often the scent changes and your nose will have to tell you just how much more or less essential oil to add to be comparable to the original formulation. This is also true in cooking and baking—sometimes recipes do not lend themselves well to doubling or enlarging.

1 troy ounce	= 31.1035 grams
12 troy ounces	= 1 troy pound or 373.24 grams
32.151 troy ounces	= 1 kilo
1 avoirdupois ounce	= 28.3495 grams
16 avoirdupois ounces	= 1 pound
1 avoirdupois pound	= 454 grams
35.274 avoirdupois ounces	= 1 kilo

See your dictionary for more weights and measures. Be sure to look up both USA measures and British measures, which differ.

Table 4
Amounts of Essential Oils for Blends

⅛ oz	= ¾ teaspoon	= 3–4 milliliters	= 80 drops
¼ oz	= 1–1½ teaspoon	= 6–8 milliliters	= 160 drops
½ oz	= 3 teaspoons	= 13–15 milliliters	= 320–400 drops
1 oz	= 6 teaspoons	= 25–30 milliliters	= 600–650 drops

As you can see, these are approximate measurements. But for the home aromatherapists they are quite adequate. The chemist would use a very careful and calculated scale of milliliters in order to measure a new perfume or aromatherapy blend.

360–400 drops = ½ ounce

20–25 drops per dropper

Use about 20–25 drops per ounce of carrier oil or product for therapy.

Table 5
The Only Measurement You Need to Know

Droppers come in various sizes with various size openings. A drop is usually exactly the same amount of liquid no matter what size the dropper, but essential oils are both very, very thin and lightweight and very, very thick and heavyweight, and so thick Patchouli weighs more in less space than thin Tea Tree. But generally:

1 dropper holds 20 drops which is 1 milliliter

½ dropper yield 10 drops which is 0.5 ml.

Table 6
Pathways of Essential Oils & Where They Go When Inhaled

In Table 6 we see why inhalation therapy works.

Essential oils are volatile substances; that is, their molecules when released into the air form a gaseous vapor. In inhalation therapy this vapor is *inhaled* and the vaporized molecules are absorbed into the blood stream via the lungs as well as absorbed by the olfactory nerves through the nose. The vapors affect the limbic system, which consists of several structures in the forebrain that deal with the integration and expression of feelings, learning, memory, emotions and physical drives.

By inhaling odor through the nose, feelings and memory are affected. The vaporized molecules are excreted via secretions of the endocrine glands.

By inhaling through the mouth, essential oils are absorbed through blood vessels in the lungs, which affects the entire respiratory system.

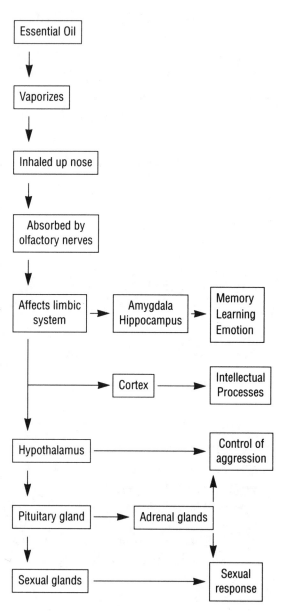

From *Aromatherapy: To Heal And Tend The Body* by Robert Tisserand. Reproduced with permission.

Table 7
Essential Oil Path to Treat Mind & Body & Where They Go When Applied Externally or Taken Internally

In Table 7 we see why external applications of essential oils work. When essential oils are applied externally, the molecules are absorbed through the skin via the small blood vessels. The oils are carried to the muscle tissue and joints and via the blood stream the molecules are carried into all the tissues and organs. Excretion takes place through the kidneys and bladder, skin, and exhaled through the lungs. So you can see that essential oils can be applied externally and will reach all parts of the body.

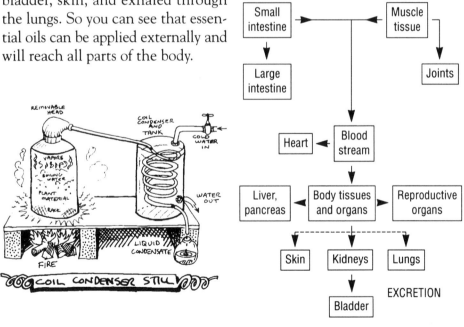

From *Aromatherapy: To Heal And Tend The Body* by Robert Tisserand. Reproduced with permission.

157

Table 8
Aromatic Constituents & Their Properties

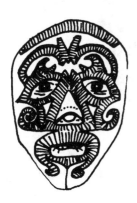
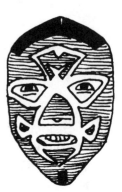

This is just a very brief outline of the constituents of essential oils and their general properties. There is much much more to learn, but since this is not a chemistry text, we will be brief and generalize.

Aldehydes	Anti-infectious and sedative, calming when inhaled and irritating used externally. Citral is an example.
Azulene	Prevents discharge of histamine from the tissues by activating the pituitary-adrenal system, causing the release of cortisone. Could be useful in asthma. Azulene causes histamine release-activating cellular resistance and speeding up the process of healing. Azulene also stimulates liver regeneration. It is anti-inflammatory as well.
Bisabolol	The strongest of the sesquiterpene alcohols is Bisabolol. It is anti-inflammatory, antibacterial, antimycotic and ulcer-protective (preventative). A fixative. Contained in Chamomile oil.
Borneol	Antiseptic and energizing, possibly anti-cancer.
Carvacrol	Antiseptic and energizing, strong bactericidal.
Cineole	Anesthetic, antiseptic and expectorant.
Citral	An aldehyde, is anti-infective and sedative and sometimes anti-viral. *Example:* The application of Melissa oil topically on herpes simplex.
Esters	"The compound resulting from the reaction of an alcohol with an acid. The reaction is called *esterification* and is accompanied by the yield of H_2O along with the

TABLE 8

ester. The reaction is fully reversible. Since esters are not very soluble in water, water can be added to the distillate, and then water plus alcohol are removed. Upon redistillation the ester soon distills off pure."* Esters are soothing, calming, and fungicidal. Geranium, Lavender and Orange Flower (Nerol) have high ester content.

Eugenol   From the phenyl-propane group, is very antiseptic and stimulating, strong properties, sometimes toxic to the central nervous system (CNS). Cinnamon leaf is distilled to retrieve the eugenol.

Flavonoid   Exerts beneficial effects on the capillaries. In Chamomile by inhibiting methyl transferase, epinephrine effects are prolonged and the pituitary-adrenal axis is stimulated.

Farnesol   Is has a very distinctive odor like Lily-of-the-Valley. It is anti-inflammatory, bacteriostatic, dermatophile (from the Latin, having an affinity for skin), good for mucous membranes, and prevents bacterial degradation of perspiration.

Farnesene   A terpene.

Ketone   Use with caution, sometimes toxic, stimulates cell regeneration and duplication. They promote the formation of tissue and liquefy mucus, are mucolytic and neurotoxic. Use in dry asthma or colds and flu with dry cough.

Limonene   Strong anti-viral properties.

Linalool (Linalol) Antibacterial, relieves discomfort, diuretic, tones without irritating, stimulates the immune system, sedating.

Monoterpenes Include pinene, camphene, sabinene, limonene.

---

*Van Nostrand's *Scientific Encyclopedia,* 7th edition. New York: Van Nostrand Reinhold, 1989.

Phenols Antiseptic and kills bacteria, such as cresol, thymol or carvacrol in Thyme. Toxic.

Sesquiterpenes Antiseptic, antiallergic, liver and gland stimulant, anti-inflammatory. They include caryophyllene and valencene.

Terpenes Provoke accumulation of toxins in certain organs, especially the liver and kidneys.

Terpene Alcohols Diuretic, anti-bacterial, tones, stimulates the immune system. They include borneol, citronellol, nerol, geraniol and terpineol. Gattefossé considered terpineols to be decongestant.

Terpene Hydrocarbons Antiviral. Limonene, pinene and sebanine are examples.

Thujone Toxic and can derange the central nervous system. Neurotoxic when taken internally. An example is the thujone content of the banned drink Absinthe. Can also be inhaled to relieve respiratory distress.

Thymol Strongly antiseptic and not as toxic as phenol.

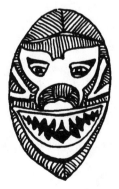

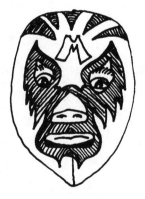

Table 9
Herbs to Improve the Sense of Smell

"Rich and varied scents enhance beauty and prolong life" is an Oriental proverb. Use the following herbs as teas or food to improve your ability to distinguish different odors and to improve your sense of smell.

You can mix the teas according to your discretion, $\frac{1}{2}$ ounce per day of mixed herbs with 1 quart of water simmered, steeped, strained and drunk. This taken over the course of a month should improve your ability to discern odors.

Asafoetida root (*Ferula foetida*) is used in curries and Indian foods. It has a sedative action and affects all the senses, reduces bronchial and nasal mucus,* soothes the nasal passages, and is used to soothe the nerves and the pain of mastoid infections.

Asparagus (*Asparagus officinalis*) is eaten as a food. It heals and is considered a nutriceutical, that is, a food having therapeutic value. The stalks can be used as tea. It is aperient (mildly laxative), diuretic and mildly stimulating to the kidneys. It has a sedative or soothing effect on the heart. Asparagus syrup can be taken for rheumatism. Asparagus stimulates the sense of smell and can be used to clear up nasal congestion.

Blood Root (*Sanguinaria canadensis*) is used as a tonic and stimulant, and has a specific action on the nose. It can cure a runny nose when the juice is snorted. It is a stimulant for all the respiratory passages. Take as a tea. Leyel mentions it as a right-sided remedy (for the right side of your body).

Camphor (*Cinnamomum camphora*) is a gum used to stimulate the function of the mucous** membranes of the respiratory tract. Look at any over-the-counter medication and you will probably find Camphor as one of the ingredients. It is pain killing and sedative. It is inhaled or applied externally in rubs for muscular aches and pains or any condition of the respiratory tract. It is also anti-inflammatory.

---

*Mucus is the slimy, snotty stuff that you expel from your nose, throat or lungs.
**Mucous is an adjective that describes a look, that is, covered with mucus or relating to mucus.

Caper Spurge *(Euphorbia lathyris)* seed is used in Chinese medicine as a tea for edema (for retention of fluid), for lack of the menstrual period, for constipation and urinary retention, and as a remedy for ulceration of the mucous membranes of the nose.

Cherry Bark *(Prunus avium)* is a common ingredient in herbal medicinal teas for the respiratory system. It is astringent, tonic, and soothing. It is especially used in syrups for runny nose, coughs and bronchial mucus. All parts of the tree can be used — the bark, leaves, flowers or flower stalks. Cherry stems are used in tea for their diuretic effect. Cherries steeped in wine can be used for arthritis.

Chilé Peppers *(Capsicum spp.)* are used as food or in capsules for flavor and the pungent effect on the mucous membranes. This is a hot food and a healing food and is recommended by some progressive medical doctors to be eaten at least three times a week to keep the airway passages open and clear. It is particularly good to eat in Mexican foods. This American original should be eaten daily by those with chronic bronchitis and emphysema. One-half of a Chilé Pepper, half of an Onion and one clove of Garlic per day is a good prescription for respiratory health.

Cinnamon *(Cinnamonum zeylanicum)* bark is a delicious spice that is used as food and medicine. It is warming and stimulating and acts as an antiseptic. If you have a cold and feel chilly, add the spice to soups or the essential oil to mixtures to warm you up. A drop on a sugar cube is sucked for sore throat.

Cinquefoil *(Potentilla reptans)* herb and root is used to enhance all the senses. It is taken as a tea and acts to reduce fever and as an astringent. The tea can be drunk, gargled and/or sniffed up the nose to stop a nose bleed, and used as a mouthwash to keep the gums healthy. This plant has a wonderful history in magic and is used to find the one you love and to cast successful spells.

Cypress *(Cupressus sempervirens)* leaves and cones are used in teas and massage oils as an astringent antiseptic. The essential oil is inhaled and is powerfully astringent for a runny nose and for all problems of the respiratory system. An infusion used as a footbath has long been in use to combat smelly feet.

Daisy *(Bellis perennis)* flowers, the common lawn Daisy, also called Bruisewort is used as a tea on the face to help cure all sorts of problems such as acne or

TABLE 9

boils. It is also used in massage oils for varicose veins (mix with Calendula). It can be used as a nasal snuff for a runny nose.

Duckweed (*Lemna minor*)plant is used as a specific* for the nose and can be eaten to improve both the sense of taste and smell.

Elder (*Sambucus nigra*) bark, leaves, flowers and berries are used to improve the sense of smell. This plant can be taken as tea or tisane to rejuvenate all the senses and all the tissues. The berries are infused in liqueur to make the drink Sambuca, and they are considered a specific to encourage a long and healthy life. This is a fine cosmetic plant (read *The Herbal Body Book* for uses). The Elder is much used in magic.

Elecampane (*Inula helenium*) root and plant is used as tea or in capsules. It is antiseptic, astringent, makes you sweat (diaphoretic), loosens mucus (expectorant) and a tonic. This is good medicine to take for all serious conditions of the respiratory tract including asthma.

Eucalyptus (*Eucalyptus globulus*) leaves and the essential oil are used in all sorts of remedies for coughs, colds, bronchitis and other problems of respiration. This is a standard remedy that we all grew up with, and we all probably used it in a hot-air vaporizer to thin mucus. It is powerfully antiseptic and antibacterial.

Garlic (*Allium sativum*) cloves are a well-known popular food and medicine that have a powerful antiseptic and cleansing effect on the respiratory system. Garlic also improves the blood and increases anti-clotting factors, and is anti-inflammatory and pain relieving. Research has shown that a component, adenosine, is the primary blocker of platelet clumping in blood. Adenosine is contained in both Garlic and Onions and is not destroyed by cooking. Eat 3 ounces of Garlic, Onions and Chilé every day, say Chinese research studies, and this will reduce your chances of getting stomach cancer. Garlic crushed in water and the water carefully strained to remove particles can be snuffed into the nostrils and will cure sinusitis and blocked nasal passages. The cure needs to be done 3 times a day for 3 days—one sniff will not work. Garlic is another specific for the respiratory system.

---

*A *specific* is a common herbal term meaning that it exerts a definitive and distinctive influence on a particular part of the body.

Ginger (*Zingiber officinale*) root is a specific remedy for jet lag or digestion. It is very valuable in any mixture of herbs used for the respiratory system. It is stimulating and warming. It is said to cure an itching nose by inhalation of a drop of the oil. The essential oil is used to help memory and migraine headache by inhalation, and a drop on a sugar cube is sucked for sore throat and tonsillitis.

Goldenrod (*Solidago virgaurea*) flowers and leaves are used in the treatment of allergic asthma and hayfever. The pollen is a potent allergen, and so the Goldenrod is used homeopathically and Goldenrod honey is taken during the hayfever season. Also known as *Solidago odora*.

Hawthorn (*Cratægus oxycantha*) leaves and berries are used to treat heart conditions and chronic runny nose.

Hyssop (*Hyssopus officinalis*) flowers and leaves are used in tea and tincture for excess mucus in nose or chest.

Lesser Celandine (*Ranunculus ficaria*). Leyel recommends that the entire plant be used by sniffing the oil or tea or juice as a cure for nasal polyps.

Lobelia (*Lobelia inflata*) herb is a good remedy for the mucous membranes. It can be smoked or used as tea or in capsules.

Melilot (*Melilotus officinalis*) herb is used as an aromatic stimulant. It is a very sweet-smelling perennial clover and contains coumarin, which is an anti-clotting factor for blood. The tea is used to fragrance the body, helps to cure flatulence (when eating any food but particularly excessive Garlic), and if taken over a period of time helps to improve the sense of smell.

Mustard (*Brassica spp.*) flowers are delicious when eaten in salads, and the flowers and leaves are used in tea or tincture to stimulate the appetite and improve the sense of smell. Mustard seeds are the well-known component of the food mustard. Oil of Mustard (the infused, ground Mustard seeds in Olive oil) is used as a snuff to relieve pain in the nose. Mustard plasters are an old-time remedy for chest congestion.

TABLE 9

Myrrh (*Commiphora myrrha*) gum is traditionally used in mouth-care products and perfumes, and as incense in church and in cleansing magical ritual. The scent is a specific to help cure asthma and all conditions of the bronchi. It is best to use the distilled oil in treatment of the lungs, and to use the resin for incense.

Nasturtium (*Tropæolum majus*) flowers and leaves are used as food and expressed for the juice, which is snuffed for polyps in the nose. The seed pods can be pickled and eaten like Capers.

Onions, Leeks & Shallots (*Allium spp.*) are ancient foods and excellent remedies for the lungs. Onions, Garlic and Chilé Peppers will stimulate the lungs, reduce cholesterol and improve heart health. Onions contain a powerful disinfectant. Tea or Onion soup is a remedy for inflammation of the nasal passages with a constant runny nose. Onions are also an excellent poultice for an earache and a remedy for measles or for a disease in which sensitivity to light is a factor. Onions are a great remedy for hayfever. Onion soup is good for a cold and will cure a hangover.

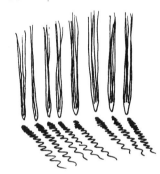

Peppermint (*Mentha piperita*) herb is used as a tea and infusion for coughs and colds. If you have a cold with fever and feel hot, this will cool you down. Peppermint contains menthol and is cooling. Peppermint oil is a common ingredient in many over-the-counter cold remedies. Mrs. Leyel states that Peppermint "is a remedy for the nose especially when the tip is sore to the touch."

Pine (many species) needles are an excellent remedy for a runny nose. Pine needle tea will totally clear a runny nose but should not be taken for more than 3 days. Tired or debilitated patients with respiratory problems are often cured by regular walks in a Pine forest. The fragrance is healing and balsamic. Pine needles infusion is a good addition to any bath to wake you up, and it helps a cold or lung congestion.

Pomegranate (*Punica granatum*) seeds are a delicious food, and the rind of the fruit is used as a remedy for tapeworm. It is very astringent, and the tea of the rind can be snuffed to stop a bleeding nose.

Ragwort *(Senecio jacobæa)* herb is a powerful allergen. So as "like cures like," it is used in tincture to cure allergic asthma or for hayfever.

Shepherd's Purse *(Capsella bursa-pastoris)* herb is used as tea and the juice is snuffed to cure a bloody nose.

Squills *(Urginea scilla)* bulbs are used as tea or tincture. They act as a diuretic and to cure constant sneezing. Now known as *Drimia maritima.*

Star Anise *(Illicium verum)* seeds are lovely and fragrant and used as tea. It mixes well with many other herbs. An infusion is taken for serious inflammation of the nose and bronchi and helps with reducing the mucus.

Thuja *(Thuja occidentalis)* leaves are used in tea or tincture for chronic runny nose or as an external application for scabies or lice. The oil is used on warts. Thuja is also a homeopathic remedy for warts.

Yarrow *(Achillea millefolium)* leaves and flowers are used as tea and snuffed for a bloody nose. The effect is astringent and should be taken in small doses every 30 minutes.

There are other herbs in the materia medica of Chinese herbalism as well as Ayurvedic herbs and treatments that would help to improve the sense of smell. The herbs listed are all good herbs to be taken consistently to improve the ability to distinguish odors and to heal the respiratory system. Besides the nutriceutical foods such as Onions, Garlic, Chilé Peppers, Asparagus, and Nasturtium and Mustard flowers, drink your *Sense of Smell Tea* every day. Go outside every day and smell everything. Open up your nostrils and let the nasal cilia quiver with the joy of new-found scent, describe what you smell, smell all the essential oils that you can get your hands on—teach yourself to appreciate the 10,000 odors that exist.

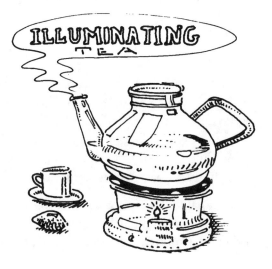

TABLE 9

A good tea mixture is . . .

Tea to Improve the Sense of Smell

1 ounce each of Star Anise, Melilot, Peppermint,
Orange Peel—all cut and sifted
½ ounce each of Cloves, Ginger, Cinnamon—ground
Pinch of Cayenne powder (Chilé Pepper)

Mix the dried herbs together. Store in a light-proof container. Use 1 Tablespoon mixed herbs per large cup of boiling water. Steep at least 5 minutes. Strain and drink daily, savoring the taste and inhaling the fragrant aroma.

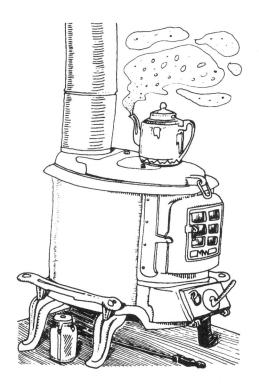

Note: Source for plants, names and correct spelling: D. J. Mabberley. *The Plant Book*. Cambridge: Cambridge University Press, 1989.

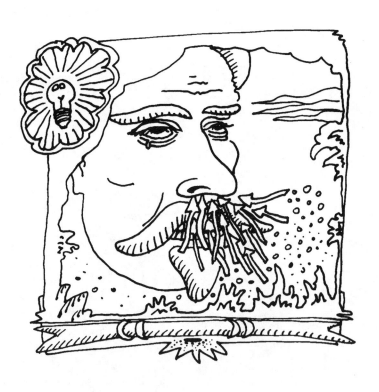

Chapter V

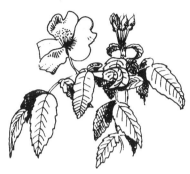

How to Do It!

Foggy Summer
> *Gray daze*
> *Foghorn blues a note*
> *Cobweb tightrobe holding a recalcitrant fly*
> *Fragrance of Lavender and Rosemary lifting up to incense the sky*
> *Prickly Rosebush catches and gently holds my hair.*
> *Moist, wet steps leading to a private place.*

—Jeanne Rose, 1991

Aromatics & Equipment

Do you want to get started using the essential oils? All you really need is a small enamel saucepan, some water and some Olive oil, and of course, a collection of essential oils.

Start with the simplest, most useful oils such as Rose oil, Rosemary oil, Peppermint oil, Tea Tree oil, Lemon oil, Eucalyptus oil, Lavender oil, Sandalwood oil, Juniper oil and Rose Geranium oil. With these basic ten, you can do just about anything.

With a pot and water, you can make an inhalation. With your palm, some Olive oil and a few drops of your oil blend, you can heal just about anything. Use Chapter I to find out what particular oil you can use for the problem that you are having, read about the oil in Chapter III, find out where to buy your oils in the source list of Chapter VI.

And then just do it. There really are no secrets to using the oils—just use them. Inhale their fragrance and you will find out just how they affect you mentally. Use them therapeutically for any problem that comes up.

When you get a bit of expertise you may wish to purchase some more sophisticated equipment such as the

AromaLamp or
Aroma Diffusor

The AromaLamp is a pottery shell enclosing a light bulb or hollow space with a little cup on top. You put water and essential oil into the cup and burn a candle below it, or plug in the light bulb. The heat from the candle or light warms up the water, the essential oil volatizes into your atmosphere, and you inhale the scent to affect you mentally or physically.

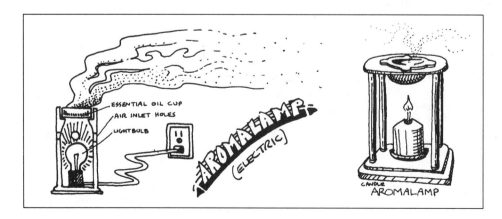

To use more advanced equipment, purchase a diffusor. This wonderful and rather newish apparatus is an ingenious device that breaks down essential oils into a micromist that disperses into a room to create a clean and healing environment. It works like a vaporizer but is cleaner and safer to use.

Someone asked me recently if the oil in the diffusor would harm furniture. My answer is, if you are worried then place a saucer or placemat under the diffusor in case of leaks or spills. Since essential oils are so concentrated and since some of them do act as solvents, it is possible that continued contact of oil dropping on a piece of furniture might do some damage. But I have used several different kinds of diffusors over the last ten years or so and have yet to damage any furniture—although I have melted a rubber stopper or two.

There are many kinds of diffusors available: hand-held ones that you can use traveling, complicated glass diffusors with exotic-looking nebulizers, simple diffusors that make a lot of noise, diffusors that you can hook up to timers so that they go on and off at intervals. Simply write to several sources in the Aromatherapy Source List in Chapter VI and look at the pictures. They all work quite well. The finest diffusor—the one that is the most quiet and works most efficiently—is Biorégène, available from a California source. However, it costs about $150.00. This diffusor is expensive. But I have used others that cost as little as $30.00. So shop around before you buy.

The Art of Distillation

Essential oils are obtained from plant material by steam or steam and water distillation. Distillation in its simplest form is the process of driving off gas or vapor from liquids or solids by heating the liquid and then condensing the vapor. Essential oil distillation from plants begins by collecting the plants, whether it is the flowers (Ylang-Ylang), flowering tops (Lavender), rhizomes (Ginger), seeds (Anise), bark (Cinnamon) or fruit (Nutmeg); preparing them by drying, crushing or breaking in order to break up the glands that contain the essence of the plant; heating the plant part over water or having steam forced through the plant, which further breaks open the oil glands, releasing the volatile essential oil as a vapor; then cooling the vapor and collecting it.

Warm air holds more moisture than cold air, and so the air above the plant and liquid is heated as well as the liquid itself. The art of distillation is in knowing the exact time to collect the plant in order to have the maximum amount of the essential oil available, and knowing as well how much heat to apply and how long to keep the plant on the still. Some plants such as Dill (*Anethum graveolens*) produce different components in their oil depending on distillation time.* After one hour on the still, the Dill distillate contains mainly carvone (about 90%) and 10% limonene, while after six hours the limonene steadily increases and the distillate will be about 35% limonene and the rest carvone. Studies such as these are only now regularly being made, and in the years to come much more knowledge will be gained regarding the appropriate time needed to obtain essential oils with desired qualities.

The goal of distillation is to extract from the plant the maximum amount of essential oil. To do this we take plant and water and heat them in a closed container. The liquid in the leaves vaporizes, taking along with it the essential oil; this is collected as a condensate, which is water and the plant's essential oil floating on top. The essential oil is then removed in some manner.

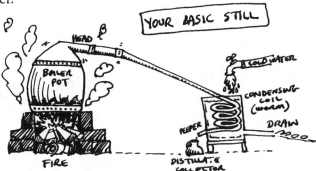

There are many kinds of stills. One of the simplest is the solar box still invented by the Egyptians. A flat bowl is placed in a tight box with a slant-

---

*"The Influence of Some Distillation Conditions on Essential Oil Composition," by A. Koedam in Volume 7 of *Aromatic Plants, Basic and Applied Aspects*. 1982: Martinus Nüyhof Publishers.

ed glass lid; this is set in the hot sun. Desert heat vaporizes the liquid, the vapors rise and collect on the inside of the cool glass, and as more moisture collects, droplets form and run down inside the glass into a trough. The Egyptians did this with their beer and by the end of the day, the distillate was a potent high-content alcohol. Several types of home stills are described here but for a fascinating account of distillation and its home use please read Secrets of the Still by Grace Firth, EPM Publications, Box 490, McLean, VA 22101. This book unfortunately is out of print but you may find it available in your local library. It is a wonderfully written and personalized account of the art of distillation.

How to Make a Home Still

Do you want to distill your own hydrosols? It is not expensive or difficult or dangerous. A simple teapot still can be made at home.

Get a copper tea kettle and a length of rubber or plastic tubing from the hardware store. Fill the teapot loosely with herbs or flowers. Rosemary is a good one to start with because the herb is available pretty much the year around. This teapot is called the *cucurbit*. If you have very smooth, very clean stones they should be placed in the bottom of the cucurbit to keep the plant material off the bottom surface.

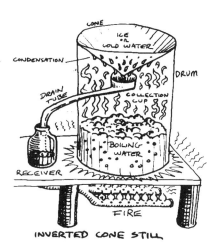

INVERTED CONE STILL

Add enough water to cover the botanicals. Use clean spring water, distilled water or deionized water. Attach enough rubber tubing to the teapot spout so that the center part of the tube can rest in a pan of ice water and then go on to empty into a small bowl. The small bowl is called the *receiver*. The receiver should be kept cool and so should be about 1–2 feet away from the cucurbit. Ideally the tube that rests in the ice water should be level with the top of the cucurbit, and the receiv-

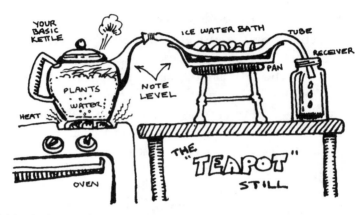

er should be below. Why, you ask? Steam rises, breaking open the cell structure of the plant and releasing the essential oil that goes through the tube, condensing in the tube where it rests in the cold water, and then dropping into the receiver, where the essential oil and water separate.

Bring the teapot to a boil and then turn the fire to low and simmer until at least half of the water has boiled off, vaporized into steam, and condensed into droplets in the ice water bath, which then collect in the receiver. This is your Flower Water or hydrosol (water solution) of Rosemary (that is, if you started with Rosemary herb). You can separate the essential oil from the water but why bother? Use the liquid as a facial spray, or to heal wounds. Lavender flower water would be excellent for this. If your hydrosol does not smell strong enough, just add a few drops of essential oil of whatever herb you started with. Since Lemon Balm is so easy to use, wouldn't it be nice if you made your own Melissa water . . .

A Simple Sand Still

Sand stills are perfect for desert terrain. The same principle operates here but Mother Nature and feminine Sun supplies the energy. A medium-sized container can serve as the cucurbit, attached by a length of *glass or metal tubing* to a receiver. Glass and metal are preferable to rubber or plastic because glass or metal will heat up in the hot sun and assist in the process of distillation.

174

The cucurbit is filled with the botanical materials, and water is added to cover them. The cucurbit is set on the surface of the ground in the hot sun. The receiver is buried in the desert sand, at least 1 to 2 feet deep. Cucurbit and receiver are attached by the tube. As the sun heats the cucurbit, the liquid evaporates and moves up the tubing and then down into the buried receptacle. When it reaches the buried receptacle, it is condensed again into liquid by the cool underground environment. And this liquid contains the vital essence of the herbs and flowers that was in the cucurbit.

A full day in the sun should suffice, and at dusk, as your still sits cooling in the shadow of the day, you can dig up your liquid buried treasure.

In both these stills it is very important to have a water-tight seal between the cucurbit and the tube, and sand-tight between tube and receiver.

A Country Still

Fragrant oils are often produced on the surface of plants, on their leaves and flowers. Rosemary is one of these, as is Lavender. There are others. Take a large, fat, clear wine bottle. Hang freshly cut flowering stems of either of these two plants upside down in the bottle. Place where the warmth and heat of the sun can shine on the bottle for at least eight hours. Check the bottle daily. Within a few days oil and water from the now-wilted branches will have collected by condensation in the bottom of the bottle. Two things to remember: have a tight seal at the top and start with a very clean bottle.

I wonder if the simple Country Still would be good for the extraction of Rose fragrance and water?

Distillations from the rose *are especially efficacious. Milto suffered a hideous tumour. She offered to Venus the flowers of her garden. The goddess appeared to her in a dream and prescribed the distilled waters of Roses to heal the tumour and return her beauty . . .*

175

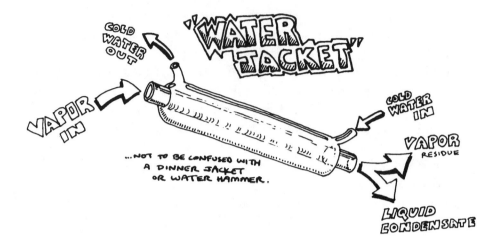

The Aromatherapy Treatment Kit is a very handy way to learn to use aromatherapy without a lot of study or expense. The kit contains a number of preblended essential oil mixtures and a wonderful chart describing their usage. John Steele and Avraham Sand have graciously allowed me to reproduce the chart in this book as well as their introduction to it.

Aromatherapy Treatment Kit

by John Steele of Lifetree and Avraham Sand of Tiferet*

The inspiration for developing this kit is our awareness of the growing need for a more complete and systematic method of aromatherapy treatment that is highly effective and ready-to-use. Aromatherapy is the ancient art of the therapeutic and cosmetic use of the earth's botanical medicines — in the extracted form of essential oils — for health and well-being. Essential oils are the highly concentrated aromatic substances found in many wild or cultivated plants, present in tiny droplets in the leaf, flower, seed, wood, root or resin. They are extracted primarily by steam distillation or mechanical pressure. The oils are thought of as being the life-force or "soul" of the plant, containing all of its special properties including characteristic fragrance and therapeutic effects.

---

*John Steele, Lifetree Aromatix, 3949 Longridge Avenue, Sherman Oaks, CA 91423; 818/986-0594; and Avraham Sand, Tiferet International, 210 Crest Drive, Eugene, OR 97405; phone 503/344-7019.

Essential oils can be used in massage, bath and inhalations to treat a broad spectrum of conditions including physical, mental and psychosomatic stress problems. This natural healing approach can help to remedy most common ailments, and combines very well with most other forms of holistic practice.

By placing carefully formulated blends and complete information into the hands of the practitioner or interested layperson, we are confident that a beneficial treatment can most often be effected. Use of the Aromatherapy Treatment Kit will allow a health practitioner to begin using Aromatherapy immediately; with progressive treatment experience the therapist will get "hands-on" training; and with supplementary reading and a course of technical study, one can in due time become a professional aromatherapist.

Ongoing formulation adjustments are welcome and subject to feedback from your treatment experience. For this purpose and for your own benefit as well, we ask that you *keep records of your treatments noting observations and results.* Special Treatment Report forms have been designed and can be requested from us at the address listed. Send us copies of your reports for product discounts (please inquire), and keep original records for future reference in your treatment work. In general, we encourage and support an interactive process of co-operative future development in all aspects of the kit. Your comments and suggestions are most helpful and greatly appreciated.

How to Use the Kit

The kit contains twelve treatment blends that consist entirely of 100% pure essential oils of high therapeutic quality. The products are full strength; no carrier has been added to extend the oils. The blends are designed for use in massage, bath and inhalation treatments. Specific treatment information is provided in the **Treatment Chart** [next pages].

It cannot be overemphasized that background knowledge is indispensable in achieving greatest success in treatments. As much as possible, read up on the subjects of aromatherapy, massage technique, and reflexology. In addition, complete courses in aromatherapy practice are available, including correspondence courses. [See *The Aromatherapy Book*, Chapter VI.]

Evaluating a client's condition accurately and completely before treatment is obviously paramount to attaining beneficial results. Reliable diagnostic methods must be studied and mastered, taking into account the mental and emotional condition of your client as well as physical symptoms. The primary focus of aromatherapy is to treat the *whole person* and the actual causes of imbalance while strengthening the affected muscles and organs involved. Techniques for diagnosis should include a complete consultation with your client, a thorough examination, and preferably the use of acquired skills such as reflexology, iridology, or applied kinesiology (muscle testing).

Contra-Indications

Before beginning any treatment, always check the Treatment Chart for possible contra-indications. These are conditions where treatment with any particular blend could prove harmful to your client and should be avoided. This includes all forms of treatment: inhalation, bath or massage.

Be especially careful in treating pregnant women. Most of the blends should not be used during pregnancy, either because they involve a risk of miscarriage, or they may be toxic to the fœtus. We can provide these Contra-Indicated Blends safely adjusted for pregnancy (although slightly less effective) as a special service.

Also be careful in cases of highly sensitive skin, asthma or epilepsy. Some essential oils can cause uncomfortable irritation to sensitive skin; others can provoke an unwanted reaction in those who suffer from asthma or are prone to epileptic attack.

Always keep essential oils away from the eyes, and be especially mindful of this whenever you do a face massage. Should essential oil get into the eye, wipe gently with a drop of olive oil on a clean tissue.

Do not take these or any other essential oils internally, unless you are under the guidance of a professional aromatherapist. Internal use can be one of the more hazardous ways of using essential oils, and is a method seldom used by many professional aromatherapists.

Keep in mind that every person is biologically unique, and will respond somewhat differently to the same blend. Attentively note your client's response to the blend you have selected *both before and during* the treatment. Never use or continue with a blend that is not well received. In such situations where for any reason the originally selected blend would not be usable, see the Chart under "Secondary Uses" for a possible alternative. Most of the blends have additional applications for which they are also quite effective. This may lead to the choice of a much better blend for the treatment.

Different blends can also at times be combined very effectively in treatment. For example, one blend might be chosen for bath and another for a follow-up massage. We have indicated on the Chart which blends might optimally be combined. You may also come up with other combinations that work well. Be creative.

Whenever possible, it is more effective to combine the different methods of treatment. Baths may be done before but preferably not right after a massage: the oils applied in the rub absorb slowly through the skin and will continue to provide benefit for several hours, as long as they are not partly washed off in a bath or shower. An exception can be made in the case of an acute problem, such as muscular pain. You may first apply massage oil to the affected area before getting in the bath; then massage the area again

Inhalations, when indicated, can be done at any time and will often be valuable during sleep. Herbal teas after a treatment can be a very rewarding therapy, and Bach Flower remedies are also an excellent complement to aromatherapy practice. After some experience in designing treatments your intuition will help to guide you.

Keep your blends fresh by leaving the bottles tightly capped and away from excessive heat or cold. Store away from children.

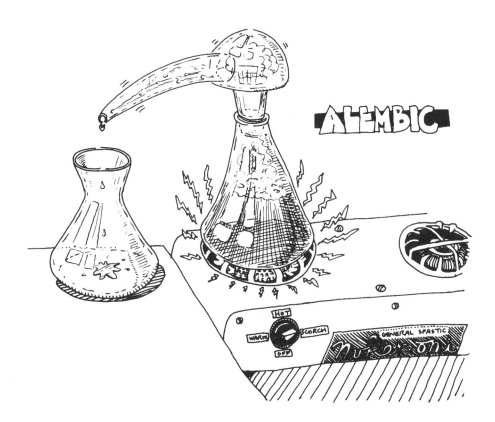

ALEMBIC

Tiferet–Lifetree Aromatherapy Treatment Chart

Blend #	Blend	TREATMENT				Contra-Indications
		Primary Uses	Inhalation	Bath	Massage 3%=10 drops in 15 ml 6%=7 drops in 5 ml 6%=7 drops in 5 ml	
1	Everyday Balancer	General balancer of nervous system. Treats low blood pressure.	5–10 drops	6–8 drops	Full Body @ 3%	Pregnancy; epilepsy; sensitive skin
2	Relaxing	Relaxation of nervous system: treats stress, tension, anxiety, depression, insomnia	5–10 drops	6–8 drops	Full body or face @ 3% or 6%	Use low concentration with pregnancy, sensitive skin
3	Pain Reliever	Treats muscular pain, cramp, strain, and sprain. Treats muscular tension, especially neck and shoulder		6–8 drops	Full body @ 3%, or locally @ 6–9% for severe pain	Pregnancy; Use low concentration with epilepsy, sensitive skin
4	Deep Joint Reliever	Treats arthritic and rheumatic pain in joints. Lubricates joints, helps repair damaged tissue.		6–8 drops	Full body @ 3%, or locally @ 6–9% for severe pain	Pregnancy; Use low concentration with epilepsy, sensitive skin
5	Headache/Migraine	Treats headache and migraine conditions. Treats tension and stress.	5–10 drops	6–8 drops	Locally @ 3–9% on forehead, temples, back of neck, shoulders; Full body @ 3%	Pregnancy
6	Respiratory	Treats a broad spectrum of conditions, including congestion, cough, cold, bronchitis, sore throat and sinus.	5–10 drops	6–8 drops	Locally on back and chest @ 3–9%	Pregnancy; Use low concentration with allergies, asthma and epilepsy
7	Digestive	Digestive disturbance, upset stomach, constipation, sluggish digestion, gas, lack of appetite.	5–10 drops	6–8 drops	Locally over stomach @ 6–9%; full or part body @ 3–6%	Epilepsy
8	Moon Time	Treats menstrual cramps and lower back pain. Helps to regulate menstrual cycle and excessive bleeding.		6–8 drops	Full body or locally @ 3%	Pregnancy; Use low concentration with sensitive skin
9	Invigorating	Stimulating. Treats low energy and fatigue.	5–10 drops	6–8 drops	Full or part body @ 3–9%	Pregnancy; Use low concentration with epilepsy, sensitive skin
10	Circulation	Lymphatic drainage for sluggish blood.		6–8 drops	Full body @ 3%, or locally @ 3–9%	Sensitive skin
11	Cellulite	Reduces and eliminates water retention.		6–8 drops	Full body @ 3–6%, or locally @ 3–9%	Pregnancy, epilepsy
12	Dry Skin	Treats dry skin conditions, sunburn and eczema.		6–8 drops	Full body or locally @ 3%	Low concentration with pregnancy; 1–2% on arms, legs and face

Secondary Uses	Supplementary Treatment with Blend #	Composition	Notes
Calming; period problems	**3, 4, 5, 7, 8**	Geranium, Melissa, Lavender, Hyssop	A general purpose Blend that can also be used as a Perfume.
Headache; period problems; skin treatment; balancer	**1, 5, 8**	Lavender, Ylang Ylang, Melissa, Bergamot	Can be used as a Perfume.
Rheumatic and arthritic pain; headache; invigorating	**1, 2, 4, 8**	Coriander, Ginger, Juniper, Lemongrass, Rosemary, Birch, Blue Chamomile	Can also be used in a compress.
Muscular pain; headache; invigorating	**1, 2, 3, 8**	Pine, Benzoin, Ginger, Cypress, Rosemary, Juniper, Oregano, Blue Chamomile, Birch	Can also be used in a compress. In cases of acute pain, use locally @ 9%.
Pain reliever	**1, 2, 3, 7, 8, 10**	Lavender, Marjoram, Aniseed, Niaouli, Peppermint, Basil	Eases constricted blood vessels.
Asthma; headache/ migraine; pain reliever	**2, 3, 5, 10**	Pine, Frankencense, Myrrh, Lavender, Hyssop, Bergamot, Eucalyptus, Peppermint, Myrtle, Lemon, Thyme, Clove	After Massage, a Hot Compress can reinforce the treatment.
Pain reliever; invigorating	**1, 2, 5, 10**	Tarragon, Coriander, Spearmint, Fennel, Ginger, Roman Chamomile	After Massage, a Hot Compress can amplifythe treatment.
Circulation; anti-depressant	**1, 2, 3, 5**	Melissa, Ylang Ylang, Rose, Geranium, Clary Sage, Blue Chamomile, Mugwort	For treating a delayed period, massage lower back.
Circulation	**1, 2, 12**	Petitgrain, Lavender, Benzoin, Rosemary, Thyme, Nutmeg, Basil	Stimulates "Sympathetic Response" System.
Headache; water retention; invigorating; period problems; balancer	**5, 6, 11**	Grapefruit, Lemon, Geranium, Cypress, Lemongrass, Black Pepper	Most effective with a Lymphatic Tissue Massage. Great for that plugged-up, toxic feeling.
Circulation; invigorating; pain reliever	**8, 9, 10**	Fennel, Mandarin, Juniper, Lavender, Cypress, Grapefruit, Rosemary	Use for PMS water retention. Also good for deep connective tissue work (use a lotion base).
Skin irritation; calming	**1, 2, 3, 5, 7, 8**	Palmarosa, Lavender, Rose, Sandalwood, Roman Chamomile, Frankencense	Can be used as a Perfume. For best results add 400 IU Vitamin E to the Massage oil.

Enfleurage at Home

Enfleurage is the elegant, old-fashioned method of extracting the scent from thick-petaled flowers such as Roses, Jasmine, Tuberose, Honeysuckle, Iris, Ylang-Ylang and others. It is a cold process that generally yields a superior result. It is done indoors.

Buy some ridged glass from a glass or window company. You will need several sheets that are about 2 feet by 2 feet. Clean them carefully and with a spatula spread on the fat. You can use Crisco, clean goose fat, carefully rendered beef fat or even solid Coconut oil, although this latter is not recommended. I have also used Jojoba oil (wax) solidified with beeswax. Spread the fat on the sheets of glass and then add just-picked flowers that have been picked at their appropriate time—Jasmine at night and Roses in the morning, for example. Completely cover the sheets of 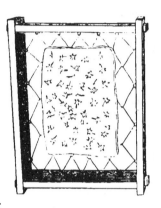 fat-covered glass with flowers. Stack two pieces of glass together, fat side to fat side, and leave for up to 36 hours. (Leave them until the flowers are descented. This depends on the warmth and wetness or dryness of the weather.) Keep the sheets in a warm, dry place. At the end of the time needed, carefully remove the flowers. Repeat the process several times, adding new flowers until the fat is completely scent-saturated. (The flowers that you have removed from the fat can then be soaked in alcohol to make a flower tincture or cologne. The alcohol removes the scent from the fat that is still on the flowers and it can be separated.)

When the fat is completely scent-saturated, it is then scraped off the glass sheets, placed in a clean glass container and pure 95% alcohol is added. Over a period of several weeks, the alcohol will absorb the scent from the fat. The alcohol is then separated from the fat and filtered.

Some points to remember:

(1) Don't throw anything out. Each step of the process leaves some of the flower scent behind.

(2) Cleanliness in this case is next to scentual godliness. Keep your hands, the glass, containers, technique—anything that you use—clean.

(3) The spent flowers can be used as a compress or soaked in alcohol and then strained out to make a lightly scented aftershave or cologne. You can also add water to the alcohol to reduce proof.

Enfleurage is easy but it does take some practice to get it just right. Every season is different, so it does no good to give you exact quantities of flowers or fat or alcohol to use.

How to Extract a Scent
& When Is the Proper Time to Apply Scent

There are many methods to "get" the scent out of a plant and these have been detailed in several books including my own Herbal Body Book and Kitchen Cosmetics. But one method that I have used to great effect was described by that great English herbalist, Mrs. C. F. Leyel, as follows:

Fill a large jar three-quarters full of good-quality Olive oil. Fill the jar up with the flowers of the Jasmine and any other sweet-smelling flowers (a nice time to extract the muscle-healing scent of the Wall-flowers). Small flowers should be chosen, and they should all be stripped of their stalks and leaves to make room for as many flowers as possible. Leave them to macerate (*to steep or soak* with warmth, in this case, sun or heat) for 24 hours. Then pour the contents of the entire jar into a black bag (or jelly bag) and squeeze the oil from it into another jar, to which more flowers must be added and the process repeated for twenty days, according to the strength of the scent required. Then the oil must be mixed with an equal quantity of strong, deodorized alcohol, and the mixture must be shaken every day for a fortnight. By that time the spirit should be highly scented, and it can be poured off, looking clear and bright.*

The Magic of Herbs, A Modern Book of Secrets by Mrs. C. F. Leyel, Jonathan Cape, London, England, MCMXXVI.

I should add to this recipe that the Olive oil should be the best Italian quality that you can obtain; California Olive oil will not do, it's too "green"

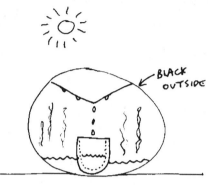

EMERGENCY SOLAR STILL

smelling. If you want your end result to be one flower scent then you must start and finish with the same flower since this recipe yields a perfume rather than an extract or infused oil. The alcohol should also be the kind that you can drink if you intend to take this flower oil therapeutically as well as using it externally in massage or as a perfume. You can start with good quality vodka or get pharmaceutical-grade alcohol to blend with the essential oils extracted.

In most states pure alcohol is available through laboratories—check your Yellow Pages. It costs about $8.00 + $30 per gallon which includes federal taxes. Also, some states sell what is called "spring water" and this is often pure alcohol. If you do take your oils internally for medicinal purpose, realize that the end result is a highly concentrated product representing an enormous amount of flowers and should be taken rather like the Bach flower remedies, that is, only a *few drops* of the tinctured oils in a bit of water.

There is an art to the extraction of scent from flowers. This art is probably much older than distillation, evidence of which has been found in ancient sites. Distillation through a solar still or something like it is thousands of years old, scent extraction at least 10,000 years old. Distillation is generally used for the green herbs, but home extraction methods will yield a good quality of tinctured or infused oil of flowers if care is taken.

When to Apply Scent or Essential Oils for Therapeutic Value

The lung time is 3–5 A.M. according to Worsley and this is indeed the best time to use aromas as therapy for therapeutic or healing purposes. If this seems a little early for you, remember that morning time is better than any other time for aroma-massage or therapy.

Other proper times for applications or inhalations of essential oil as therapy for particular parts of the body are as follows:

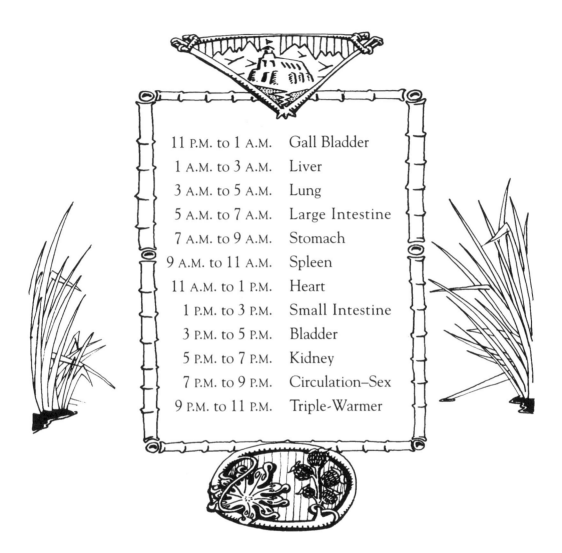

11 P.M. to 1 A.M.	Gall Bladder
1 A.M. to 3 A.M.	Liver
3 A.M. to 5 A.M.	Lung
5 A.M. to 7 A.M.	Large Intestine
7 A.M. to 9 A.M.	Stomach
9 A.M. to 11 A.M.	Spleen
11 A.M. to 1 P.M.	Heart
1 P.M. to 3 P.M.	Small Intestine
3 P.M. to 5 P.M.	Bladder
5 P.M. to 7 P.M.	Kidney
7 P.M. to 9 P.M.	Circulation–Sex
9 P.M. to 11 P.M.	Triple-Warmer

Aromatherapy Massage

Massage is very appropriate to use and to aid in the absorption of essential oils through the skin of the body. The deep thumb pressures of shiatsu; the pressure of deep tissue massage that is intended to reach nerves, ligaments, tendons; the soft tissue work called Swedish massage; and the slow, gentle, rhythmic movements of effleurage massage that are so appropriate for pets, infants and the infirm—all are used in aromatherapy massage. The total

185

effect should be harmonious, and not jar in any way. England has many schools that teach various methods of aromatherapy massage, and by reading the books of the English authors you can learn their techniques. However, some massage is counterproductive if used with oils, such as a massage to help ease the discomforts of menopause or hot flashes. In this case the simple application of essential oils mixed with cold water and sprayed on the face or body is a better method. Use your common sense when applying, or massaging in, or ingesting of essential oils.

Deep tissue massage should be done gently rather than vigorously. Swedish massage should be consistent and deep enough to affect the soft tissues but not so vigorous that it is painful. The purpose of aromatherapy massage is to aid in the penetration of the oil, to stimulate the body to relax, to treat local problems, to soften and diminish scar tissue, to stimulate nerve supply, and to treat via reflex or meridian.

Get a chart showing the spinal nerve roots and you will notice that there are five distinct sets of vertebrae. Have a friend massage along the indentation that occurs on either side of the spine. If you are a beginner, just rub gently up and down this spinal gutter in small circular motions using the thumbs. Massage to loosen up the area, then apply essential oils or infused oil and massage again. Specific oils can be used on specific nerve roots to affect specific organs. Certain general oils can be applied along the entire body for a relaxing, stimulating, sedating or uplifting effect. See Chapter I for a list of the specific oils.

General Oil Qualities (Refer to Table 1)

Rose Geranium oil is especially useful along the cervical vertebrae and affects the skin. Bergamot-infused oil is good along the entire dorsal vertebrae, as this oil has an antispasmodic effect on all the internal organs. Fennel oil is useful along the upper lumbar vertebrae, as it causes the intestine, especially the large intestine, to release trapped gas and in general acts as a tonic. Jasmine oil is very relaxing for the entire body and especially useful along the lumbar vertebrae over the 1st chakra—it can act to release certain sexual tensions. A massage using oil of Rose is generally balancing, useful to improve meditation, and works from the 7th around to the 1st chakra ↺. Peppermint-infused oil is stimulating to the entire body and especially useful along the cervical vertebrae to reduce brain fatigue or headache.

Specific Oil Qualities for Massage

Basil oil extracted from the herb is especially useful for respiratory difficulties such as bronchitis, and can be mixed with Hyssop and *Ammi visnaga* oils. Basil oil acts as an antispasmodic and expectorant. It is useful for nervous tension and headache. A useful mixture to detoxify the nose to *relieve stuffy sinus* is to mix

> 1 part Juniper Berry oil
> 2 parts Eucalyptus oil
> 2 parts Basil oil

Add 12–15 drops of this mixture to the well of a hot vaporizer and allow the warm moist air to flow in an enclosed room. Eucalyptus oil has an antisep-

---

Specific Oil Mixtures to Use in Massage Therapy

Acne • Bergamot oil, Lavender oil and Sandalwood oil

Allergies • Chamomile oil, Mullein oil, *Ammi visnaga* oil

Asthma • Eucalyptus oil, Marjoram oil, Lavender oil

Colds or **Bronchitis** • Basil oil, Eucalyptus oil, Lavender oil, Rosemary oil

Earache • Mullein-infused oil, Black Pepper oil, Rosemary Verbenon oil, Tea Tree oil

Fevers • *that make you hot and sweaty:* Peppermint oil

Fevers • *that make you chilled and cold:* Cinnamon oil

Headache • Moroccan Jasmine oil, Rosemary hydrosol

Hysteria • Basil oil, Clary Sage oil, Chamomile oil, Marjoram oil, Neroli oil, Jasmine oil, Rose oil

Mental Exhaustion • Peppermint oil, Rosemary oil, Basil oil

Obesity • Fennel oil, Juniper oil, Patchouli oil, Lemon oil

Rejuvenation • Rose oil, Melissa oil, Neroli oil, Jasmine oil, Frankincense oil, Patchouli oil

Skin Care • Lavender oil, Chamomile oil, Rose Geranium oil

Painful Cramps in Pregnancy • Carnation-infused oil, Wallflower oil

---

tic, deodorant, expectorant effect and works especially well on the respiratory system to relieve thick mucous secretions and fevers. These three oils work well together.

Fennel oil is useful for any sort of digestive disturbance or flatulence. It is also an excellent diuretic and helps to heal the bladder and clear the urine. A good way to take the oil is to place a drop or two of it in a half glass of water and drink in the morning before breakfast. Add the juice of half a Lemon. This is very effective against the queasiness of morning sickness or for a stumbling "hangover." Juniper Berry oil acts on the skin, digestion, urinary tract, the blood, and the nerves. Along with Sandalwood oil it is one of the classic diuretics and remedies for urinary tract infections.

Use Chapter I, Table 1 and Table 2. These comprise a fabulous reference guide to essential oil use.

Please check the columns in Chapter I of this book for skin care as well as Chapter 1 of Jeanne Rose's *Herbal Body Book*.

This is an extremely brief description of aromatherapy massage and how to use it. The use of the aromata is just one part of the path that leads to total health and beauty. Remember that good nutrition, exercise, clean water and clean air form the rest of the prescription.

Ivan Popov puts the prescription to good health in another way in his book *Stay Young*. He says that a long and happy life involves the following:

(1) have a happy marital and sexual situation;

(2) there should not be a great abundance of food eaten;

(3) clean fresh air, clean fresh water, and clean fresh natural food should be consumed; and

(4) food should emphasize fresh fruits and vegetables and the fermented stuffs such as sauerkraut, kefir, yogurt, etc., and it should deemphasize meat.

Remember that your essential oils need to be *natural* to be effective. That is, they must actually be extracted from a plant material. Synthetic oils are simply not acceptable.

Keep Smiling!

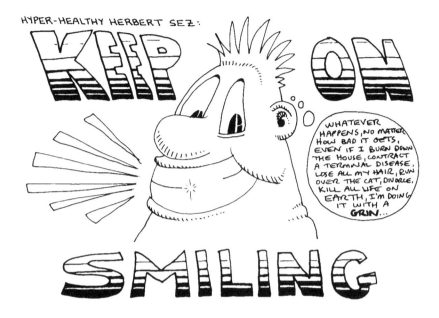

Essential Oil Path to Treat Mind and Body

The chart that follows has been partially explained in the preceding Tables 6 and 7. Here you will see the entire picture of the way essential oils affect the mind through inhalation and the body through inhalation and application.

Essential oils are applied to the skin as a liquid or by the inhalation of their vaporized molecules. When inhaled via the mouth the vapors are absorbed by the blood vessels in the lungs and proceed into the bloodstream. When inhaled through the nose the vapors are absorbed through the olfactory nerves and affect the limbic system, which is composed of cortex, temporal lobe, thalamus and hypothalamus (the home of the memory, drives and expression). From the limbic system in the brain, memory and emotion are affected as well as the intellectual processes and the cortex. Here the hypothalamus, which is responsible for the integration of many basic mechanisms and behavioral patterns that involve correlation of neural and endocrine function, absorbs the tiny molecules of oil. The hypothalamus appears to be the single most important control area for the regulation of the human internal environment.* It is the location of short-and long-term

---

* *Human Physiology* by Vander, Sherman and Luciano. McGraw Hill, 1970.

memory and the inhalation of essential oils stimulates this area and this is why we say that *scent is the most memoristic of the senses*. The hypothalamus also has an effect on aggression control, and affects the pituitary and adrenal glands. Via the pituitary the sexual glands are affected, which is why scent can be an aphrodisiac. Excretion of the essential oils is via the endocrine glands and exhaled air.

When essential oils are applied to the skin, they are absorbed by muscle tissue and blood vessels. The circulatory system goes throughout the body and the small molecules affect all aspects of the body—the joints, the digestive process, all tissues and organs—and are excreted via the skin, kidneys, bladder and lungs.

It is easy to see why essential oils can have such an important part in all aspects of human health and well-being.

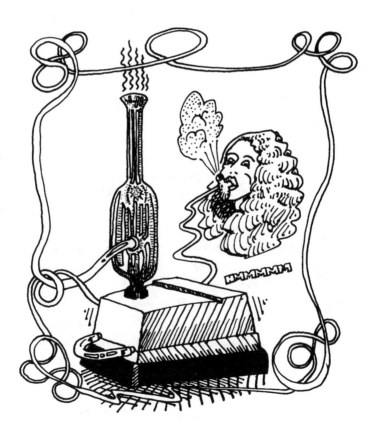

Table 10
Essential Oil Path to Treat Mind and Body*

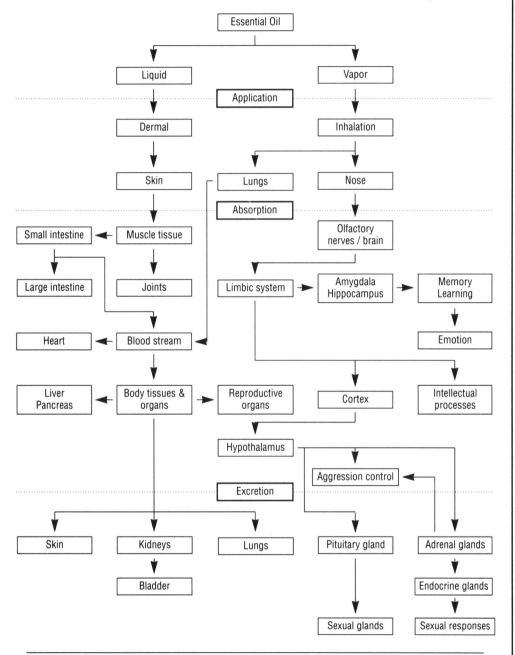

*From *Aromatherapy: To Heal And Tend The Body* by Robert Tisserand. Reproduced with permission.

Chapter VI

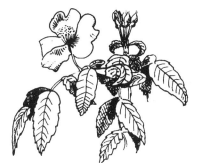

Source List

Where to Buy the Best Essential Oils, Aromatics and Fabulous Products
Where to Get Information
Journals & Schools*

AT = Aromatherapy
EO = Essential Oil
PEO = Pure Essential Oil
Ste AT/JR = Reference Code

Where to Get Information

The first thing that we should talk about in this chapter is how to get information. Many companies will send you information and a catalog based on a simple request written on a postcard, but because of the increasing cost of postage and the desire to not waste paper and printing, many companies require that you send them an SASE. Remember these initials because SASE means Self-Addressed Stamped Envelope. These initials occur over and over again in herbal literature and advertising. And should you write to any of the people named in this chapter, they often get bushels of letters daily and will answer first and sometimes only the letters that include an SASE.

---

* See end of chapter

There are many, many outlets for essential oil (EO) products and for pure essential oils (PEO), and many businesses that advertise "the best," the "purest," the "most fabulous true essential oils," but in my search for the truth among these many claims I found out that one's sense of smell and the depth of the pocketbook was the only reliable way to determine quality. Good smell? Probably a good oil. Expensive price? Probably but not necessarily a determinant. Many growers supply a few distilleries that sell to as few as half-dozen source distributors that furnish dozens of wholesalers who in turn supply the retail trade and then on to the consumer. All the oils that are now available in the United States come from the same few original sources.

I called the president of a major supplier of essential oils, a wholesale supplier of fine-quality product in Bloomfield, New Jersey, and asked him about these many claims to quality. His response was very enlightening regarding the dynamics of getting essential oils from field to consumer: "Take for instance, Citronella oil—a few growers in a particular province in China grow this plant. Then along comes the representative of the factory where the plant will be steam-distilled for its oil. The factory representative negotiates with the farmer and buys the entire harvest. There may only be one distillation factory where the many different farmers and their Citronella crop will go. From the still it goes to the government representative who allots or sells the oil to wholesalers all over the world. So even though there were many farms, probably with different growing conditions, the finished oil comes from only one or two stills. And this is what we all [the distributors] sell. Price differences come from being able to buy in quantity and then passing this savings on to the wholesaler, who then prices the oils accordingly."

It seemed to me also that this explanation might negate the big sell of the so-called chemotype oils. Many responsible people have very definite ideas about the value of chemotype oils.

Chemotypes are particular plants all identical with the parent plant because they are produced by cloning rather than from seed. But a chemotype from one year's planting may be dramatically different from another year's planting due to adverse weather or varying soil conditions or time left on the still. An essential oil that is sold at a very high price because it is considered a chemotype of a particular plant will probably not be identical in its type and the quantity of components (in the resulting essential-oil content from one field to another or one year's product to another year's). These oils should be treated just like fine wines which are identified and labeled accordingly by chemotype, variety, county and particular vineyard, as well as the year the plant was grown, processed and bottled. I feel that if you are going to pay a premium for an essential oil that is labeled as a particular chemotype, then it too should be fully labeled accordingly. All this should appear on a high-priced chemotype oil to justify the price: genus, species, variety, chemotype, county, country, planting area or farm, year harvested and bottled. My advice is to buy good quality oil from a reliable wholesaler who is willing to disclose source.

Most of the major sources are listed in this directory. Use mail-order as most stores cannot carry or will not carry fine quality oils for your most cherished cosmetic or magical usage. *Synthetic oils will not work* as either a healing or a ritual ingredient in a product. Synthetic oils may smell up a potpourri or make a candle smell strongly—and they are even used in perfume; but if you want to tap into the healing quality and the nourishing vitality of oils, or plants for that matter, then you must use *pure essential oils* (PEO) that are actually distilled from the plant after which they are named. Do not be misled by wordy advertising. Rosemary oil that costs $10.00/ounce is probably identical to that sold for $5.00 or even $2.00/ounce. Be an educated consumer. Educate your nose by smelling and even tasting the oils. Synthetic oils often smell that way—synthetic. Pure essential Rose oil smells like sitting in a room filled with Roses, while synthetic rose smells rather soapy and "curls your nose."

When you wish to purchase fine aromatherapy (AT) cosmetics or essential oils (EO or PEO) for making your own products, please check this directory. Send postcards or letters to the companies that interest you and ask for a catalog. Do not forget to include any charges for the catalog and where you found their name. If you are writing to a person, enclose an SASE. Unfortunately, people move and businesses close. If the postcard is returned try using the Yellow Pages of your phone directory or call information to secure the phone number or for an updated listing. Use the Yellow Pages. They really work. I am always amazed at how seldom people use this wonderful phone service. When you receive a few catalogs, compare prices. Buy a small sample of the same oil from several different stores. Compare the color, compare the price, compare the scent of the oils. Once you have determined who is selling a good quality oil then buy oils based only on price differences. There is one company that I know of that buys oils from Europe and then inflates the price hundreds of times by telling customers they are buying something that they can get nowhere else. The poor deluded saps buy!

This person is making a fortune on the gullibility of consumers who are entranced with anything European. The consumers still live in small rental houses and the European has been able to purchase a home in one of the most exclusive sections of the United States.

You can buy fine-quality cosmetics and cosmetic ingredients from many different places. I have been amazed and pleased at the number of stores and mail-order houses that sell truly wonderful AT products. Before I researched this section I thought that I would find maybe a dozen companies that sold quality AT goods. I have been pleasantly surprised that I have found ethical companies, in every state and many countries, that produce quality AT goods. Knowing your source is the best education that a consumer can have. And the sources are listed here. I personally have tried the products that are individually named and have also sent many of the products out to "testers" who have rated them based on certain criteria. Following is one of our sample test sheets so that you can see how we rated and scored many of the products.

To find products, use this directory or first find sources as listed in the Yellow Pages of your phone directory, or look in the catalog section of the many herbal journals that are now printed.

General Headings in your directory or phone Yellow Pages:

    Aromatherapy
    Botanicals
    Cosmetics
    Cosmetic Ingredients
    Essential Oils
    Health Food Stores
    Herbs
    Nature or Natural Ingredients
    Oils
    Perfumes
    Pharmacies, Natural or Homeopathic
    Sachets
    Soaps
    Spices

Use a sample cosmetic test sheet. You may copy the one following or make up your own to test products.

Sample Test
on available aromatherapy (cosmetic) products

Number of Sample _____

Type of Sample _____

Actual Name of Sample _____

Producing Company or Manufacturer _____

_____

_____

_____ Phone number _____

Feel _____

Smell _____

Texture _____

Color _____

Action _____

Personal Opinion _____ Tester's name _____

Any Other Information You Feel Is Important _____

_____

_____

_____

_____

pH if available _____

Wt. or Size Available _____

Cost _____

Number of Uses _____

Packaging _____

Fine quality cosmetics and pure essential oils (PEO) that I have tried include products from the following listed companies. Some products that I tried are not listed because quality was poor, or the so-called essential oils were diluted, or the advertising was deceptive or incorrect in nature. Please note that people go in and out of business constantly and we have found that this is about 10% of companies per year. It pays to send request post cards. And it pays to make your own products for really fresh aromatherapy care.

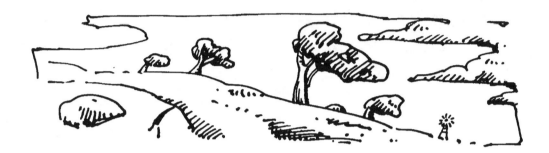

Nationally

There are several companies that once were small specialty essential oil and product companies but have since grown to such a size that they are now nationally distributed throughout malls and department stores across the country. This includes companies such as AromaVera, Aura Cacia, now owned by Frontier Company, Aveda, Bath and BodyWorks, Bare Escentuals, Origins, Tisserand Aromatherapy and The Body Shop which has a few AT products. These companies have some nice products and generally good essential oils. Check them out in stores.

Arizona

Janca's Jojoba Oil and Seed Co., Ste AT/JR • 456 Juanita #7, Mesa, AZ 85204. No charge for catalog. A long list of essential oils and vegetable oils and some cosmetic products. This is a good source for jojoba oils and various vegetable butters.

Lotions & Potions, Ste AT/JR • 422 S. Mill Avenue, Tempe, AZ 85281. 200 essential oils, natural vegetable oils, massage oils and assorted bath products.

Windrose Aromatics, Ste AT/JR • 12629 N. Tatum Blvd., Suite 611, Phoenix, AZ 85032. No charge for the mail-order catalog. Complete line of essential oils, aromatic body-care and accessories as well as literature. Custom blends available with special terms for aroma practitioners. I particularly like Composure, a combination of Geranium, Ylang-Ylang and Patchouli, which is calming with antidepressant qualities.

California

Abracadabra, Ste AT/JR • 10365 Highway 116, Forestville, CA 95436. This is a wonderful company with many product lines including botanical mineral bath salt mixtures that are scented with both synthetic oils and pure essential oils. If you want only PEO in your bath salts, order their simple bath salt mixture unscented and then scent it yourself for you and your customers. I especially like Abracadabra's "Wintergreen Sport Therapy™ Bath." They have a new product line called Earth & Body Care. A portion of all sales from this line goes to save endangered species. This is wholesale only, no retail except in your favorite stores. Write and ask for a price list and a sample or two.

Acme Vial and Glass Co., Ste AT/JR • 1601 Commerce Way, Paso Robles, CA 93446. 805/239-2666. Now carries blue and green glass. For more description, see page 229. Tell them Jeanne Rose sent you.

Archangel Herbs, Ste AT/JR • P. O. Box 778, Boyes Hot Springs, CA 95416. Patricia Dunn-Serota has invented and perfected a wonderful new way to make and apply massage "oils." She calls them "Annointments" and they are semi-solid salves made from organically grown herbs, AT oils and flower essences. I have been massaged with her Annointments™ and have been very pleased. The texture and fragrance is harmonious. I particularly like "Italian Lemon" which smelled like an Italian Lemon Ice. And yes, she has a brochure and it's free.

Aromatherapy Chart, 219 Carl Street, San Francisco, CA 94117. A unique full-color chart listing color, aroma and sound healing attributes and corresponding them for use. This is a wonderful and beautiful chart. $13.50 includes shipping charges. Wholesale available, prepay $6.60, minimum 10. Add $2.00 for every ten charts for shipping.

Body Love, Ste AT/AA • P. O. Box 7542, Santa Cruz, CA 95061. A wonderful line of bath and body products. Our favorites are the Aroma Bath Beads and the Aroma Lotion. All products are very well formulated. The owner of this company has said that she was inspired by Jeanne Rose's work, especially *The Herbal Body Book.* She also carries Love Mits for Shower, Goddess Blends and the Fragrant Farmacy - 12 beautiful EO with droppers. Elizabeth Jones is teaching AT classes in the Santa Cruz area.

Dry Creek Herb Farm, Ste AT/JR • 13935 Dry Creek Road, Auburn, CA 95603. Offers several formulations using wild-crafted and organically grown herbs and made by hand in tune with natural cycles. Shatoiya's Eye Kare looked interesting. Classes also!

Elements Aromatherapy, Ste AT/JR • 1415 Abbott Kinney Blvd. #144, Venice, CA 90291. Carries a collection of aromatic oils for bath and body, AromaLamps from Aromaland, misters, EO and a product line of EO blends that harmonize in the five elements.

Energy Essentials, Ste AT/JR • P.O. Box 470785, San Francisco, CA 94123. Carries over 100 different EOs primarily for the small manufacturer.

Essential Aromatics, Ste AT/JR • 205 North Signal St., Ojai, CA 93023. Julia Meadows does AT Massage and while analyzing you she will test 12–15 essential oils. This essence testing results in a personal oil blend that the client uses thereafter. She has wonderful products, fabulously scented candles and wonderful lotions and does AT counseling and teaching.

Essentiel Elements, Ste AT/JR • 2039 Green Street, San Francisco, CA 94123. Wonderful AT mineral salts for the bath. The mixtures of mineral salts are deeply drenched with PEO to create a product that is both pleasant to use and healing. I use them with a bit of food coloring in the water. Blue for Rosemary and yellow for Citrus.

Feather River Co., Ste AT/JR • 133 Copeland, Petaluma, CA 94952. Distributes 150 lines of cruelty-free body-care products including many herbal lines and AT products. "In the west, this one's best." I personally have used hundreds of products that appear on their list. My favorites? Seaweed Bath (thank goddess it is non-foaming); Paul Penders St. John's Day Cream; Bath Therapy from Para Labs; Sport Therapy from Abracadabra; Air Therapy Orange Spray for refreshing and purifying the air; Alexandra Avery's Day Cream and perfumes; Weleda Rose Petal Day Cream; Olba's Bath from Penn Herb; Sea Kelp Scrub from Rachel Perry; the Radius toothbrush; and my 18-year-old son is crazy about Tom's Peppermint Baking Soda toothpaste. I like the simpleness of the Home Health products (most of which could just as easily be made at home). Remember Feather River is a wholesale distributor only and their catalog is free to all retail stores. First order is about $100.00 minimum. If you have a retail store, this distributor is one of the best.

Flower Essence Services, Ste AT/JR • P. O. Box 1769, Nevada City, CA 95959. Free catalog. Flower essences, hand-crafted herbals, EO literature and oils, AromaLamps, classes and field trips. I loved the Self-Heal Flower Essence Skin Creme—it has a rich fragrance, sharp and sweet as young innocence. The herbal oils I have found to be particularly fine, and I especially liked the St. John's Wort Flower Oil and Calendula Flower Oil for use on children. These herbal oils are useful as carrier oils for essential oils in massage and on the skin. The Bergamot EO seemed of especially good quality.

H2B, Ste AT/JR • 610 22nd Street, Suite 247, San Francisco, CA 94107. Wonderful eye pillows. Send for their catalog.

Herbal BodyWorks, Ste AT/JR • 219 Carl Street, San Francisco, CA 94117. This company went into business in 1965 as NewAge Creations, primarily as a clothier making organically designed 100% pure cotton, wool, linen and silk garments for the Rock and Roll stars of the '60s. By 1968 the business had evolved into 100% pure "the only real organic, body-care & natural cosmetics on the market. Absolutely pure, natural herbs and oils. NO synthetic scents, NO . . . chemical preservative, NO additives . . . Beautiful cosmetics gathered from the earth and good enough to eat" [from an original catalog of products dated September 1973]. The same is true to this day, although the number of products has been greatly reduced.

Also, a new line of "perfect body-care and for complete ritual" products called Ritual Works! has been introduced. Each type of product comes in each of the seven colors of the spectrum and have been made with correlating PEO aromas.

Bruise Juice is one of the original products, a medicinal oil that is still being made in the old-fashioned healthful way using organically

201

grown herbs and enhanced with therapeutic quality PEO. This product is a formula dating from 1650 and reduces bruising, heals insect bites and plant rashes. Also this company was the first to make AT and color therapy coordinated products, massage oils and potpourris. $2.50 for catalog.

Herbal Studies & Aromatherapy Course/Jeanne Rose (same address as Herbal BodyWorks). Where the BodyWorks is run by employees, the Herbal Studies Course is Jeanne Rose. 2800 pages of instruction that includes 5 texts. All homework and questions are personally answered by Jeanne. Includes 200 pages of AT work (more than some courses at $400). Includes *All Things Herbal*. Seventy percent of graduates are already working in various herbal fields. $2.50 for gift and brochure.

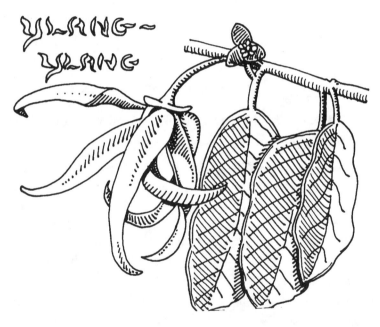

Herb Products, Ste AT/JR • 11012 Magnolia Blvd., North Hollywood, CA 91601. So what can you say about a company that has been in the same location with the same friendly staff for 20 years or so. And with the same high-quality merchandise—always with reasonable prices. They sell everything herbal, herbs, oils and other items. This is a wonderful company, always ethical, and always with new products. No price for the mail-order catalog. Get it and see!

Jeanne Rose Aromatherapy, *Aromatic Consultant and Creator of "Scents and the Psyche™" and "Aromatherapy: A Demonstration for the Senses," The Healing Power of Essential Oils.* Inquire at 219 Carl Street, San Francisco, CA 94117. This is a demonstration that shows the magic and the effective aromatic connections that can be made with events and feelings long ago experienced. Jeanne Rose can choose the correct scent for your home, your business, your hotel or just for you. A small and exquisite product line of rare essential oils at extremely reasonable prices as well as First Aid Kits, each containing four essential oils named First Aid Kit; for Minor Emergencies, Women's Kit, Stress Relief, and Meditation.

Joseph Mack, Ste AT/JR• c/o Pacific Demand, Inc., 531 Howard Street, San Francisco, CA 94105. This is the oldest Dwarf Pine distillery in the world. Their product line includes EOs, medicinal bath additives, embrocations, and an inhalator that will help you economize your essential oils.

Karl Lee Design, Ste AT/JR • Partington Ridge, Big Sur, CA 93920. Phone 408-667-2492. Producer of high-quality hand-distilled EO primarily of wild-crafted origin, spagyric oils and tinctures, consultation and distillation classes. Specialist in azulene-producing plants.

Lavender Lane, Ste AT/JR • 6715 Donerail Drive, Sacramento, CA 95842. A quality line of hard to find herbal ware and glass ware.

Leydet Oils, Ste AT/JR • P. O. Box 2354, Fair Oaks, CA 95628. Victoria Edwards, founding member of the American Aromatherapy Association, owns this company. She produces wonderful custom blends including all sorts of fine facial products, and she also teaches terrific classes and gives seminars. She is importing her own oils and bottles from Europe that finally give aromatherapy enthusiasts a choice different from the "same old oils" we've known so far. So if you want to try some really fine-quality therapeutic PEO and not the same average quality stuff everybody else sells, write to Leydet for a catalog and enclose $2.00.

Lifetree Aromatix, Ste AT/JR • 3949 Longridge Avenue, Sherman Oaks, CA 91423. Mail-order only. $2.50 for catalog. John Steele is an aromatic consultant and he makes a truly dandy, handy AT Treatment Kit. It costs about $175.00 but contains everything you need to treat mind and body both externally and internally. I highly recommend this beau-

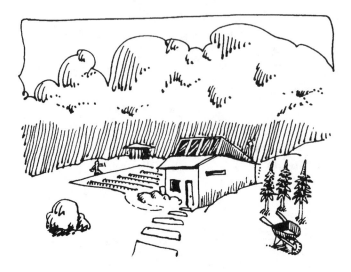

tiful product. The blends allow a beginner to practice AT massage without a lot of study regarding the properties and uses of each oil and without a lot of expense buying oils. This will give the beginner or home
user plenty of time to learn while using aromatherapy.

Medicineflower, Ste AT/JR • 3026 Azahar Court, Carlsbad, CA 92009.
Carries Egyptian perfume bottles for EO and oils.

Mountain Rose Herbs, Ste AT/JR • P.O. Box 2000 Redway, CA 95560. No
charge for the mail-order catalog that lists herbs, books, oils and bottles to package your own products and original medicinal tea blends.

Nature's Herb Company, Ste AT/JR • 1010 46th Street, Emeryville, CA
94608. Now owned by Barry Meltzer since its esteemed former owner
Nathan Podhurst passed away, the company has been moved to
Emeryville from San Francisco. We all miss Nathan and Emma here in
SF but Emma is still at Nature's Herb Company and if you phone she will
send you a free mail-order catalog. The parent company is San Francisco Herb & Natural Food. Retail and wholesale bulk herbs, teas, spices,
essential oils, tinctures, extracts, etc.

Oak Valley Herb Farm, Ste AT/JR • 14648 Pear Tree Lane, Nevada City,
CA 95959. Send $1.00 for mail-order catalog. AT body-care products and
oils. Literature regarding herbal use and AT usage. Kathi Keville is owner and also edits the American Herb Association quarterly newsletter.

Oceans of Lotions, Ste AT/JR • 842 Cole Street at Carl, San Francisco, CA 94117. Cruelty-free, natural cosmetics, perfumes, hair accessories, fine soaps, massage oils and more. Step in and look around.

Of The Jungle, Ste AT/JR • Box 1801, Sebastapol, CA 95473. A family owned business dedicated to the preservation and propagation of favourite beneficial plants and botanical products that are not listed in any other catalogs. They also carry an herbal blend called the Cosmic Caffeinator, made up of all known species containing xanthine components "a cup a day is all you need!"

Original Swiss Aromatics, Ste AT/JR • P. O. Box 606, San Rafael, CA 94915. Mail-order only. Sells a very exclusive line of good PEO oils and products and a diffusor that works better than any other I have tried. Asthmatics should know that they carry *Ammi visnaga* oil. Kurt Schnaubelt is one of our better teachers, see page 230.

The Oshadi Collection, Ste AT/JR • 15 Monarch Bay Plaza, Suite 346, Monarch Beach, CA 92629. A good quality line of PEO distilled from the wild, organic biodynamic, and from carefully selected plants. Also, a wide variety of very nice products.

Palmetto, Ste AT/JR • 1034 Montana Ave, Santa Monica, CA 90403. Head to toe natural skin and bodycare products. Very strong on AT. Carries a full line of PEOs from several producers plus books and blends.

Prima Fleur Botanicals, Ste AT/JR • P.O. Box 3471, San Rafael, CA 94912. Suppliers of high quality EO for manufacturers of AT products. Many of the oils are wildcrafted and/or organic. They work directly with distillers to ensure quality and supply. Carries some oils found nowhere else. Write for their complete catalog. Say JR sent you!

Quan Yin, Ste AT/JR • P.O. Box 2092, Healdsburg, CA 95448. Carries an interesting selection of products including Aroma Pillows, Aroma Lockets, fabulous bath treatments, massage oils, etc. They also do private parties featuring personalized EO blends!

Sunburst Bottle Co., Ste AT/JR • 7001 Sunburst Way, Citrus Heights, CA 95621. Hard to find bottleware for all you wonderful EO blends.

Thursday's Plantation, Inc., Ste AT/JR • P.O. Box 5613, Montecito, CA 93150. 1-800-848-8966. Sells all grades of Tea Tree oil from bath use to therapeutic quality. Will also supply copies of scientific documents and certification papers if you request.

Time Laboratories, Ste AT/JR. P.O. Box 3243, South Pasadena, CA 91031. Owned by Ann Marie Buhler. This is a respected company that has been in business for over 30 years. The EOs are guaranteed to be 100% pure and natural. They also offer custom manufacturing and product development.

Vitae, Ste AT/JR • 576 Searls Ave. Nevada City, CA 95959. An esoteric line of blended essential oils.

Vital Essence, Ste AT/JR • P.O. Box 956 Topanga, CA 90290. Carries EO, AT kits, a skin and hair care line.

Whole Herb Co., Ste AT/JR • 8th Street East, Sonoma, CA 95476. Wholesale EO and herbs. Wonderful selection of potpourri ingredients.

Zia Cosmetics, Ste AT/JR • 300 Brannan Street, Suite 601, San Francisco, CA 94107. Zia is the author of six good books on skin care. Her line of botanically based skin care products includes a nice selection of aromatherapy treatments and products. Zia also publishes the newslatter *Great Face*, in which she examines the pros and cons of new skin care products and treatments.

Colorado

Breh Laboratories, Ste AT/JR • Box 18116, Boulder, CO 80308. They make a number of botanical sea bath creations using AT, herbal therapy, and thalassotherapy (therapy using seawater or in this case sea salts). The sea crystals are from an ancient unpolluted sea bed. The testers especially liked Respiratory Rescue.

Herbal Reign, Ste AT/JR • Sunshine Mesa Ranch, Box 900, Hotchkiss, CO 81419. Many years ago I received a gorgeously designed box in the mail that contained a truly elegant mixture of bath potpourri herbs. These bath herbs came to be sold in many elegant shops but as with most pioneers, Kathryn McCarthy was years ahead of the times. Hers is one of the few companies that has given recognition to the fact that she has read a Jeanne Rose book and given credit publicly to the knowledge that she gained and put this fact on the label. But she took the concept of bath herbs to a new refinement. Her mixtures and packaging are first rate. Unfortunately, not enough people recognize quality when they see it and Herbal Reign went out of business for a while. But now with the resurgence of AT and the use of herbs and EO for body care, Kathryn's company has come back and will again supply us with her wonderful products. Write to Herbal Reign and she will send you a brochure.

Quintessence Aromatherapy Inc., Ste AT/JR • P. O. Box 4996, Boulder, CO 80306. Carries a number of EO and various blends including crystal chakra blends. Teaches seminars and a correspondence course.

Resources, Ste AT/JR • 1445 Balsam Ave., Boulder, CO 80304. AT consultations, massage blends, classes and workshops taught by Laraine Kyle.

Connecticut

Herban Lifestyles, Ste AT/JR • 84 Carpenter Road, New Hartford, CT 06057. A wonderful newsletter with a regular aromatherapy column. Edited by Christine Utterback, this is worth subscribing to. $18.00/year.

Judith Jackson, Ste AT/JR • 10 Serenity Lane, Cos Cob, CT 06807. Author of Scentual Touch, has a wonderful line of facial and body products. She is a licensed massage therapist. All of her blends are slightly fragranced and perfect for massage use.

Delaware

Sandy Hollow Herb Company, Ste AT/JR • 1717 Delaware Avenue, Wilmington, DE 19806. The complete herbal resource center. Spices, herbs, botanicals, extracts, EO, Dr. Haushka and Weleda products, and culinary blends. Classes and workshops are offered.

Florida

Essential Products, Ste AT/JR • No. 5018 N. Hubert Ave., Tampa, FL 33625. I was confused when I first looked at the price list until I realized they carry two lines of oils: the first is a very fine, high-quality therapeutic type. One would only use this type if interested in serious healing potentials for application, ingestion or deep inhalation. The second line is also of high quality and is used for massage, or for fine products and perfume. I was able to examine several of the oils and thought all were quite distinctively special, including *Ammi visnaga,* which smelled fresh and pure (in comparison with other brands I have checked). Write for information.

EuroHealth & Beauty, Inc., Ste AT/JR • 4981 SW 74th Court, Miami, FL 33155. Wonderful products, Moortherapy, Phyto-Aromatherapy, Thalassotherapy, Algotherapy and a quiet diffusor as well as diffusor blends. Carries Remy Laure products.

Rumors, Ste AT/JR • 16018 Saddle String Drive, Tampa, FL 33618. Sylla Hanger offers aromatics, a full-service salon, and her oils are of truly excellent quality from the Essential Oil Cooperative. $2.00 for the mail-order catalog.

Hawaii

Alexandra Avery, Ste AT/JR • 42 Palione Place, Kailua, HI 96734. Formulator of Purely Natural Body Care, licensed aesthetician. In addition to her Aromatherapy Facial practice called Facial Pleasures, she combines Jungian-based psychotherapy with aromatherapy consultation, a delightful harmony of mind and body relaxation and rejuvenation. Heaven meets earth at the one-week Aromatherapy Treatment Retreat she offers at her beach home. Write for details. Alexandra has recently published a book, *Aromatherapy and You: A Guide to Natural Skin Care.*

Hawaiian Islands School of Massage, Ste AT/JR • P.O. Box 390188, Kailua-Kona, HI 96739. Essential oil blends in unique formulations for therapeutic effects. Large quantities of Almond, canola and essential oils available. Week-long certification courses in Aromatherapy held in Hawaii every January. No charge for the catalog.

HeartScents, Ste AT/JR • Box 1614, Hilo, HI 96720. Take an enchanting and refreshing break from the real world with a visit to the "home of heartscents." Special recipes for pampering and in addition to products, owner Barbara Irwin will pamper you personally with a delightful, elegant foot-bath. $1.00 for catalog.

Idaho

The Peaceable Kingdom, Ste At.JR • 8375 Rapid Lightning Creek Road, Sand Point, ID 83864. This wonderful company is owned by Lois Wythe who produces a quarterly newsletter, sponsors herbal and AT workshops and sells herb things by mail.

Illinois

Fragrant Fields, Ste AT/JR • P.O. Box 160, Dongola, IL 62926. Herbal and dried flower wreaths, potpourri, essential oils, books, herbal gifts and plants. No charge for catalog.

Herb 'N' Renewal, Ste AT/JR • R.R. One, Laura, IL 61451. Carries a standard line of EO and a selected line of AT bodycare from many sources as well as books, herbs, herbal stationary and gift tags, and herbal and aromatic jewelry.

Sensory Essence, Ste AT/JR • P.O. Box 87, Island Lake, IL 60042. Jan Salco carries only very high quality Rose oil from Bulgaria that comes in a hand carved and painted wooden container.

"IRON STOMACH"

Indiana

Indiana Botanic Gardens, Ste AT/JR • P. O. Box 5, Hammond, IN 46325. This has always been one of my favorite herb stores. I have been doing mail-order business with them for 20 years and have never been disappointed. It really shocked me when I found out they had moved to Hobart—thankfully they have maintained a mail-order address in Hammond. They have a recipe for *real marshmallows* using Marshmallow root. Write for a free catalog and enjoy yourself—plenty of herbal reading to entertain you.

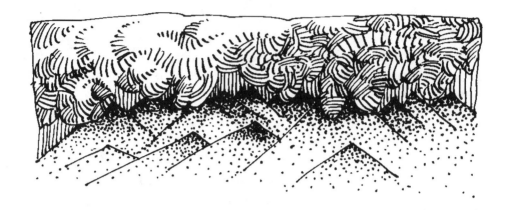

The Lebermuth Co., Ste AT/JR • P. O. Box 4103, South Bend, IN 46624. They are one of the world's largest distributors and direct importers of botanicals. They offer a large variety of EO, fragrances and flavors. Their prices are good.

Iowa

Amrita Quality of Life Products, Ste AT/JR • P. O. Box 2178, Fairfield, IA 52556. Carries a variety of products including the Biorégène Aromatic diffusor and skin-care line. Lovely products and excellent EO synergies.

The Herb & Spice Collection of Frontier Cooperative, Ste AT/JR • P. O. Box 118, Norway, IA 52318. Iowa means "a beautiful place" and I was pleasantly surprised at just how beautiful this land of rolling hills and lush growth truly is. Frontier offers a large stock of essential oils from many different distributors, herbs, spices, great herbal mixtures, and potpourris made with those unpleasantly colored wood chips and dried flowers. My testers noted that the Combination Skin–Steam Facial was clean, simple and real. And I very much like their quality selection of essential oils. This is an honest and reliable source of supply, and with the order will come reams of good information. No charge for the catalog.

Herbs-Liscious, Ste AT/JR • 1702 S. 6th Street, Marshalltown, IA 50158. Over 250 varieties of herb plants, dried herbs and potpourri. Offers an unusual service: locating and obtaining unusual or "difficult to find" herb plants, herb seeds and herb-related products for customers. Send them $1.00 for their catalog, refundable when you buy something.

Maryland

Phybiosis, Ste AT/JR • P.O. Box 992, Bowie, MD 20718. This is a new source of top quality EO at wholesale prices as well as wonderful healing clay distinguished by particular colors of green, red, yellow, pink, white. They also have a good quality diffusor and AT and herb products. Write for a catalog and tell them Jeanne Rose sent you.

Massachusetts

Blessed Herbs, Ste AT/JR • 109 Barre Plains Road, Oakham, MA 01068. Wildcrafted and organic herbs. This is one of the best! No charge for catalog.

Carol Corio Precious Jewel Box, Ste AT/JR • 460 Indian Camp Lane, Lincoln, MA 01773. A number of products not carried elsewhere such as a car diffusor and a lovely box to hold your precious essential oils.

Michigan

Herbal Endeavours, Ltd., Ste AT/JR • 3618 S. Emmons Avenue, Rochester Hills, MI 48307. Owned by Colleen K. Dodt. She has PEO, pure AT potpourri, custom blending, workshops and AT personalized gem essences. $2.00 for catalog.

Minnesota

The Business of Herbs, Ste AT/JR • Rt. 2, Box 246, Shevlin, MN 56676. A bi-monthly journal for the herb business and serious herb enthusiasts with news, views, growing and marketing hints, sources of materials and supplies, and much more. This is one of the best of the herb journals. Write for a free brochure. At this time subscriptions are $20/year.

Herb Gardeners Resource Guide, Ste AT/JR • Rt. 2, Box 246, Shevlin, MN 56676. Contains a wealth of information useful to anyone interested in herbs: unusual plants, international plant selection, heirloom seeds, accessories made of herbs, garden supplies, natural pest controls, body-care products, restaurants with an herbal ambience, botanical gardens and more. $8.50 for the guide.

Missouri

Cheryl's Herbs, Ste AT/JR • 11953 Meadow Run Court, Maryland Heights, MO 63143. Makes made-to-order shampoos with PEO. You need to fill out a form for them, listing your special conditions or problems. Also carries PEO blends for a variety of problems or situations. A very interesting catalog is yours by request.

The Herb Shoppe, Ste AT/JR • 111 Azalea, Duenweg, MO 64841. Offers many services. Carries over 700 jars of bulk items, oils, soaps and books. No charge for mail-order catalog.

Willow Rain Herbal Goods, Ste AT/JR • P. O. Box 5, Grubville, MO 63041. AT massage oils, aroma consulting for the body, PEO diluted by carrier oils, amulets, etc. A very ethical company. Free catalog.

Nevada

Libations by Loridonna, Ste AT/JR • 1050 Whitney Ranch Road, # 2021, Hendersen, NV 89014. PEO and wonderful bath blends and body oils containing EO. Write for free catalog.

New Hampshire

Baudelaire, Inc., Ste AT/JR • Forest Road, Marlow, NH 03456. *Once upon a time, there lived a monk who was an expert herbalist. His masterpiece was a blend of essential oils and herbal extracts . . .*
These products produced by Anton Hubner are imported by Baudelaire. My favorites are the therapeutic bath oils that include revitalizing Dwarf Pine, stimulating Horse Chestnut, and Thyme for congestion. The Hubner line of bath oils are 10 in number. Besides the Moor Bath and Kniepp bath oils, these are definitely my favorites for bathing therapy. What makes them stand out is their high percentage of PEO and their purity. Baudelaire also carries the Faith in Nature soaps from England and combination bath oils from C. A. Gregory

Aromatics Ltd which include Winterset to cheer you (the four oils are Juniper, Lavender, Eucalyptus, Geranium), and five other oil combinations. Send for a free catalog.

Internatural, Ste AT/JR • P. O. Box 680, South Sutton, NH 03273. Carries many different lines of personal care products and PEO. Free catalog.

New Jersey

Berjé, Ste AT/JR • 5 Lawrence Street, Bloomfield, NJ 07003. A wholesale only supplier of PEO. One of the best companies because they always openly and honestly discuss their oils and content. Call 201/748-8980 for wholesale information.

Ecco Bella, Ste AT/JR • 6 Provost Square, #602, Caldwell, NJ 07006. Many beneficial products for people and the environment. Carries several lines of skin care products and AT beauty oils for bath and massage. A wonderful free catalog with lots of goodies in it.

Elisabeth Woodburn, Ste AT/JR • Booknoll Farm, P.O. Box 39, Hopewell, NJ 08525. Years ago when I was first collecting my aromatherapy books and years before there were any books called aromatherapy, I wrote to Elisabeth for help and through the next few years was able to amass quite a library. She has recently passed away but her husband and a helper continue the business. They have a good comprehensive herb catalog/book catalog.

Louise Beebe Wilder wrote a wonderful book called *The Fragrant Path*, among other books, and I have Louise Wilder's personal copy (with bookplate) of *Myths and Legends of Flowers, Trees, Fruits, and Plants* by Charles M. Skinner. This is one of my most treasured books and I purchased it from Elisabeth. Thank you Elisabeth and I hope heaven is full of plenty and books.

New Mexico

AromaLand, Ste AT/JR • Route 20 Box 29, Santa Fe, NM 87505. EO, diffusing lamps, reference cards and more.

Native Scents, Ste AT/JR • Box 5763, Taos, NM 87571. This is AT in the spiritual way. The best ceremonial objects that are available by mail order. They carry Indian perfume sachet bags made with 100% natural herbs harvested in New Mexico, incense wands and wonderful smudge sticks as well as Sweetgrass braids and ceremonial Blue Corn. This company supports American Indian work. No charge for catalog.

Santa Fe Fragrance, Ste AT/JR • P. O. Box 282, Santa Fe, NM 87504. Christine Malcolm does much in the field of AT: consulting, fragrance blending, natural product development incorporating the use of PEO and absolutes, workshops and lectures, and olfactory perception. Her company also offers a line of natural botanically based skin care and AT products including the Ascent line of EO blends and bath oils, colognes and anoints. She sent me some samples of her products that my testers described as having superb quality and were a stand-out among the many items tested. I very much enjoyed sampling these products but became even more enthused one dreary afternoon when I put one of her blends into the diffusor. Shortly, the day turned bright and cheery and I walked around humming and singing. I can only describe the feeling as *joyous*. The actual name of the blend was "Meditation"; but I certainly did not feel like meditating— rather more appropriately I felt delighted and happy with my state of life. I strongly recommend that you write for this wonderful free mail-order catalog and ask for Jeanne Rose's favorite blend. Stock up on Santa Fe Fragrance's definitely wonderful products.

As an addendum, Christine says, "an essential oil contains the life force of the plant from which it comes and because they are organic, essential oils they tend to work in harmony with the body and give a sense of balance and well being."

New York

Aphrodisia, Ste AT/JR • 264 Bleeker Street, New York, NY 10014. A complete herb store which carries bulk herbs and spices, bath blends, EO, and synergy blends. No charge for mail-order catalog.

Enchantments, Ste AT/JR • 341 E. 9th Street, New York, NY 10003. A huge catalog (80 pages) of goddess items, books, herbs, jewelry, EO, candles, cards, ritual objects, classes, workshops and lectures. There is just lots and lots and lots of wonderful products and enchanting ritual goodies. This catalog just contains everything you ever thought that you wanted and best of all—the pure EO are carefully separated from the fragrance oils. $2.00 for mail-order catalog.

E-Scentially Yours, Ste AT/JR • 24 E. 38th Street, New York, NY 10016. PEO , AT blends, products, and herbal products as well as books and charts.

Essensa, Ste AT/JR • P.O. Box 450 Radio City Station, New York, NY 10101. Represents Potter's (Herbal Supplies) Ltd. in North America, and the wonderful Essensa line from England.

The Fragrance Foundation, Ste AT/JR • 145 East 32nd Street, New York, NY 10016. This honest, ethical organization located in the United States can give you reliable aroma-chology information regarding research. Also, you can order booklets and articles from a mail-order catalog listing publications. The executive director is Annette Green, the doyenne of aromatherapy information and the one who invented the word aroma-chology.

Industrial Aromatic, Ste AT/JR • 184 Furnace Dock Road, Peekskill, NY 10566. Wholesale only. Aroma speciality is artificial Civet. Sells many pure resins such as Balsam Peru and Tolu, as well as Labdanum, Mastic, Styrax, etc., and also essential oils of these. They have been in business for 67 years as manufacturers of natural raw materials. I have personally tried all of these balsams and resins and was very much impressed.

Kato, Ste AT/JR • One Bradford Road, Mt. Vernon, NY 10553. A direct source of oils for aromatherapy as well as blends and extracts.

Kiehls, Ste AT/JR • 109 Third Avenue, New York, NY 10003.
    A long-term supplier of PEO and body-care products. I remember the original owner and his men friends sitting in high-back chairs watching the customers. One time, years ago, this man had me picked up at the airport in a limousine and brought directly to Kiehls to look around. This is a long-time supplier of natural and synthetic essential oils, blends and body-care products. The variety of oils is immense and many of them can be used for effective AT treatments.

Kneipp Herbal Baths, Ste AT/JR • Available in many stores.

I have used all the Kneipp baths and they are one of the three companies that make a truly herbal bath using therapeutic amounts of essential oils. (The other two brands are Anton Hubner which is imported by Baudelaire in New Hampshire and C. A. Gregory Aromatics in England.) Father Sebastian Kneipp (1821–1897) was the founder of what has come to be known in Germany as Kneippism—a comprehensive system of water therapy with herbs. Father Kneipp studied the beneficial effects which water therapy and essential herbal oils have on coping with the stresses and strains of everyday living. The Kneipp botanical extracts are manufactured according to specific formulas and include baths of Hops, Rosemary, Meadow Blossom, Juniper, Spruce and Pine, Camomile, Lavender, Eucalyptus, Melissa and my latest favorite, the Linden and Orange Blossom Bath for calming and relaxing. The only negative aspect to these products is the artificial colors that are used to color the products.

Norimoor Company, Inc., Ste AT/JR • c/o La Maison Française, 5th Avenue, Box 5222, New York, NY 10185. The Moor Bath is a healing, therapeutic product made of peat from the Scottish moors. This ancient, dark-brown, condensed, compressed plant residue makes the bath water so dark you are unable to see any part of your body when submersed. It leaves no ring around the tub and the residue is easily rinsed away. Has great therapeutic benefits and should be used in a series of baths, taken at night before bedtime. I used six series of seven baths separated by five days between series to help heal a respiratory condition. I also used some essential oils to increase the efficacy of the baths. The Moor Bath is *very* relaxing and detoxifying and should only be taken in the evening before bed. Write or call for local distributors of this product, or they might sell direct. My testers loved the healing quality of these baths.

Sederma, Ste AT/JR • 7110 Fort Hamilton Parkway, Brooklyn, NY 11228. Wholesale plant extracts suitable for fine cosmetics. I have particularly enjoyed using the Wild Pansy and Horse Chestnut extracts among the many that have been incorporated into products.

Weleda, Inc., Ste AT/JR • P. O. Box 769, 841 S. Main Street, Spring Valley, NY 10977. For twenty years I have been writing glowing reports of this company. Weleda body-care products begin with purely grown plants wild-crafted or naturally grown with compost and companion planting, and proceed to quality products whose plant ingredients are chosen for their unique "personality" with consideration for the plant's beneficial properties. All products can be fully recommended with special mention to the baby-care line. The company began in 1924, the name suggested by Rudolf Steiner, meaning "the wise virgin" or the "much knowing one." No charge for the mail-order catalog.

North Carolina

Ch-Imports, Ltd., Ste AT/JR • P.O. Box 18411, Greensboro, NC 27419. Carries the complete line of Fleurom EO. Wholesale only.

Complete Body Shop, Ste AT/JR • P. O. Box 1324, Hamlet, NC 28345. The $2.00 cost for the catalog is refundable with first purchase. Susan Chavis sells original design, beautiful "Herbal Bouquet" T-shirts in 100% cotton and poly/cotton. She is also very involved in local environmental issues and her recycled paper catalog and cellulose packaging reflect this concern for the environment. Offers wonderful soaps, T-shirts and other body-care products.

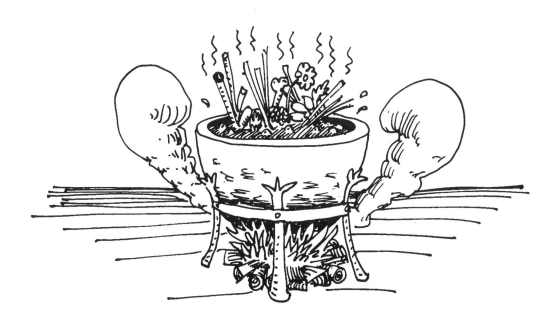

Rasland Farm/The Farm Shop, Ste AT/JR • NC 82 @ US 13, Godwin, NC 28344. Herb plants and all sorts of herbal supplies including wreaths and bouquets. Special gifts include Garlic braids and Apple stacks. The main purpose of their business is listed as education. $2.50 for mail-order catalog that also lists tours and the southeast Herb Fest.

Ohio

Barbara Bobo Soap, Ste AT/JR • 1920 Apple Road, St. Paris, OH 43072. Barbara makes the finest natural soaps using simple ingredients and pure essential oils. Try the soap named Jeanne Rose Seaweed Soap, Frankincense & Myrrh and Pacific Mist. My favorite for washing fine lingerie is called Windsor.

Oregon

Essence Aromatherapy, Ste AT/JR • 1760 West 34th Avenue, Eugene, OR 97405. A wonderful line of AT products using natural essential oils (PEO). I am particularly fond of the candles, which incorporate the finest principles of Aroma, Color, Crystal and Flower Essence to enhance particular emotions and feelings. A fabulous product to burn during rituals, as the fragrances are not so overpowering that one would feel asphyxiated. Susan Leigh is also an aromatic consultant and educator. These are products for Body/Mind/Spirit.

The Essential Oil Company, Ste AT/JR • P. O. Box 206, Lake Oswego, OR 97034. They clearly state which oils are pure and which are not. They also carry a few cosmetic ingredients such as Cocoa Butter and lanolin. No charge for catalog.

Lady of the Lake, Ste AT/JR • P.O. Box 7140, Brookings, OR 97415. EO bath products, AT blends. Mail-order catalog.

Liberty Natural Products, Ste AT/JR • P. O. Box 66068, Portland, OR 97266. A wholesale supplier of essential oils, both culinary and medicinal. Some body-care products including a wonderful breath freshener, TIBS (Toothpick In a Bottle). The prices are competitive.

Pacific Botanicals, Ste AT/JR • 4350 Fish Hatchery Road, Grants Pass, OR 97527. Organically grown herbs and spices sold both dried and fresh. No charge for the price sheet. A fine company.

Purely Natural Body Care, Ste AT/JR • 4717 SE Belmont Street, Portland, OR 97215. This is a nice collection of fine quality bodycare using PEO and clean ingredients. For more information see the listing for Alexandra Avery in Hawaii. Free catalog.

Tiferet International Aromatherapy, Ste AT/JR • 210 Crest Drive, Eugene, OR 97405. Avraham Sand is the owner. Many quality essential oil products, natural AT blends and treatment blends. I really liked the fact that Avraham clearly stated in his catalog that the rare AT oils such as Attar Rose and Jasmine could be purchased pure as well as diluted with carrier oils so that regular people can afford them. Who can afford $200 for a few drops of the precious Rose-Maroc? But you can afford precious oils if you buy from a reliable firm that lists the dilutant. Tiferet Rose-Maroc dilutes 1:4 in a fine-quality carrier oil for $20. My tester loved the Rose and commented on the golden yellow color and fine quality of the scent, not knowing it was diluted. We both liked the products. No charge for the catalog.

Pennsylvania

Celestine Gifts and Books, Ste AT/JR • 254 High Street, Pottsdown, PA 19464. Full line of fabulous essential oils, great books, candles, wonderful products, certified aromatherapy and herbal classes. Request a catalog or phone 610/970-8050.

3000 BC, Ltd., Ste AT/JR • 7946 Germantown Ave., Philadelphia, PA 19118. Owned and perated by Korin Korman, this is one of the most beautiful AT stores I have visited with a mesmerizing display of fabulous AT products from many different manufacturers. Write for her catalog.

Village Herb Shop, Ste AT/JR • Box 173, Blue Ball, PA 17506. Full line of herbs for cooking and fragrance. Essential oils and classes on growing and using herbs and herb-related gifts. No charge for catalog.

Rhode Island

Meadowbrook Herbs & Things, Ste AT/JR • Whispering Pines Road, Wyoming, RI 02898. Herbs, spices, essential oils, garden supplies and fine fragranced herbal cosmetics. Carries the full line of fine-quality Dr. Hauschka products for the body as well as Weleda Herb Products. I like the seasonal tonics by Wala.

Texas

Active Organics, Ste AT/JR • 11230 Grader St., Dallas, TX. Supplies active and aromatic herbal extracts to companies which wish to make herbal products. I have had experience using many of the extracts in cosmetic products and like them very much indeed. Probably wholesale only.

China Bayle's Thyme and Seasonings Herb Company, Ste AT/JR • Pecan Springs, TX. One of my testers attests to this shop. They carry a variety of products and seeds as well as all the books written by China Bayles.

Fredericksburg Herb Farm, Ste AT/JR • Mail-order address is: P. O. Drawer 927, Fredericksburg, TX 78624. This is the type of store and bed & breakfast that I wish had been available when I was younger and wilder. A beautiful store filled with exquisite herbal products and a bed & breakfast that is very elegant and comfy, with Sylvia's delicious herbal breakfasts that come in the morning. They also sponsor classes and lectures. If you are in the area do not pass this place by—besides this is Lyndon B. Johnson country which is incredibly beautiful. $1.00 for catalog

Vermont

Geremy Rose Fresh Cosmetics, Ste AT/JR • P. O. Box 1947, Brattleboro, VT 05301. I was delighted when I found these products. Now several years later I see them in every herbal products store. My cosmetic tester and I both noted that the products really looked and smelled like fresh fragrant Roses. We like the products enormously and feel that they are a truly good addition to any herbal product shelf. These are unique products with wonderful herbal extracts and essential oils. My favorite is the Creamy Rose Cleanser. Write and ask them for a price list and the distributor in your area.

Meadowsweet Herb Farm, Ste AT/JR • 729 Mount Holly Road, Shrewsbury, VT 05738. Wreaths, Cinnamon-stick centerpieces, old-fashioned hats with herbal sprays, tussie-mussies (nosegays that convey messages), herbal wedding bouquets, hundreds of varieties of herb plants, gift baskets, herbal hot pads, and essential oils. No charge for catalog.

Rathdowney, Ste AT/JR • 3 River Street, P. O. Box 357, Bethel VT 05032. They carry a full line of herbal products from the usual to the unusual. They have gift baskets for babies to pets. Lots of wonderful culinary herbal mixtures. This full-service herb/apothecary shop also has display gardens and herb walks. A very informative newsletter goes to those on the mailing list. No charge for the catalog.

Virginia

Tom deBaggio Nursery, Ste AT/JR • 923 N. Ivy Street, Arlington, VA 22201. Has an incredible selection of plants including many cultivars of Lavender and Lavandin. No mail order, but certainly worth a visit.

Washington

Elazar's Olive Oil Lamps, Ste AT/JR • Box 1384, Long View, WA 98632. I love his lamps! They are absolutely beautiful. They are an ancient way of obtaining heat and light through the use of olive oils as a high quality, clean burning fuel., The AT lamps are quite effective, and work very well to diffuse EO.

The Herb Farm, Ste AT/JR • 32804 Issaquah-Fall City Road, Fall City, WA 98024. I have really enjoyed this catalog and the products that I tried. The Herbal Sea Salt with essential oils was exceptional in its varying shades of green and its gentle scent. It felt good on my skin. The Calendula Cream smelled like Calendula and it certainly sealed in moisture in the testers' dry skin. They also carry over 450 herb plants and a large selection of dried herbs as well as essential oils. They carry many herb books, have a restaurant, display gardens, and offer over 175 classes. No charge for this wonderful, informative mail-order catalog.

Island Herbs, Ste AT/JR • Waldron Island, WA 98297. Certainly not strictly AT but if you didn't know of this herb company before then you are in for a pleasant surprise. Sea plants are the specialty but they also have available aromatic Northwest wild-crafted herbs such as Mugwort, Yarrow and Grindelia. An SASE is needed for the mail-order catalog. I am especially drawn to the naturally harvested Sea Lettuce, a green algae with excellent nourishing properties for your insides and outsides.

Nu Essence, Ste AT/JR • P. O. Box 30152, Seattle, WA 98103. Incense and per-fume made in accordance with Cab-balistic and astrologic considerations, and elegant custom blending for per-sonal needs. This is truly the best incense maker in the United States. Twenty-five 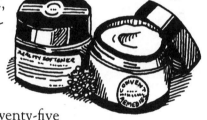 years ago I collected all the then-known resins and made incense, but after the initial experimentation ended, these resins that get richer and more fragrant with age sat upon my shelves until I heard of Kirk Bergman. I requested some personal incense which, when it arrived, was so fabulous that I immediately realized I had met a master incense alchemist. So I sent Kirk all my true resins. You can absolutely count on the quality of his product—after all, I supplied some of his more unusual ingredients. No charge for the small brochure.

Wonderland Herbs • Teas • Spices, Ste AT/JR • 1305 Railroad Avenue, Bellingham, WA 98225. Linda Quintana is the owner and runs and harvests the Alpine Herb Farm, a totally organic farm. Carries bulk herbs, essential oils (Tiferet), body-care products, herbs and incense. $1.00 for mail-order catalog.

Wisconsin

Soap Opera, Ste AT/JR • 319 State Street, Madison, WI 53703. Carries many interesting products including the full line of Herbal BodyWorks Aromatherapy massage oils and bath oils that contain therapeutic-quality aromatherapy oils.

Wood Violet Books, Ste AT/JR • 3814 Sunhill Dr., Madison, WI 53704. A full-service retail book service specializing in herbs and gardening and an out-of-pring book search service. $2.00 for catalog.

Wyoming

Wyoming Wildcrafters, Ste AT/JR • Box 874, Wilson, WY 83014. Wildcrafted and organic herbal tinctures and salves, ceremonial herbs and essential oils. Their catalog shows that they have many interesting medicinal herbals. I have used their Arnica Oil (a blend including Arnica extracted in Almond oil). No charge for catalog.

International Aromatherapy Suppliers

Africa

Africana Herbal Service, Ste AT/JR • 22 Sankone Avenue, University of Ibaday, Ibaday, NIGERIA. Essential oils, especially Citronella and Lemongrass, with Palm Kernel and Jojoba as carrier oils. Offers a consultancy service on herbal preparations. No charge for catalog but I imagine it would help if you included some international postage orders.

PLANTER BOX

Australia

The Fragrant Garden, Ste AT/JR • Portsmouth Road, Erina, NSW 2250. An extremely extensive listing of herbal items in their mail-order catalog. They sell books, bathroom products, dried herbs and flowers, essential oil blends including a very popular version of Breathe Easy blend, essential oils, scented balls, floral waters, and other miscellaneous items. Many of these intriguing products are very Australian sounding in nature. Maybe they will invite me for a visit someday. $2.00 for the mail-order catalog.

Pennyroyal Herb Farm, Ste AT/JR • Penny's Lane, Branyan, Bundaberg, Queensland 4670. Carries potted herbs, potpourris, essential oils, herb books, and is the Queensland agent for the Fragrant Garden products. $2.00 for mail-order catalog. Owned by Ian & Di Waters.

Canada

Charisma by Linda Diamond, Ste AT/JR • 319 15th Avenue SW, Calgary, Alberta T2R 0R1. Specialty facial treatments for women and men as well as teens. AT oil-essence blends and customized skin care. Carries European skin-care products. No catalog so you will just have to stop in. I hope that in the future they will carry the other more elegant essential oil blends.

Jean Adams Aromatherapy, Ste AT/JR • 74-1175 Haro Street, Vancouver, BC V6E 1E5. Carries the same essential oils that other AT salons have. The service is great—hopefully they will carry other brands of essentials soon. Also offer AT and natural product skin-care workshops. A personal service salon. Stop in when you are in Vancouver.

Naturissimo Enterprise, Ste AT/JR • It would pay to use the telephone directory in Canada to find them. Carries the Ecologicair, a diffusor in two models, an electric as well as manual style. The manual style is very handy when traveling.

True Essence Aromatherapy, Ste AT/JR, 1910 Browness Road NW, Calgary, Alberta T2N 3K6. No charge for this wonderful mail-order catalog. They have everything, although it would be nice if they carried a greater variety of brands of essential oils. This company is run by Rae Dunphy, a warm and ethical human being. Custom blending, personal consultations and AT facials, as well as massages, classes, seminars and an interest in children's health using the best principles of AT. Carries a hand-held diffusor.

England

Aromatherapy Associates, Ste AT/JR • 7 Wardo Avenue, London SW6 6RA. Offers essential oils and specialized bath and body oils. Courses accredited by IFA (International Federation of Aromatherapists) are taught.

Aromatherapy Quarterly, Ste AT/JR • 5 Ranelagh Avenue, London SW13 0BY. A very informative journal. Please write for subscription information. £12/year.

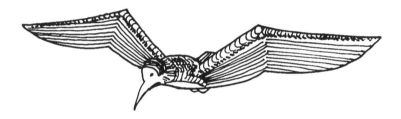

Aromatherapy Supplies, Ltd., Ste AT/JR • 52 St. Aubyns Road, Fishersgate, Brighton, Sussex BN4 1PE. Features Tisserand pure essential oils. Since the English have been using AT longer and more therapeutically than the Americans it stands to reason that they would probably have better oils. The Americans are catching up but for a while yet we should look to Europe for the finest quality oils.

C. A. Gregory Aromatic Oils Ltd., Ste AT/JR • 78, Princedale Road, Holland Park, London W11. Wonderful skin oils that are blends of natural oils and contain pure essential aromatics. Their products come packaged with booklets that describe methods of massage and skin oils. Very, very nice products.

Culpeper the Herbalist, Ste AT/JR • Hadstock Road, Linton, Cambridge CB1 6NJ. Culpeper was formed in 1927 by Mrs. C. F. Leyel, who also founded the Herb Society. Products take their name from the herbalist Nicholas Culpeper who believed in the healing power of herbs. These products are as natural as possible, have not been tested on animals, and have a world-wide reputation for quality, simple yet attractive packaging and excellent value. Extensive range of natural full-strength essential and vegetable oils available by mail order. All credit cards accepted. Try their sleep pillows. $1.00 for catalog. London address is 21 Bruton Street, Berkeley Square, London W1X 7DA.

Czech & Speake, Ste AT/JR • 244/254 Cambridge Heath Road, London, E2 9DA. Fine-quality aromatic toiletries and luxury bathroom fittings and accessories. $3.50 for brochure of items available by mail order. To burn essential oils they provide *porcelain* rather than metal rings for light bulbs. The oils burn more slowly as well as more evenly while not altering the fragrance.

Danièle Ryman Aromatherapie, Ste AT/JR • Park Lane Hotel, 107 B Piccadilly, London, W1Y 8BX. A wonderful line of AT products designed by one of the earliest proponents of this practice.

Essentia • Shirley Price Aromatherapy, Ste AT/JR • Upper Bond Street, Hinkley, Leicest, LE10 1RS. I had the opportunity to meet Shirley Price and found her, her information and most importantly her AT-based skin-care products to be wonderful—simply wonderful. She has an efficient mail-order service. Send her $1.00 for postage. You won't be disappointed and more importantly your skin won't either.

Fleur Aromatherapy, Ste AT/JR • Pembroke Studios, Pembroke Road, London N10 2JE. Offers a comprehensive range of pure essential oils available by mail order.

International Federation of Aromatherapists, Ste AT/JR • 4 Eastmearn Road, West Dulwich, London SE21 8HA. An independent professional body with members all over the world. This is the United Kingdom's governing body of aromatherapy. Recommends fully qualified AT persons to the general public. The newsletter is very informative and membership costs lb/15 in the UK and lb/20 elsewhere.

Les Senteurs, Ste AT/JR • 227 Ebury Street, London, SW1W 8UT. Owned by Betty Hawksley, this business has essential oils, bath products and a mail-order catalog.

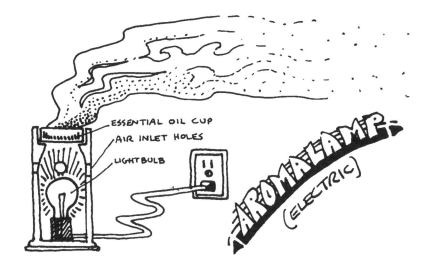

ESSENTIAL OIL CUP
AIR INLET HOLES
LIGHTBULB
"AROMALAMP"
(ELECTRIC)

Norman & Germaine Rich, Ste AT/JR • 2 Coval Gardens, London SW14 7DE. Suppliers of essential oils. This is a family business established at the turn of the century.

Universal Flavors, Ltd., Ste AT/JR • Bilton Road, Bletchley, Milton Keynes, MK 1 1 HP, UK. A complete selection of EO both regular and terpene free. Has American outlets. Write for information.

France

Biorégène, Ste AT/JR • 1 rue Montholon, 75009 Paris. Wholesale source of fine quality essential oils and diffusors.

Hasslauer, Ste AT/JR • 10 rue De L'Ancienne Marie, 92100 Boulogne. Very fine high quality EO.

Maître Parfumeur et Gantier, Ste AT/JR • 84 Bis rue de Grenelle, 75007 Paris. Carries perfumes, bath oils, soaps and potpourri supplies. Jean François LaPorte creates lovely perfumes in the elegant French tradition.

Pranarom, Ste AT/JR • La Courtête, Belvèze Du Razes. Wholesale source of especially fine-quality therapeutic oils. (68) 69.07.13.

Remy Laure • Laboratoires France Beauté, Ste AT/JR • Z.I. 1re Ave— 1re Rue, 06515 Carros Cedex. A fabulous line of 100% natural beauty care. I particularly like the products made from Moor which is an organic mud formed 30,000 years ago when water flooded immense forests of plants and medicinal herbs. When applied regularly, or if you bathe regularly in Moor bath waters, youth is preserved and regeneration can occur.

Secoma, Ste AT/JR • sarl au capital de 50.000 F Z.A.P. du Lattay, 53240 Andouillé, France. A full line of quality essential oils.

Sunarom Laboratory • This company is located in the Toulouse region of France. Look for correct address Very fine-quality therapeutic essential oils.

Synarom, Ste AT/JR • Z1 Beaulieu, 6 Rue Charles Tellier 2800, Chartres. Essential oils.

New Zealand

Apothecary Shoppe, Ste AT/JR • P. O. Box 4451, Auckland. Books, charts, wonderful body-care supplies, organically grown herbs, essential oils and more. The catalog is free. Associated with the Australasian College of Herbal Studies.

Switzerland

Laboratories Kart, Ste AT/JR • S.A.-CH-1052 Le Mont, Lausanne. One of the primary distributors of fine essential oils.

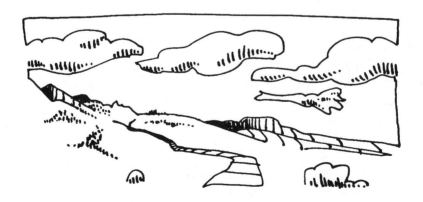

Other Aromatherapy Products

Fine-quality carrier oils are produced by Simplers Botanicals in California, Shirley Price in England and Jeanne Rose Herbal BodyWorks in San Francisco, California. From experience I know that 8 ounces of Shirley Price Calendula-infused carrier oil is about $28.00 and that Calendula-infused carrier oil by Jeanne Rose is $14.00 for 8 ounces. There is a great disparity in the price of the oils because Shirley Price imports her oil, and shipping costs from France are expensive, while Jeanne Rose buys organically grown Marigold (Calendula) flowers and cold-processes them with fine-quality Olive oil in the cool weather of San Francisco. Both are fine-quality products. Herbal BodyWorks is at 219 Carl Street in San Francisco, CA 94117.

AromaLamps and Diffusors are wonderful instruments to use to volatize essential oils and vaporize them for inhalation. They are listed throughout this directory. Add here AromaLamp at 1-800-933-5267. These are wonderful porcelain and clay burning pots to use with electricity or a candle. They are reasonably priced and gently fragrance the air. A glass diffusor is available from Leydet in California, 916/965-7546, and this is one that I personally prefer to use when not using the AromaLamps. However, it is expensive and probably not useful in a home with small children.

Glass Containers in various sizes can be obtained from laboratory and glass supply companies, as well as Acme Vial and Glass, 16012 Commerce Way, Paso Robles, CA 93446; Beatson Clark Containers, call 1-800-433-6417, a customer hotline for sources or Berlin Packaging, 111 N. Canal Street, Chicago, IL 60606; and Lavender Lane, 6715 Donerail Drive, Sacramento, CA 95842—a source of hard-to-find herbalware.

Aroma Jewels are lovely gemstones with a drilled space for an essential oil. They are really beautiful and a way to keep the essence of a plant near your 4th or 5th chakra. Write P. O. Box 662, Graton, CA 95444.

Aromatherapy Jewel Boxes are specially designed to store essential oils. They are made of natural pine and walnut woods. Call 1-800-688-8343 and say Jeanne Rose sent you.

Listing of Aromatherapy Schools and Correspondence Courses

Aromatherapy & Herbal Studies Course, Ste AT/JR • 219 Carl Street, San Francisco, CA 94117. Taught by Jeanne Rose, this extensive correspondence course is full of "All Things Herbal and Aromatic." Jeanne has been writing and lecturing about Aromatherapy since 1972. She also travels around the nation frequently, doing seminars, lectures and AT intensives. Phone 415/564-6785 and leave your address.

Pacific Institute of Aromatherapy, Ste ATJR • P.O. Box 6723, San Rafael, CA 94903. Correspondence course, seminars, retreats, EO analysis & research. Good on AT chemistry. Taught by Kurt Schnaubelt.

Australasian School of Herbal Studies, Ste AT/JR • P.O. Box 57. Lake Oswego, OR 97034. Home study courses in herbs, AT, bodycare, etc. Write for a prospectus. Taught by Dorene Petersen.

Quintessence Aromatherapy, Ste AT/JR • P. O. Box 4996, Boulder, CO 80306. This has been written by Ann Berwick, who has been practicing holistic aromatherapy for ten years.

Atlantic Institute of Aromatherapy, Ste AT/JR • 16018 Saddle String Drive, Tampa, FL 33618. Seminars, correspondence course, consultations and blends. No charge for catalog. Taught by Sylla Hanger.

Aromatherapy Seminars, , Ste AT/JR • 3379 S. Robertson Pl., Los Angeles, CA 90034. The Certification Course costs $750.00 which includes a Home Study Course and a 4-day seminar. The Home Study Course is very nicely done with audio tapes, a video tape and 22 samples although there are only 250 pages of written material.

The New England Center for Aromatherapy, Ste AT/JR • 25 Plante Street, Norton, MA 02766. Courses, seminars and correspondence course, consultations and blends. No charge for catalog. Taught by Jade Shutes.

Laraine Kyle, Ste AT/JR • 3072 Edison Court, Boulder, CO 80301. Aromatherapy for nurses. Write for information.

A General Listing of Fragrance Materials Suppliers
Supplier Address Guide

A-Aroma Tech Inc., 162 Hwy 34, Exec Ste 95, Matawan, NJ 07747.

Alpine Aromatics International Inc., Edison Industrial Center, 51 Ethel Road, W, CN-1348, Piscataway, NJ 08854-1348.

American Aromatics Inc., 1295 Northern Blvd, Manhasset, NY 11030.

Aroma Globe Inc., 171 E. Second Street, Huntington Station, NY 11746.

Arylessence Inc., 1091 Lake Dr., Marietta, GA 30062

BBA Aroma Chemicals, Div Union Camp Corp, 7 Mercedes Drive, Montvale, NJ 07645.

Belle-Aire Fragrances Inc., 1600 Baskin Road, Mundelein, IL 60060.

Bell Flavors & Fragrances Inc., 500 Academy Drive, Northbrook, IL 60062.

Belmay Inc., 35-02 48th Avenue, Long Island City, NY 11101

Berje Inc., 5 Lawrence Street, Bloomfield, NJ 07003.

BPS Fragrances Srl, Via Della Resistenza 34/F, Buccinasco (Milano), 20090, Italy.

Camilli Albert & LaLoue, 230 Brighton Road, Clifton, NJ 07012.

Charabot & Co., 83 Cedar Lane, Englewood, NJ 07631.

Chemessence Inc., 180 Sunny Valley Road, Unit 15, New Milford, CT 06776

C M Aromatics Inc., 159 Dwight Place, P. O. Box 1228, Fairfield, NJ 07006-0225.

Creations Aeromatics, 61-12 32nd Avenue, Woodside, NY 11377.

Creative Fragrances Mfg Inc., 10420 Piano Road, Dallas, TX 75238.

Custom Essence Inc., 67-10A Veronica Avenue, Somerset, NJ 08873.

de Laire Inc., 950 Third Avenue, New York, NY 10022.

Dragoco Inc., Gordon Drive, Totowa, NJ 07512.

Elias Fragrances Inc., 999 E 46 Street, Brooklyn, NY 11203.

Felton Worldwide, 599 Johnson Avenue, Brooklyn, NY 11237-1388.

Flavor & Fragrance Specialties, 530 Commerce Street, Franklin Lakes, NJ 07417.

Florasynth Inc., 410 E 62 Street, New York, NY 10021.

Fragrance Resources Inc., 275 Clark Street, Keyport, NJ 07735.

Fritzsche Dodge & Olcott, 76 Ninth Avenue, New York, NY 10011.

Givaudan Corp, 100 Delawanna Avenue, Clifton, NJ 07015-5034.

Global Aromatics, 340 W Channel Road, Benicia, CA 94510.

T Hasegawa USA Inc., 5351 W 144 Street, Lawndale, CA 90260.

Intarome Fragrance Corp, 71 E. Palisade Avenue, Englewood, NJ 07631.

Intercontinental Fragrances Inc., 800 Victoria Drive, Houston, TX 77022.

International Flavors & Fragrances, 521 W 57 Street, New York, NY 10019.

Manheimer Inc J, 47-22 Pearson Place, Long Island City, NY 11101-4481.

Novarome Inc., 30 Stewart Place, Fairfield, NJ 07006.

Orchid Laboratories Inc., 1525 Brook Drive, Downers Grove, IL 60515.

Penta Mfg Co., P. O. Box 1448, Fairfield, NJ 07007.

Quest International, 400 International Drive, Mount Olive, NJ 07828.

Robertet Inc., 125 Bauer Drive, Oakland, NJ 07436.

Roure Inc., 1775 Windsor Road, Teaneck, NJ 07666.

Shaw Mudge & Co., 16 Dyke Lane, P. O. Box 1375, Stamford, CT 06904-1375.

Synarome Corp of America, 200 Hudson Street, New York, NY 10013.

Takasago International Corp (USA), 11 Volvo Drive, Rockleigh, NJ 07647.

Ungerer & Co., 4 Bridgewater Lane, Lincoln Park, NJ 07035.

Universal Fragrance Corp., 124 Case Drive, South Plainfield, NJ 07080.

Ve Vonque Inc., 132-15 Atlantic Avenue, Richmond Hill, NY 11418.

Via Semeria 18, P. O. Box 716, Genova, 16131, Italy

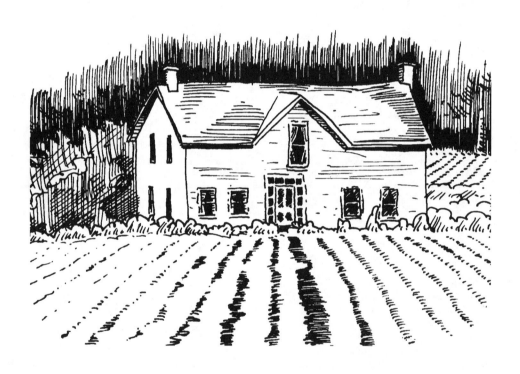

Part II

The Recipes

Inhalations
& Applications

FRAGRANCE affects her
She sees the azure sights from her alien sky
She sees the lolling hills
    and an emerald scented sea.
Her past sheds its carefree perfume around her
And the secrets fade away as the scent of
    the Violet
                    —Anonymous

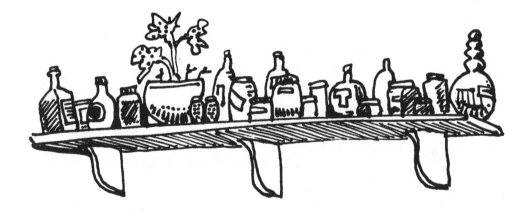

Introduction

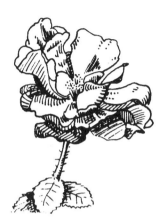

Aromatherapy & Skin Care

by Joni Loughran*

A romatherapy and the use of essential oils can open up an exciting new world for the professional aesthetician. Essential oils are extraordinary gifts from nature. Their profound effect in skin care is due to their ability to penetrate the skin. When applied topically, their small and simple molecular structure allows them to easily pass into the fluid surrounding the cells beneath the skin's surface. From here, they enter the lymph ducts and capillaries, pass into the bloodstream and circulate through the body. [See Table 10.] Because essential oils are so active, care must be taken with their use and education should precede their introduction into a professional skincare practice.

Essential oils are extracted from many parts of the plants. Depending on the species, the oil may come from the leaf, stem, flower, seed, root, bark or resin. Because the practice of aromatherapy is enjoying a renaissance, a vast array of essential oils has become available. Amongst these, there are a few that stand out for their effectiveness and multiple applications in the aesthetic world. Lavender, Chamomile, Geranium, Rose, Sandalwood, Tea Tree and Ylang-Ylang are superb cosmetic essential oils.

---

*Joni Loughran, used by permission, 1991

235

Lavender is considered to be the most useful and versatile of all the essential oils. Its soothing, antiseptic, anti-inflammatory and balancing qualities make it invaluable for skin care. Lavender is one of the few oils that can be applied undiluted (neat) to the skin, and few people are allergic to it. It is excellent for the treatment of acne because it inhibits bacteria, soothes the skin, helps to balance the over-active sebaceous glands, and helps to reduce scarring by stimulating the growth of healthy new cells. It is beneficial for all types of skin, including aging skin.

Chamomile's properties are soothing, calming and anti-inflammatory. It is an analgesic, disinfectant and gentle in nature. Chamomile is especially good for dry, sensitive skin, and because it has the ability to shrink small blood vessels it can help reduce the redness due to enlarged capillaries. (This may take months of regular applications.)

Geranium is an astringent, antiseptic and promotes speedy healing. It is excellent for balancing the production of sebum, so it is well-suited for all types of skin, especially combination skin with patches of oily as well as dry areas.

Rose is considered the "queen" of essential oils. It is a gentle yet powerful antidepressant. It soothes the nerves and is renowned for its aphrodisiac qualities. In skin care, Rose is good for all types of skin, but especially for dry, sensitive or aging skin. It is an excellent antiseptic and can help diminish enlarged capillaries. Rose is the least toxic of all the essential oils.

Sandalwood is good for all types of skin. It is excellent for dry, dehydrated or old skin and beneficial for oily and acne skin as well. It is soothing, inhibits bacterial growth and is slightly astringent.

Tea Tree (Ti-Tree) oil is unique in that it is active against bacteria, fungus and viruses. It is also a powerful immune system stimulant. It can irritate the skin, so care must be taken not to use it on sensitive skin and to dilute it properly. Tea Tree oil is excellent as a wash for acne, and a small drop can be applied undiluted on pimples to help clear them quickly.

Ylang-Ylang has aphrodisiac, anti-depressant and sedative qualities. For skin care, it is suitable for both oily and dry skin and has a balanced effect on the secretion of sebum.

The practical application of essential oils for aestheticians will fall into four categories during a skin-care treatment: masks, massage oils, compresses and washes. Before preparing these, allow your client to smell your chosen oil or blend. Ask them to close their eyes and gently inhale the aroma. If it is is especially disagreeable to them, it is wise to choose another. Patricia

Davis, principal of the London School of Aromatherapy, feels so strongly about the sense of smell's input to our psyche that she suggests if the smell is distasteful, it is an indication that it may not be effective for that person and to not use it.

Masks are primarily designed to draw, tighten, moisturize, soothe, nourish and help clear blemishes. The essential oil or oils you choose will be added to a mask base. Clay is especially well-suited to work with essential oils. All of the aforementioned oils can be used in a mask. Use approximately 3 to 5 drops.

Massage oils can be used on the face, neck and shoulders, the entire body. The essential oils can be added in a 2% solution (or less, if need be). To mix an approximate 2% solution, add twenty-five drops of the essential oil in two ounces of the base oil. Shake well. The amount of essential oil can vary depending on the oil, its intended use and the type of skin it is going to be used on.

Compresses (folded cloths) are used during a facial with cold water to contract the tissues and with warm water to relax the tissues. Essential oils may be added to the water in which the compress is dipped to impart their qualities to the compress. Use only the gentlest oils for this method such as Lavender, Chamomile or Rose. Use approximately four drops of the essential oil (again, this amount can vary) in a basin of water, stir well and then immerse the cloth. Wring it out well before applying it to the skin.

A facial wash is used as a toner or a conditioner, depending on the skin type and the need. It can be made by mixing five drops of an essential oil in one cup of pure water. (This amount may vary.) Shake vigorously, wet a cotton ball until damp and wipe the skin. Tea Tree oil is an excellent wash for acne. Lavender, Rose, Chamomile and Geranium are good for all types of skin.

Another way that an aesthetician might use essential oils is to add them to existing products. Essential oils blend well into fatty substances such as moisturizers and cleansers and into any products containing alcohol. In these cases, it is recommended to start with simple, unscented products and follow the same guidelines for proportions.

The safety of essential oils has become a concern in the world of aromatherapy. Because essential oils are pharmacologically active, they can be toxic to the body if used incorrectly. Chronic toxicity can be caused from dermal (skin) application when a small amount of a potentially hazardous oil is used repeatedly over a long period of time. Gradual kidney or liver damage could occur. However, Robert Tisserand, author of *The Safety Data Man-*

ual for Essential Oils, states that "the risks of toxicity are relatively easy to tackle. The essential oils that present risks are, in most cases, easy to identify, and those that present a high risk should be avoided altogether in aromatherapy."

Aside from toxicity reactions, there can also be irritation and allergic reactions. Skin irritations can occur with almost any essential oil because they are so concentrated; the problem is solved by diluting the oil. The more the oil is diluted, the less irritating it will become. Tisserand states, "Those who use undiluted essential oils directly on the skin are playing with fire, while almost anything diluted to less than 5% will be safe to use."

Allergic reactions are a risk when using essential oils, though it is not common. However, in this case, diluting the oil will not prevent the problem. Allergic reaction most often occurs in people with sensitive skin. Though they will not react to all essential oils, care must be taken in oil selection as well as in dilution.

In any case, the aesthetician preparing to work with aromatherapy would be well-advised to study one or more of the many books now available in order to understand the subtleties and contraindications of using essential oils. The essential oils that I have mentioned here are safe to use in the suggested format.

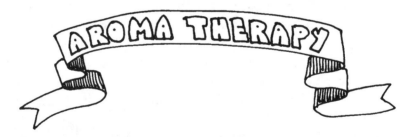

All professional aestheticians will, in time and with experience, develop a philosophy that is unique to their practice. And because of this, they will attract a certain clientele. My own niche is as a natural skin-care aesthetician and my philosophy is based on four principles.

(1) Wholistic approach. All aspects of the client's lifestyle are taken into account. Do they smoke? Do they get enough exercise? Are they eating a wholesome diet? Anything that may be affecting the condition of their skin is reviewed.

(2) High standard of quality. Only the finest domestic and imported skin-care products are used. They do not contain any mineral oil, artificial

colors or artificial fragrances. Special treatments are formulated with natural raw ingredients such as clay, herbal extracts and pure essential oils.

(3) Continued education for the aesthetician. It is a "dangerous" mental attitude to think one has learned all one needs to know. It stops learning and mental growth. The aesthetician must continuously study some aspect of their work as well as keep an open mind to new ideas that will benefit the practice.

(4) Client education. The client must be educated about skin care as it pertains to them. A guided, at-home program supports the work of the aesthetician.

These four principles come into play as I work with each client on an individual basis. My goal is to work toward solving their cosmetic skin problems, provide support for a positive self-image (I never tell someone that their skin is "bad"), and establish a program they can live with using affordable natural skin-care products. It is my belief that how we relate to each other can be as valuable as the skin-care treatment itself. I want all my clients to know that they are "in good hands" and that I care about them. The treatment should be an enjoyable experience that will allow them to unwind, de-stress and feel pampered.

Aromatherapy plays an active role in my skin-care practice and is in keeping with my basic philosophy. Though each treatment may vary slightly, I follow a general format that begins by using an essential oil diffusor to disperse tiny droplets of essential oil into the air. The diffusor is on ten minutes just prior to the appointment and gives the room a delightful fragrance that pleases the nose as well as the psyche. After the client has changed into a gown and is sitting in the facial chair, the feet are placed in a warm aromatherapy foot bath. During the remainder of the treatment, I will use aromatherapy compresses, massage oils, and will custom-blend a facial mask using essential oils chosen for their skin type.

The initial skin-care treatment lasts two hours. The major portion of that time is spent relaxing the client. The face is cleansed, toned, steamed and nourished with three different facial masks keyed to the complexion, while soft peaceful music is played in the background. A reflexology hand and foot massage are included. In the last portion of the time the client begins to revitalize. Cool compresses are used with either Rosemary oil or Lemon oil, which have uplifting qualities, and a *stimulating* foot massage is given. At the end of the facial, the client sits up and receives a drink of water and then a small glass of Dr. Hauschka's elixir. While sipping the elixir, one client smiled and dreamily said, "I feel like I have been on a journey." Clients will react differently to this comprehensive skin-care treatment. That comment was one of my favorites.

Because of my background in wholistic health sciences and cosmetology, my work as an aesthetician has combined these two areas. As a result, I draw from a variety of alternative therapies and cosmetically apply them in my treatments. I use principles from acupressure, reflexology, herbalism, nutrition, polarity and, of course, aromatherapy. At this point in my professional work, I believe that there is no *one* way to work with a client and no *one* cosmetic line to use for everyone. The treatment designed for a client may even vary from visit to visit. Because this has been my experience, I want available to me as much information from as many schools of thought as possible that will benefit the client. I am, to be certain, an eclectic in my approach to skin care, and am proud to offer an intelligent, natural approach for men, women and teenagers.

For the Aesthetician:
Using Essential Oils in the Salon

At the beginning of an aromatherapy skin-care treatment, the first role of the essential oils is to relax and calm the client. I use basically the same group of essential oils for everyone during this process: relaxing oils diffused in the room, relaxing oils in the foot bath and relaxing oils in the massage oil. There are a variety of single essential oils as well as blends that can be used to 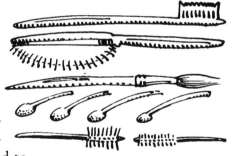 treat each skin type: dry, oily, normal, combination, sensitive, couperose, ageing and problem (acneic). There are also a variety of ways to use these oils during the treatment. How and why you use the essential oils will depend on the client's needs. During the first part of the treatment, uplifting and sometimes stimulating oils are used to bring the client "back to reality" so they will leave in a state of mind that is ready to face the world again.

Diffusion

The first opportunity available to use essential oils is in the waiting or reception area of the salon. My facial room was within a natural food store. The store frequently has an AromaLamp in use, diffusing a scent into the store. Lavender oil seems to evoke more responses from customers than any other scent. "Mmmmmmmm, what smells so good?' Other popular scents are the citrus oils such as Orange, Lemon or Tangerine. They have a very clean and fresh appeal.

The next opportunity is in the treatment room. You will need to purchase a good essential oil diffusor. For the treatment room, my preference is the nebulizer type with the glass expansion chamber. In your diffusor, use an oil that will promote relaxation such as Lavender, Bergamot or Marjoram and let it run in the treatment room for about fifteen minutes prior to your client arriving. I never have the diffusor going while I am giving a treatment. I do this for two reasons. If it is on too long, it is overpowering for the client. Second, if it is on throughout my treatment, which lasts for two hours, I become too affected and cannot stay focused on my work. If your client is particularly in need of relaxing, you can offer her a tissue with a few drops of calming-relaxing oil or blend on it. She can sniff it periodically through the treatment, at her own discretion.

The diffusor is a wonderful opportunity to use special or favorite blends. Once you get to know a client, you might even have special blends that you use just for them. There is a variety of wonderful commercial blends available. I use both purchased blends (from reputable sources) and blends that I have made myself. Two of my favorites are:

Diffusor Blend #1		or	**Diffusor Blend #2**	
Lavender oil	5 drops		Clary Sage oil	6 drops
Bergamot oil	2 drops		Lavender oil	2 drops
Clary Sage oil	1 drop		Ylang-Ylang oil	1 drop

I have deliberately given these formulas to you in very small quantities so that you can test them before you commit a large amount of oils only to discover that you do not care for the fragrance. If you *do* like it, simply increase each ingredient proportionately.

Remember, the attraction or repulsion of any specific oil or blend is entirely subjective and very personal. So powerful is this message that I believe if the aroma of an oil displeases you, particularly in a treatment that is meant to relax, it is an indication that it will not benefit you and it should not be used. So, it is important to take some time and experiment with essential oils to discover the ones to which you resonate and then experiment blending your own.

At the end of the treatment, when you are bringing your client out of the relaxation mode, you may put a few drops of Basil or Rosemary oil on a tissue and allow them to sniff it. These both have a wonderful, mind-lifting effect.

Baths

As part of my skin-care treatment, an aromatherapy foot bath is given. This is another opportunity to continue the relaxation process. I fill a large stainless steel bowl with very warm water. Depending on the client and my inclinations, I will either use:

(1) an aromatherapy mineral/bath salt mixture;

(2) an aromatherapy bath concentrate (essential oils combined with sulfonated castor oil, which disperses in water); or

(3) 2–4 drops of a single essential oil mixed with a small amount of grain alcohol. The alcohol is used as a solvent to dilute the essential oils so they will evenly disperse in the water. This prevents "hot spots" in the foot bath that may irritate the skin. Any single oils or blends that are for relaxing can be used in the foot bath. I most often use lavender but will also choose from Geranium, Bergamot or Clary Sage.

Massage

Massage is often considered the best way to use essential oils and for the aesthetician, it can be incorporated into a skin-care treatment in a variety of formats. Consider its use, using an aromatherapy massage oil, on the feet, the lower leg, the hands, the arms, the back, the upper chest and the face. Not only does the client benefit from the qualities of the essential oils, she/he benefits from the energy and healing qualities of the human touch.

In my practice, I give an extensive foot massage at the beginning of the treatment. Applying reflexology techniques, I cover the entire foot and pay extra attention to the areas that will affect the organs that are most closely related to the skin. Again, I use the relaxing oils. I mix 25 drops of an essential oil, usually Lavender, into 2 ounces of a carrier oil. You can also use the same blend that you use in the diffusor.

You may choose to massage the hand in the same manner.

I massage the neck, the upper chest and the upper back after I have applied a facial "mask." For this massage, my oil of preference is Rose massage oil. Though it is expensive, there is not a more wonderful massage oil to be used while massaging over the heart. After all, the Rose is for love and it is, spiritually, excellent for the heart. If you choose not to use Rose, again, any of the relaxing oils would be appropriate.

I do not massage the face, though I know qualified aestheticians that do. My training in skin care as well as my instincts have directed me to be very gentle with the face. Too vigorous a massage can overstretch the tissue and as the skin ages, it loses its elasticity. If it is over-stretched too often, it will begin to sag. Instead, after I apply an aromatherapy facial oil, I use acupressure points to stimulate the facial tissues without massage. I have found this method to be the most effective.

Compresses

I use aromatherapy compress twice in my skin-care treatment. The first time is right before I cleanse the face. It serves the purpose of continuing to relax the client, it warms and softens the facial tissue and is a pre-cleanse treatment. I begin by filling the basin with warm water (the temperature depends on the type of skin). For this I only use the very gentlest of essential oils—either Lavender, Rose or Chamomile. Put 4 drops in the basin and stir well. If you are concerned about "hot spots," mix with a little alcohol first or choose a commercial product that has been formulated to mix well with water. I apply about 10 compresses to the face and upper chest before I begin the cleansing process.

The second time I use the compress is at the end of the facial. In this instance, cool water is used to facilitate the uplifting process. I use one or two drops of Rosemary or Peppermint to a full basin of water. Care must be taken not to irritate the skin, which is now in a very clean and vulnerable state. Be aware that if you have done any active exfoliating, you should not follow with anything that contains essential oils, unless you are certain it will not irritate the skin. In this case, simply use cool compresses in plain water and give the client a tissue to sniff with one of the uplifting oils.

Compresses can also be employed for the hands and the feet.

Masks

Most skin types will benefit from a mask. I follow these guidelines with my clients. Clay masks are excellent for oily skins, blemished skins and young normal skins. Cream masks are generally indicated for sensitive and mature skins. However, wonderful masks can be made using both clay and creams. The possibilities are extensive and essential oils lend themselves beautifully to aid in the purpose of the masks.

For normal skin (not yet ageing):
    2 tablespoons of green or rose clay
    1 teaspoon of honey
    2 drops of Geranium oil
Use *Aloe vera* juice or water to make a paste

For dry skin:
    1 tablespoon of rose clay
    1 tablespoon of instant oatmeal or finely ground regular Oatmeal
    1 teaspoon of honey
    1 teaspoon of Almond oil
Use enough water to make a paste
    1 drop of Rose oil
    1 drop of Lavender oil

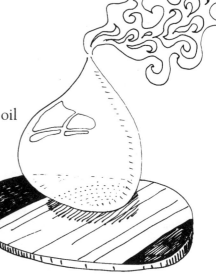

For oily skin:
    2 tablespoons of green clay
    1 teaspoon of *Aloe vera* juice
    ½ teaspoon of vegetable oil or Jojoba oil
Use enough water to make a paste
    1 drop of Bergamot oil
    1 drop of Lavender oil

For sensitive skin:
    1 tablespoon of rose clay
    1–2 teaspoons of Avocado oil
    1 drop of Rose oil
    1 drop of Roman Chamomile oil
Use water, if necessary, to make a paste. Use a little more clay if too runny.

For mature or ageing skin:
    1 tablespoon of rose clay
    1 tablespoon of instant Oatmeal or finely ground regular Oatmeal

1 teaspoon of honey
1 teaspoon of Avocado or Almond oil
Use water to make a paste.
1 drop of Frankincense oil
1 drop of Neroli or Lavender oil
1 drop of Rose oil

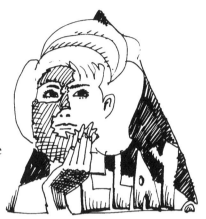

When using essential oils with masks, they can be combined with raw ingredients, such as described above, as well as mixed with a commercial product. If you choose to mix the oils with a pre-made commercial product, choose one with a very simple formula and no other added fragrances or essential oils.

Facial Washes or Water Sprays

The facial wash or water spray can be used as a toner or a conditioner during the skin-care treatment. It can be used any time you need to moisten the skin or a skin-care product that is on the face, such as a mask. I use these frequently during the treatment. Simply put about 5 drops of a chosen essential oil in one cup of water that is in the misting spray bottle. For this, I most commonly use Rose or Lavender, but Chamomile and Geranium are also good because they are good for all types of skin. If you want to individualize the facial sprays, the same essential oils that are used in the masks can be used in the spray bottle. It is important to remember to shake the bottle vigorously before you spray—this breaks up and disperses the essential oils into the water.

Following is a description of Joni's current skin-care practice as written on her brochure.

Joni Loughran brings to her profession a unique expertise that is the result of fifteen years of experience in the health and beauty field. Joni is a licensed cosmetologist and cosmetology instructor. She has a doctorate degree in wholistic health sciences and has a diploma in the highly regarded Dr. Hauschka method of skin care. She has worked as a consultant for health spas, designed and directed facial programs, instructed seminars and has written numerous published articles on natural hair and skin care. Joni currently has a private skin care and consulting practice and authors the "Aesthetician Column" for the American

Aromatherapy Association. Joni's work reflects her commitment to a high standard of quality, continued education and wholistic approach to meet the cosmetic needs of today's men and women. Write to Joni at P.O. Box 751150, Petaluma, CA 94975.

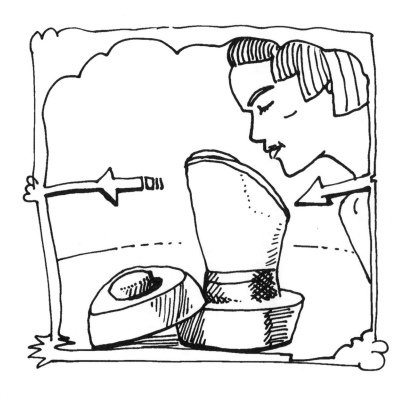

Chapter VII

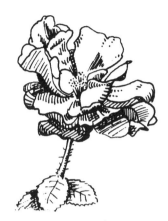

Carrier Oils

What to Use as a Base
for Your Aromatherapy Products

EO = Essential Oil
PEO = Pure Essential Oil

Carrier Oils are the oils that you would choose to be used as a carrier or receptacle for fine essential oils, e.g. PEO, quintessential oils, volatile oils. In the years since 1972 when first I became acquainted with aromatherapy I have tried every single essential and fixed oil mentioned in Chapter III plus a few that aren't mentioned. In the *Herbal Body Book* on pages 332–333 is a list of oils considered non-drying or drying. Non-drying oils are useful for dry skin. Semi-drying oils do not have much linolenic acid but more of the saturated acids. They dry slowly on contact with air and are suitable for normal to oily skin. Drying oils are high in unsaturated glycerides and especially linoleic and linolenic acid. These are temperate-climate oils and the most suitable for oily skin.

Dry Skin Oils	Dry–Normal–Oily Skin Oil	Oily Skin Oil
Almond oil Castor oil Cocoa butter *Olive oil Palm oil Peanut oil	*Calendula-infused oil Corn oil *Jojoba oil Sesame oil Soybean oil	*Grapeseed oil Hazelnut oil most nut oils *Sunflower oil *Walnut oil
*Best to use		

Of these oils, several are not to be recommended because they go rancid so quickly: most notably, Peanut oil, Cottonseed oil and generally the ubiquitous Soybean oil. Others can't be recommended because such a high quantity of pesticides are used when they are grown, including Cottonseed oil. Others are not recommended because they are supersaturated and solid at room temperature, such as Cocoa butter and Palm oil, and in cool climates, Coconut oil.

Some oils are recommended because they have specific uses, such as Walnut oil being a fine carrier oil when used in products for the hair and scalp. Sunflower oil is a fine-quality oil, especially for normal to oily skin. It is thin and light and has virtually no scent. It is also recommended for products for the genital area, and as a carrier oil for aromatic products for men. Almond oil too is a fine-quality carrier oil and can be used for virtually any product, although it can go rancid in a relatively short time. Wheat germ oil is not listed but it can be used to preserve aromatherapy products. It has a powerful smell and alters the ultimate fragrance of any product. It is recommended only for internal use and healing rather than cosmetic external use.

The best oil to use is Olive oil. The easiest preservative would be straight vitamin E oil. The best carrier is actually Jojoba oil—which is not an oil at all but rather a fine wax that has become the substitute in all formulas that used to recommend spermaceti or sperm whale oil, which is now banned.

Jojoba also has the added advantage that it does not go rancid and that it is healing and helpful of itself. It has the unique ability to get into the follicles of hair on the body and scalp, dissolving old plugging sebum and hair-strangling wax that then can be removed via the bath or shampoo. This stimulates hair growth on the scalp. For hair and scalp products, Jojoba oil (wax) has no equal.

Finally there is Calendula Carrier Oil. This is the product that results when you infuse fresh or dried Calendula flowers in oil, usually Olive oil. The resulting product can be protected from oxidation with the addition of vitamin E and can be kept in the refrigerator. I have seen this product listed in catalogs from $4.00 to 8.00 per ounce. This is a prohibitive price for something that can so easily be made at home. Calendula flowers contain lots of carotene and vitamin A, which is essential in itself for healthful skin. Vitamin A is oil soluble and will enter the base oil when the flowers are macerated. The most recent time that I made Calendula-infused oil was late 1991. I ordered fresh Calendula flowers from Montana Botanicals (see Chapter VI) at $6.00 a pound and bought a gallon of Olive oil from the corner store. Total cost was $21.00. Then I took these flowers and placed them in the top of a double boiler, added the Olive oil, and pressed the flowers into the oil with a Potato masher. I allowed the flowers to macerate in the room-temperature warm oil for 24 hours, then turned on the heat and brought the water in the bottom of the double boiler to a boil. The flowers were allowed to heat slowly in the Olive oil for 4 hours. I turned off the heat and let it cool. When cool I pressed the flowers and oil through cheesecloth, letting the oil drip into a container. Finally I bottled the gallon of oil into 16 8-ounce containers. Then I squeezed 4 vitamin E capsules into each bottle and refrigerated them. This is enough oil for me for a year of experimentation and application. The cost? 20¢ an ounce! Compare this reasonable price with $8.00 an ounce for the store-bought product.

There are approximately 120–250 flowers in 4 ounces (by weight). So to make only one quart of Calendula-infused oil, here is the recipe:

Golden Calendula Carrier Oil
(A carrier oil for All Fine Aromatherapy Products)

> 1 quart (by volume) of Olive oil or any mixture of oils of your choice
> 4–8 ounces (by weight) of fresh Calendula flowers (125–250 flowers)
> 1 double boiler with water in the bottom

Place the flowers and the oil in the top of the pot. Mash with a masher, pestle or back of spoon. Macerate (to soften and extract by steeping with heat) in the oil for 10 minutes to 24 hours (with only natural heat, that is, in a warm room). Then turn on the heat bringing the water in the bottom of the double boiler to a boil, and simmer until the oil and flowers are hot and have been gently heated for at least 4 hours. At this point your oil should have a delicious toasty fragrance. If it even begins to smell burnt or like burnt toast, you have applied too much heat and should get the flowers out of the oil immediately. But after 4 hours this delicious-smelling and gloriously golden-colored oil will have been heated enough to have extracted all the beneficence from the flowers. Also, were you to taste the oil it would have a yummy flowery taste as well. Let cool, until cool enough to handle, about an hour. Now strain through a gold-type or other fine filter or cheesecloth (whatever you have), into a 1-quart container. You may squeeze the cloth or not. If you squeeze it to extract every bit of oil, the oil becomes opaque with suspended flower matter. This delicate solid flower matter will eventually settle out. If you do not squeeze the cloth, the oil stays relatively clear and golden.

At this point, you have 1 quart of Golden Calendula Carrier Oil. You may add the contents of one 400 IU vitamin E capsule per ounce of oil (32 capsules per quart), or you may just refrigerate it until your oil is needed. Remember that this is a living product and will not last indefinitely in any circumstance. Use up your oil and make a new batch whenever you have Calendula flowers in season.

I live in San Francisco and generally these flowers never do grow well, although in the summer of 1990 it was so hot that my beautiful neighbor child Kyra grew a virtual field of Calendula flowers to enjoy just for their beauty. Normally, I buy Calendula flowers from Montana Botanicals at Box 1365, Hamilton, MT 59840; call 406/363-6683. Call around. I am sure that there are several other companies that grow and pick organically grown Calendula (Marigold) that they will sell to you. You can also grow your own. But for me, Montana Botanicals was the place easiest to find.

In a recent book that I read, Calendula carrier oil was emphasized over and over again. I called every source listed in the back of the book—of the eight sources, six did not answer the phone and two did not carry the oil. So believe me, it pays to make your own.

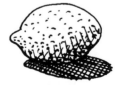

Chapter VIII

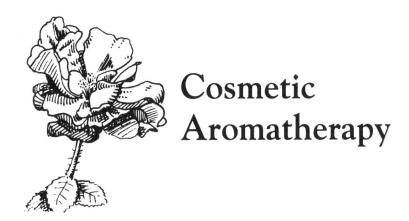

Cosmetic Aromatherapy

Applications for Hair, Head, Scalp, Face, Body

We think of the word *cosmetic* as "covering up" but it really means the *art of beautifying the body*. Beauty is not a word that we would typically use to describe what a man does to make himself and his appearance handsome— but it is the only word that we have. If you want a natural, wholesome look to your skin, of course you will want to use natural and wholesome ingredients not only upon your body but in it as well. You will want to use the clean, wholesome, natural essential oils in your body-care products to enhance their therapeutics. The word "cosmetic" comes from the Greek root word *kosmetico*, the art of beautification. The older meaning of this is from the word *kosmea*, meaning to harmonize. And this is what we want to accomplish when we make our own products with herbs and essential oils.*

There are many many formulas and recipes available listing ingredients for body-care products.* These formulas won't be repeated here, but they are new and tested on myself and friends and neighbors. No need for an extensive listing when you can easily add essential oils to products that you already own; you can use Chapter I as a basic resource for making your own

---

*adapted parially from *Kitchen Cosmetics* by Jeanne Rose. Berkeley: North Atlantic Books, 1988.

products from scratch. First you will need to know how many drops of essential oils you need to add to products to obtain their most potent results. Here is a simple chart.

The 2% Solution for Best Body-Care Results

Bottle Size			Drops of Oil Added
⅓ oz	or	10 ml	4 drops
½ oz		15 ml	.25 ml or 5 drops
1 oz		30 ml	.5 ml or 10 drops
2 oz		58 ml	1 ml or 20 drops
4 oz		115 ml	2 ml or 40 drops

Baths . . . Add 10–30 drops PEO per tub full of water, diluted in a bit of alcohol before adding to water

Facial Creams or Lotions . . . Add 10–15 drops PEO per tablespoon of cream, lotion or facial mask

Bath Oils . . . Add 10 drops PEO per tablespoon of carrier oil for one bath

Massage Oils . . . Add 10–15 drops of PEO per 2 tablespoons of carrier oil per massage

Hand Cream or Lotion . . . Add 3 drops PEO per teaspoon of carrier oil per application

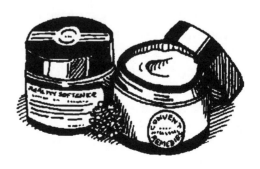

Hydrosol . . . Use pure hydrosols (water solution from distillation) for healing. Just spray and use. Keep hydrosols refrigerated.

Healing Hydro-mist for Wounds . . . Add 60 drops per 4 ounces of distilled water and keep for use (3% solution). Shake vigorously before each use.

After-Shave Lotion . . . Add 40 drops PEO to 1 ounce of Apple cider vinegar or alcohol. Shake vigorously. Add to 3 ounces of distilled water.

External Application on Zits, Acne Sores, Pimples . . . Apply 1 drop neat (undiluted) directly on blemishes.

Bath Salts . . . Add 15 drops to 1½ ounce mixed salts. Shake thoroughly. Age one week before using. Use the entire amount per bath.

Shampoo or Hair Rinse . . . Add 8–10 drops of essential oil per shampoo or rinse for a therapeutic treatment. Add only 2 drops per shampoo or rinse simply to perfume your hair.

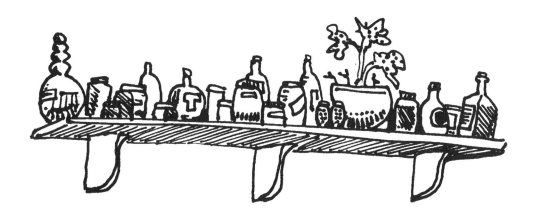

Cosmetic Aromatherapy for the Hair

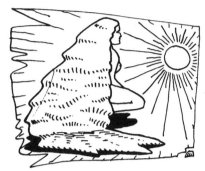

Oily Hair Shampoo . . . Add 8 drops Rose Geranium oil and 8 drops Lemongrass oil to any 8-ounce bottle of your favorite shampoo and use.

Dry Hair Shampoo . . . Add 8 drops Rose Geranium oil and 8 drops Sandalwood oil to any 8-ounce bottle of your favorite shampoo and use.

Dandruff Shampoo . . . Add 8 drops Rose Geranium oil, 8 drops Lemon oil and 8 drops Rosemary oil to any 8-ounce bottle of shampoo and use.

Normal Hair Shampoo . . . You can use any mixture of oils but a very nice combination would be 8 drops each of (1) Rose Geranium, (2) Lavender and (3) Lemon or Clary Sage, and add this to any 8-ounce bottle of shampoo and use. This mixture can be used for normal to oily hair, hair that is falling out, or for an irritated scalp. This mixture would also be very useful for smelly hair or for your pets, especially dogs.

Oily Hair Rinse . . . Make an herbal rinse* of herbs such as Lemongrass, Lemon and Rose Geranium, and add 8 drops of Rose Geranium and 8 drops of Lemon to every 8 ounces of the strained fluid. Use 2–4 ounces per shampoo. Remember that this is an herbal as well as essential oil rinse, and the herbs part will go bad within 4 days. Use this up and make fresh every 4 days. Refrigerate the excess.

Dry Hair Rinse . . . Make an herbal rinse* of herbs such as Chamomile, Red Clover and Orange peel. Strain it carefully and to the warm infusion add 8 drops each of Chamomile and Orange peel oil. Use 2 ounces in shampoo base or 2 ounces as a final rinse. Make sure to pour over the rinse, catch in bowl and pour over again as many times as possible. Remember that this is an herbal base as well as an essential oil treatment, and the herbal liquid will go bad. Use it up within 4 days and keep refrigerated between uses.

---

*Make a mixture of 1 ounce herbs to 2 cups water. Simmer a few minutes, steep and strain.

Dandruff Hair Rinse, also good for Irritated Scalp . . . Make an herbal rinse* using herbs such as Rosemary, White Willow Bark, Peppermint and Nettle. Strain it carefully and to the warm infusion add 8 drops each of Rosemary and Lavender oil, and 4 drops of Basil oil. Use 2 ounces in a shampoo base for shampoo or 2 ounces as a final rinse. Make sure to pour the rinse over the hair, catch in bowl and pour over again as many times as possible. Remember that this is an herbal base as well as an essential oil treatment and the herbal liquid will go bad after a time. Use it up within 4 days and keep refrigerated between uses.

Get Rid of That Dandruff-Shampoo or Rinse . . . In a blender grind up 1 hot Chilé Pepper and blend with 16 ounces of water. Pour this into a pot with ½ ounce Rosemary herb and ½ ounce Lemongrass or Lemon peel herb. Heat until just up to a boil. Turn off heat and steep, covered, for 15 minutes. Strain carefully through silk cloth or panty hose into a container.

At this point you have a very good anti-dandruff rinse to which you can add 6 drops of Black Pepper oil, 2 drops of Peppermint oil and 2 drops of Rosemary oil.

But you can go on with this formula and make the shampoo by adding half (8 ounces) of the hot, strained herbal liquid to 1 ounce of dried powdered castile soap. Stir together until the soap is completely dissolved. You may need to heat it up again (*gently*) for a few minutes. *Do not allow to boil.* Since you have already added the therapeutic quantities of essential oils you will now have 8 ounces of Dandruff Shampoo and 8 ounces of Dandruff Herbal Rinse. This should be enough for 4–6 shampoos and rinses.

A General Dandruff Formula . . . Wash your hair with a Scalp & Dandruff Shampoo. When hair is dry, rub hair and scalp with your palms, to which you have added a few drops each of Rosemary oil and Lemon oil. Massage into your scalp and brush with a soft hair brush. If your scalp is itchy, also add a few drops of Sandalwood oil.

A Hot Oil Formula for Glossy, Shiny Hair . . . Make a mixture of 3 drops each of Rosemary Verbenon and Lavender oil, 4 drops Lemon oil and 2 drops Sandalwood oil. Add this to 2 teaspoons of Walnut oil. After you have shampooed and half-way dried your hair, apply the oil to the scalp, rubbing gently. Try to keep the oil on the scalp rather than the hair itself. Wrap your head in a very hot towel. (I like to use real Linen tow-els.) Cover your head (not the face) with a thick plastic bag. Take a very hot shower, letting the hot water run over your head as well. After you are nice and clean and dry, remove the plastic bag and towel. Let your hair completely dry. Brush it regularly. If there is any oil residue left, leave it on the hair and shampoo again in 24 hours.

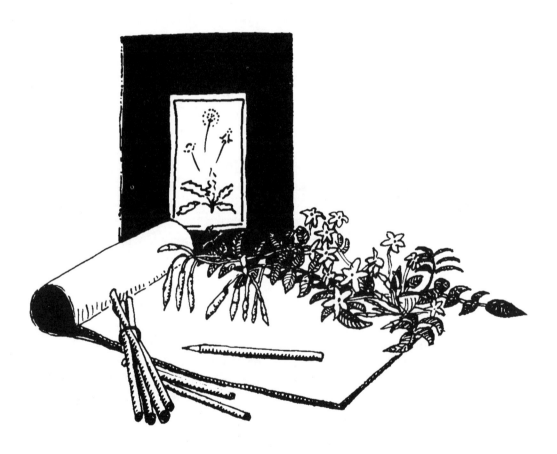

Additional Notes • Read Jeanne Rose's Herbal Body Book or Kitchen Cos-metics for many many more herbal and essential oil formulations for your hair, or add the correct essential oils to your current shampoo product using Chapter I for the appropriate essential oil combinations.

Cosmetic Aromatherapy for Skin

In the early '80s I formulated some wonderful essential oil therapies for problem skin for a well-known San Francisco firm, Skin Care Institute. These formulas are still in use and still clearing up various skin problems. They are quite simple, unlike some more recent formulations, but they are very effective.

The Basic Carrier Oil Base is composed of Calendula infused oil or Hazelnut oil with 10% Wheat Germ oil, vitamin E capsules, and 3% essential oil added. Make your base oil:

8 oz Hazelnut or Calendula-infused oil
1 oz fresh Wheat Germ oil
10 400 IU vitamin E capsules, punctured and the contents squeezed into the mixture

To every ounce of this base add about 20–25 drops of mixed essential oils for a 3% mixture. Use daily as a body oil.

Body Mask . . . A favorite formula of mine is a body mask. I take about 6 tablespoons of ionized clay (the fragmented type recommended by Neva Jensen) and mix it with a strong quart infusion of Red Clover, Calendula, Peppermint and St. John's Wort. I cover the body and thrill with the interaction of sunlight, herbs and special earth. It is truly a sensual and healing experience both on and off the body. —Paul Schulick of New Moon Extracts

Mature or Broken Capillaries . . . 10 drops Cypress oil, 5 drops Patchouli oil and 5 drops Blue Chamomile oil

Dry Skin . . . 5 drops Rose Geranium oil, 10 drops Sandalwood oil, 5 drops Rose oil

Acneic Skin . . . 5 drops each of Juniper Berry, Bergamot, Chamomile and Benzoin in the carrier oil or pulverized with enough white clay to make a facial mask.

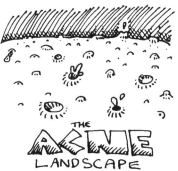

THE
ACNE
LANDSCAPE

Oily Skin . . . 5 drops each of Lemongrass oil, Lemon oil, Cypress oil, and Camphor oil or Clary Sage oil with 1 drop of Peppermint oil.

Puffy Skin . . . or as a compress for bags under the eyes. Use 5 drops each of Juniper Berry oil, Cypress oil, and Lavender oil. Fennel oil would also be nice here. Please remember: **Do not put essential oils directly into the eyes.**

Sensitive or Young Skin . . . 6 drops each of Neroli oil, Rose oil and Chamomile oil for inflammation. Rose Geranium oil is also good for regular use.

An Ancient Egyptian Remedy to Treat Wrinkles . . . is composed of equal parts of gum of Frankincense; wax, probably beeswax; fresh Moringa oil (*Moringa pterygosperma*), also called oil of Ben; and Cyperus grass. These are all finely ground together and then mixed with fermented plant juice. It must be applied daily.

—from *An Ancient Egyptian Herbal*
© Lise Manniche and British Museum Press

An Ancient Egyptian Remedy to Treat Bags & Wrinkles Under the Eyes
. . . Mix together equal quantities of clarified goose fat and kohl with ground lapis lazuli and honey. Apply gently to the eyelids and leave overnight.

Ancient kohl was a toxic mixture of antimony and fat, but a modern nontoxic version can be made with any finely ground soot from a cosmetic plant such as Marshmallow leaves or Cornflowers.

From the ancient herbal of Dioscorides comes the famous oil of Lilies that has been copied and used for centuries. It sounds very difficult and complicated, but if you halve and then halve again the ingredients you can indeed come up with a very creditable and wonderful formula for your complexion that uses herbs and oils and resins to very good effect.

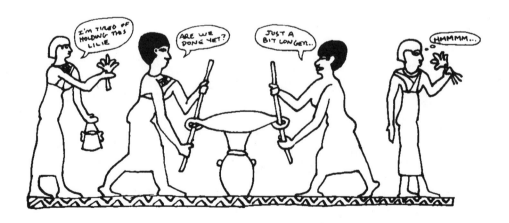

Susinon. Oil of Lilies

Mix together 9 libras* 5 ounces of oil, Calamus 5 libras* 3 ounces, Myrrh 5 ounces, in sweet-smelling wine, boil it, then let the oil run through a strainer, and add 3 libras* 6 ounces of Cardamom that has been bruised and macerated in rain water. Take 3½ libras of the thickened oil, 1000 Lilies that have been stripped of leaves and put into a broad, deep, clean vessel. Anoint your hands with honey and stir. Let stand for 1½ days. Strain carefully into another vessel. Do not let any of the water or filth into the clean, strained oil. Repeat this process adding Cardamom. It is important to use clean vessels and to keep the oil from being contaminated with water that may settle out. Take again 1000 Lilies stripped of their leaves and pour over them the clean, strained oil. Repeat this three times. "But by how much the oftener you shall macerated fresh Lillies therein, you shall have your ointment the stronger." Finally, when it seems enough, mix with 72 drachmas* of the best Myrrh, 10 drachmas of Crocus, 75 of Cinnamon. Beat it and sift it, put into a vessel with water, and pour in the ointment of the first expression: leave it for awhile, [strain or skim off the oil] and put into little dry containers that have been smeared with Myrrh gum, and with Saffron, & honey diluted with water. Repeat with the second and third expression.

This is better than that made in Egypt. It has a warming, mollifying, opening faculty and is good for inflammations of the vulva. When you drink it, "it expels choler, & it moves urine; but is hurtful for the Stomach."

—from Dioscorides Greek Herbal I.62, A.D. 512.

A Vitalizing Carrot Lotion

    3 grams Carrot oil
    2 grams Clary Sage oil
    5 grams Calendula-infused oil
    Add 50° alcohol to make 1 liter.

Mix all together and apply nightly. Carrot derivatives are rightly regarded as giving vigour and vitality to the skin tissues.

—after Gattefossé, *Formulary of Cosmetics*, 1928.

---

*The ancient libra is equal to our current 0.7221 pound and the ancient Greek drachma is our current 4.3 grams.

A Fragrant Water for Oily Hot Skin

I grow Spearmint and Tuberose and both are in full growth, and in the case of the Tuberose, full-bloom, in mid-August here in San Francisco. On those days when it is very warm and my skin feels so hot and oily, a cosmetic water of these plants is delicious and cooling. I drink it and apply it by a sprayer on my face and chest. As follows . . .

A Tea of Tuberose & Spearmint

Take 3 tops of Spearmint about 6 inches in length and place in a 12-ounce glass. Add 2 Tuberose flowers and fill the glass with warm water. Let this steep for a while and then strain off half of the water and place in a sprayer or container with a pump spray and chill. Drink the first 6 ounces as tea and spray the other 6 ounces that have been chilled, on your face.

A Cooling Spray of Fragrant Tuberose for the Skin

Take 6 ounces of chilled spring water or Ylang-Ylang water and place in an 8-ounce pump-spray container. Add 6 drops of Spearmint oil and 2 drops of Tuberose. Shake it vigorously each time before use.

The Tuberose oil and Ylang-Ylang oil are good to inhale or apply for oily skin or oily hair, to reduce depression, and to calm. It is wonderful to spray on your skin for wrinkles or to cool you if you are having a hot flash.

The Spearmint oil in water has a cooling and minty fragrance and is a good cleanser for acne or oily skin.

Facial Water for Dry or Puffy Skin

Mix together ½ ounce Fennel seeds and ½ ounce Rose Geranium leaves. Add 1 cup of water and let infuse, mashing gently with the back of a wooden spoon. Infuse cold for 20 minutes and then heat gently for 10 minutes more. Cool and strain through silk. Add 5 drops Rose Geranium oil. This mixture is delicate enough for the most sensitive skin. I have used it as a wash for my baby's fair white body as well as for my own darker skin.

For Oily Skin . . . Use a mixture of Lemon Peel, Lemongrass herb and 5 drops of Lemon oil.

For Inflamed Skin . . . Use a mixture of Chamomile and Rose herbs and 5 drops of Chamomile oil.

Gattefossé developed many lotions according to aromatherapy recipes for the care of the skin. They were used for "aromatising cold or hot water sprays, shower baths, steam baths, frictions or any other lotions that demand the use of aromatic waters or alcohols. They are usually prepared at 50° (strength of alcohol).

Tonic Lotion
7 grams Lavender oil
3 grams Clary Sage oil
5 grams Ambretta oil (substitute for 1% tincture of Musk)
5 grams Spikenard oil (substitute for 1% tincture of Civet)
5 grams Rose Geranium oil (substitute for 1% tincture of Castoreum)
This mixture can be added either to 50° alcohol or unscented white lotion to make 1 liter.

This is a tonic lotion as well as a sexual balancing agent. When applied to the face it helps to obtain a calm, relieved appearance and can be rec-

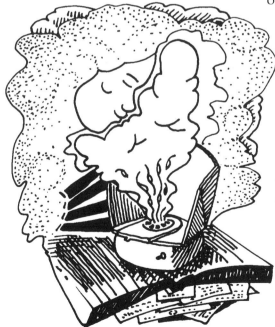

ommended for strains, overwork, and for application after disturbing nights."
—after Gattefossé, *Formulary of Cosmetics*, 1928.

Lotion for Herpes & Eczema
5 grams terpeneless Hyssop oil
5 grams terpeneless Lavender compound
Add to 50° alcohol to make 1 liter. Apply daily.
—after Gattefossé, *Formulary of Cosmetics*, 1928.

See Chapter I Table 1 for more combinations.

Cosmetic Aromatherapy for the Body

An Aromatherapy Bath for Silky Smooth Skin

You will be amazed at how smooth and silky your skin will feel after this bath. Even if you have never taken an herb bath, even if you never even considered the health and loving benefits of having velvet-soft skin, this bath will convince you. It is made up of a variety of elements including an herb bath with Seaweed, body brushing, and aromatherapy application.

(1) First you must make up an herbal formula. Soft skin will benefit from Rose, Lavender and Chamomile herbs. Men may prefer the more woodsy scents of Pine or Sandalwood. In any case use a mixture of at least 4 ounces of herbs and bring to a boil in 2 quarts of water. Immediately turn off the heat, cover the pot.

(2) The next step while your herbs are infusing is to give yourself a good body brushing using a loofah, turkish towel or soft body brush. Put a drop of stimulating essential oil on both sides of the brush. Brush from your toes up to your nose and your nose down to your toes. Brush from your fingertips to your heart. Brush in big upsweeping strokes or in great circular strokes. Now finally brush once more from toes to heart and from nose down to heart.

(3) Now take a cleansing shower with a good gritty soap like the ones that Barbara Bobo makes. (See Ohio, Chapter VI.) I particularly like the Barley Bran Soap or the Seaweed/Oatmeal Scrub.

(4) Run a nice warm bath and strain your herbal bath mixture into the water. Add a selection of oils that go well with the herbs. You must soak at least for 20 minutes to get the effects of the essential oils. Since your body is clean, the oils will actually be absorbed into the body.

A Silky Aphrodisiac Bath

1 oz each of Rose, Lavender, Sandalwood and Chamomile herbs in 2 quarts of water. The actual bath should also contain 3 drops of each of these oils: Rose, Lavender and Sandalwood.

A Woman's Bath

1 oz each of Rose, Lavender, Chamomile and Comfrey herbs in 2 quarts of water. The bath water to contain 3 drops each of Rose and Lavender oils and 1 drop of Chamomile oil.

A Man's Bath

1 oz each of Pine, Comfrey, Sandalwood and Lemon peel herbs infused with 2 quarts of water. The bath water to contain 3 drops each of Pine, Lemon peel and Sandalwood oils.

Where to Purchase: Buy your herbs from your local store or use any of the sources listed in Chapter VI. The *Herbal Body Book* by Jeanne Rose contains literally hundreds of bath herb formulations. Just remember to use the same essential oils as you did herbs, about 10 drops per bath. The Herbal BodyWorks in California makes very specific color, scented baths to stimulate particular chakras (see Chapter VI), and Barbara Bobo is the soapmaker in St. Paris, Ohio, that makes super specialty herbal soaps.

Deep Forest Bath or Potpourri Herbs

For inhaling, for respiratory health and to calm . . .
For bathing, to balance and harmonize skin function . . .

Mix together all sorts of freshly picked (if possible) Pine needles, Fir needles, Fern leaves, Cedar branches and Redwood branches. Scent each of these by sprinkling several drops of their own essential oil upon them. Fir would get sprinkled with Fir oil, Cedar with Cedar oil and so on. Use mostly brightly colored needles and very small branches. Pack into a plastic bag and then a paper bag so that the oils can become incorporated into the plant material. If you use fresh-picked plants, they must be used as soon as possible in your bath. If you dry the twigs and needles, the resulting bright-green heavily scented potpourri can be used to scent your home or in pillows as a sleep pillow. This will be very relaxing and enchanting, and a sleep pillow of the forest materials will encourage dreams that are pleasant and harmonious.

Your Deep Forest Potpourri will be enhanced if you can add dried branches of Sweet Fern or Licorice Fern as well as pieces of Sassafras. To every pound of green Fir and Pine needles add 1 ounce of Sassafras bark.

Your Deep Forest Bath herbs will be improved if to every pound of scented needles you add 1 ounce of Violet or Pansy leaf herb for skin health and Spearmint oil for added fragrant zip. The bath will be refreshing and stimulating especially if you are overtired, but will be relaxing to your mind (thought processes). So your bath can be both physically stimulating and mentally or psychically relaxing.

Relaxation Bath Oil

About 40 minutes before bed, step into a warm relaxing bath to which you have added a spray of Rose buds and 10 drops each of Lavender and Marjoram oils. Read a boring book, drink some Lemon Verbena tea. Stay in that tub for at least 20 minutes. Step out and wrap up in a nice thick flannel robe and go to bed. Keep reading, finish the tea. Rub a drop or two of Rose oil on your temples and turn out the light. You will quickly drop off to sleep and have wonderful dreams. This mixture of oils (Lavender oil and Marjoram oil) is also very good if you have any sort of joint pain or menstrual pain. It can be used in the bath or as an inhalant or mixed with a carrier oil for external body massage.

Lotion for Chapped & Cyanotic Hands
    2 grams Rosemary Verbenon oil
    1 gram Tansy oil
    2 grams Cinnamon oil
    1 gram Clove oil
    6 grams Calendula-infused oil
Add to 50° alcohol to make 1 liter of lotion.
Rub gently into hands when needed.
                             —after Gattefossé, *Formulary of Cosmetics*, 1928.

Anti-perspirant Lotion
    5 grams terpeneless essence of garden Sage
    5 grams Eau-de-cologne essence
Add to 50° alcohol to make 1 liter. Apply daily to the underarm.
                           —from Gattefossé, *Formulary of Cosmetics*, 1928.

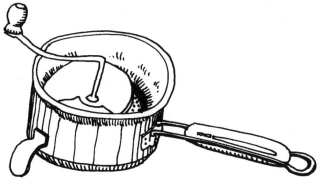

Lavender Body Powder Delight

Ingredients

    1 part powdered Blue or Black Malva flowers

    1 part powdered blue Bachelor buttons or Cornflowers

    1 part powdered Lavender buds, scented with a few drops of Lavender oil

    1 part powdered Violet leaves (optional)

Quantities . . . I like starting with 50 Lavender flowering tops (weighs about 6 grams, which is less than ¼ ounce). If the total weighs 1 ounce, you will have enough powder for 4–6 total body applications.

To Make: . . . Use dried herbs ground in a Coffee mill and sieved or buy herbs already powdered. Mix together the ground, dried herbs and store them for a few days so that the Lavender oil is thoroughly incorporated into the mixture.

To Use: . . . Simply apply with a powder puff, whenever necessary.

Why: . . . Lavender is used externally on any wound or sore or for burns or sunburns, on insect bites, and any irritation. This mixture of herbs is especially useful for sore or irritated skin, as the herbs are all considered emollient and antiseptic. This is a very soothing mixture that an athlete might use for jock itch or chafing. The scent will soothe and calm.

Feet Stink?

Make an infusion of Rosemary, Pine and Sage herbs. Soak feet in the herbal solution twice a day. Dry feet and rub with a mixture of 6 drops each of Sage oil, Pine needle oil and Tea Tree oil in 2 ounces of carrier oil. Use the herbal bath and essential oil rub twice a day for as long as necessary and don't forget to take zinc tablets.

    This formula will cure your feet of bad odor and heavy sweating.

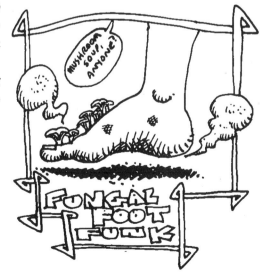

Lotion for Underdeveloped Breasts
    5 grams Verbena oil
    4 grams Caraway oil
    10 grams infusion of true Musk (1%)
Add to 50° alcohol to make 1 liter.
This can be used in morning frictions, but is preferably diluted with water. The lotion is intended to
firm the breasts and to develop them.
    —after Gattefossé, *Formulary of Cosmetics*, 1928.

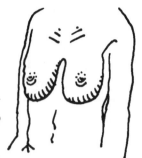

Lotion against Over-Development of Breasts
    3 grams Garden Sage oil
    2 grams Peppermint oil
    5 grams Lavender compound
    10 grams Calendula-infused oil
Use in evening as friction rub.
Add to 50° alcohol to make 1 liter.
    —after Gattefossé, *Formulary of Cosmetics*,
                             1928.

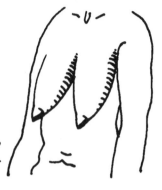

Chapter IX

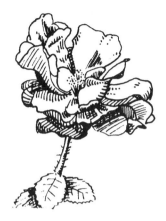

Cellulite Control

Another Phase of Cosmetic Aromatherapy

So you have fat, dimpled buttocks and thighs. You read somewhere that deep massage will help break up the ripply, dimpled, ugly mess. Do you massage with fatty oils? Of course not, for that is counterproductive. Make your massage mixtures with diluted alcohol, water-herbal infusions or herbs infused in vinegar to which you have added the perfect complement of essential oils. The way to get rid of cellulite:

(1) Drink plenty of water and no Tea, Coffee or alcohol.

(2) Eat simple nourishing foods, about 1200 calories per day. Include in your day's allowance of food 1 each of Orange, Apple, Tomato and Carrot to encourage good elimination. Eat several vegetable servings, a giant salad and vegetable or animal protein.

(3) Drink Obesity or Detoxify Tea (see below).

(4) Take daily Aromatherapy Cellulite baths.

(5) Scrub and rub the cellulite deposits daily with a loofah or hemp brush using the herbal formula given (Fennel/Orange Facial & Body Scrub).

An Aromatherapy Bath for Cellulite Control

In order for this bath to work, you must take it at least three times a week. You should also drink at least 1 liter of water daily and eat only a light diet high in vegetables and fruits.

(1) Make an herbal infusion of 1 ounce each of herbs of Lemon peel, Juniper or Pine or Lavender, Rosemary and Seaweed herbs. (4 oz herbs to 2 quarts water).

(2) Give yourself a 10-minute all-over brushing. I prefer to use an Imperial Loofah in the stimulating color of yellow (see Chapter VI, Herbal Body-Works, CA, for source). Use 1 drop of Lemon oil on the loofah.

(3) Take a brisk cleansing shower using Oatmeal/Seaweed Soap or any sort of gritty soap.

(4) Run a warm bath, pour in your strained herbal infusion and 1–2 whole Seaweed fronds if you have them. Add 3 drops each of Juniper oil, Lemon oil and Rosemary oil to a bit of alcohol. Shake and add to the bath. While you are relaxing in the tub, massage your lumpy rear-end and cheesy thighs with a washcloth or the loofah or even using a kneading motion with your hands. Rub yourself with the Seaweed.

(5) After 20 minutes in the tub, get out, pat dry and give yourself a massage using a vinegar friction rub. You may also give yourself a massage using essential oils in white lotion.* Complement the bath herbs using similar oils with the white lotion rub. A good mixture would be 1 oz of white scentless lotion* to which has been added 1 oz Calendula oil, 6 drops Lemon oil, 6 drops Rose Geranium oil and 4 drops Rosemary oil.

(6) Drink a cup of tea using DeToxify herbs.

Obesity Tea or Obesi-Tea
    juice of 1 Lemon
    finely chopped peel of ½ Lemon
    1 drop Lemon oil
    1 drop Lovage oil
    12 ounces of soda water
Stir thoroughly and drink once per day before breakfast.

---

    *White lotion is any homemade or commercial product made without grease but with vegetable oils and emulsifiers and without scent. I often use unscented Alba Botanica Very Emollient Body Lotion or make homemade Avocado lotion with lanolin and Orange flower water.

Obesity Herbal Rub

To 8 ounces of white vinegar, add 1 entire Lemon, juiced and chopped up

    1 drop Lemon oil
    1 drop Juniper oil
    1 drop Lavender oil

Steep for 10 days, shaking daily. Strain. Use this to vigorously massage your fat belly and thighs or sprinkle on a loofah or brush for a dry-brush massage. Use twice daily with the tea and a 1200-calorie per day diet. You will lose weight and gain good skin tone.

Detoxify Tea* for All Conditions

Parsley is one of several ingredients in this tea, which also includes a variety of herbs not generally mentioned in this particular book. But I feel this tea has an importance belying its seeming simplicity. The tea is used when dieting, instead of liquid when fasting, and to improve the all-over health of the body or the hair (drink it instead of other liquids during the day and see how cleansed you will feel). I prefer to have one day a week when I eat very little and drink this mixture, at least one quart a day: It acts as a mild diuretic and body cleanser.

You can easily get the individual ingredients from any herb store and mix them yourself. Use ¼ cup per quart of water, simmer 5 minutes, steep, cool and strain.

Using Dry Herbs *Can Be Mixed & Stored* *Away for Later Use*	**Using Fresh Herbs** *Must Be Used Immediately*
3 oz Parsley, CS**	1 bunch whole Parsley
1 oz Celery, CS	1 pinch chopped Celery tops
1 oz Fennel seeds, WH	1 pinch Fennel seeds, dried
1 oz Cherry stems, CS or WH	10–15 Cherry stems
1 oz Dandelion herb, CS	1 leaf chopped Dandelion
1 oz Couch grass, CS	1 pinch Couch grass
1 oz Corn silk, WH or CS	1 pinch Corn Silk
1 oz Blackberry leaves, CS	*from Red Indian Corn*
	1 Blackberry leaf

*by permission from *Kitchen Cosmetics*. Berkeley: North Atlantic Books, 1988.
**CS stands for cut and sifted; WH stands for whole herb.

Reduce Oedema Tea

½ peel of Mandarin or Tangerine
Chop or crush to break open glands in peel
1 Tablespoon Fennel seeds
1 Tablespoon chopped Parsley

Simmer 10 minutes in 10 oz water. Strain, pour into cup and add 1 drop Mandarin oil or Tangerine oil and 2 drops Fennel oil.

Fennel/Orange Facial Scrub & Cellulite Attack Powder

4 ounces of Cornmeal—best to buy whole Corn and grind it yourself to a coarse and gritty meal, but store-bought Cornmeal is okay.

4 ounces of Almond meal or Oatmeal—again, to make it gritty enough it is best to grind yourself, but it is easily purchased already ground in the health-food store. I usually buy Oat groats and grind them myself in the seed mill.

1 ounce of Fennel seed—grind coarsely in your grinder
10 drops Fennel seed oil
10 drops Orange peel oil
Other oils that can be added are Juniper Berry oil and Lemon oil.

Mix the powders together and add the oils. Stir vigorously and put away for a few days while the scents mix and meld. This is used as a simple facial scrub or body scrub.

For cellulite, rub your hips and thighs in a circular motion using a loofah and wash cloth. Take a 25-minute bath using 1 lb of Epsom salts. Stand up in the tub and take a small handful of the powder and rub the lumpy bumpy skin in nice firm circular hand motions. Rub yourself down from the waist and up from the knees. This should take at least 10 minutes. Then sit back in the tub, rinse off and rinse off again with a quick warm and then a cold shower. Use this regularly with dietary changes and the addition of drinking 2 quarts of water a day, and your cellulite should just melt away.

Chapter X

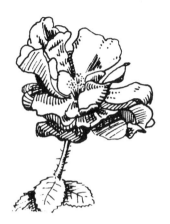

Perfume, Zinc, The Sense of Smell & Other Items of Interest

Scent . . . *"is an excursion into the world of aesthetics*
as old as the first Egyptian hieroglyphics and
ancient Chinese cultures . . .
as varied and fascinating as a stamp collector's
catalog (or baseball card collector's binder)."

—Edward Sagarin, 1945
The Science and Art of Perfumery

S mell is the most primitive and the most basic of the senses. It is the first sense. Why do we have a sense of smell? It is to pick a mate? Or to smell out an enemy? Or is it simply for pleasure—the pleasure of smelling sweet fragrance in the world we inhabit. The literature of smell is burgeoning at a rapid rate and entire books are being written on its metabolism as well as the whys and wherefores of the Sense of Smell. But one scientific fact that we do know for sure is that zinc, a trace element, plays a very important role in this sensory process. No zinc in your body? No sense of smell! Zinc is found in high concentrations in two parts of the human body—the retina of the eye and the male prostate gland. Maybe this is why having regular sexual relations is healthy for both partners through the absorption of seminal fluid in the vaginal tract. Zinc is also found in the secretions of the parotid gland. It is important in maintaining normal taste function.

Lack of zinc and you stink!

Zinc makes you think!

Zinc has been found to be of great importance in olfactory function. Patients with zinc depletion lose their sense of smell as well as sensations of taste. Zinc is present in the cells and fluids at each stage of the olfactory process and that implies some role of this trace metal at each of these stages. The role of zinc in the processing of smell information at the brain level is also unclear but of obvious importance.

Zinc is found in high concentrations in the hippocampal area of the brain, an area in which olfactory information is integrated into the brain.

How much zinc do we need daily to have an acute sense of taste and smell? No one really knows but it has been speculated that taking one 30mg zinc table every evening before bed is very helpful.*

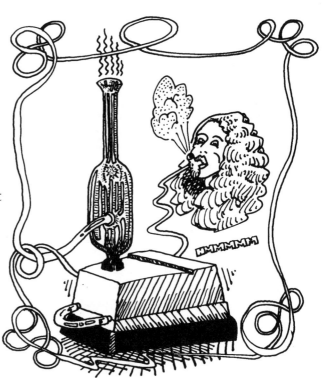

So we have the ability to discern odors for pleasure. We need zinc in our systems to ensure this ability. And we use perfume and fragrant oils to attract a mate or at least a mating partner.

Perfumes often retain their scent for centuries. An archæological team found a flask of perfume balsam near the Dead Sea Scroll caves. It is a pottery flask, holding 1½ ounces of balsam, that was covered in palm mat-

---

*For more information: see *The Journal of Olfaction*, Issue 1, 1978, "Why Do We Have a Sense of Smell?" by Dr. Robert I. Henkin and edition 2, 1979, "Zinc Metabolism and the Sense of Smell." Both of these issues are very valuable reading and available through the Fragrance Foundation (see Chapter VI, Source List, for address in New York).

ting. The only remaining residue of scent is oily and musky and it matches a description of the perfume called Persimmon oil as described by Pliny in A.D. 50. This oil was probably solar-distilled from a small bush-like plant that once grew on the edges of the Dead Sea. Persimmon oil was the most costly luxury in the ancient world and the ancient Israelites made the most famous of these oils, the formula of which was a carefully guarded secret.

To please Cleopatra, the Roman general Antony acquired an entire orchard of the precious Persimmon (Balsam) tree so that he would always be able to supply her with this favorite fragrance. It was costly and precious and worth twice its weight in silver.

Today the only surviving flask of Cleopatra's favorite scent is kept in a locked and padded box in the Israel Museum.

And what about the flowers—why do they have these volatile oils? I remember reading *The Secret Life of Plants* almost 20 years ago and being attracted by the following description, "Like animals and women, flowers exude a powerful and seductive odor when ready for mating. This causes a multitude of bees, birds, and butterflies to join in a Saturnalian rite of fecundations. Flowers that remain unfertilized emit a strong fragrance for as many as eight days or until the flower withers and falls; yet once impregnated, the flower ceases to exude its fragrance, usually in less than half an hour. As in humans, sexual frustrations can gradually turn fragrance into fetor."*

Scents have been subjected to odor classification since time began. Everyone seems to have their favorite method of organization. One of the more interesting was the "odophone" created by Septimus Piesse in *The Art of Perfumery* in 1867. The odophone was designed to be played like a glass harmonica with the fingers rubbing the glass bells, each of which would be scented with a particular odor. The fingers would release the scent and a fragrant symphony would result. A very exotic idea for that time as well as now.

The Secret Life of Plants by Peter Tompkins, New York: Harper & Row, Publishers, 1972.

273

Odor Classification

Septimus Piesse created an "odophone." He says that odors are like sounds, and a scale called "The Gamut of Odors" can be created from the lowest or heavier smells to the higher or sharper smells. Each odor corresponds to a key, a perfect mixture is called a bouquet. Some odors have neither sharps nor flats. To make the bouquet, the odors must be harmonious. As an artist would blend his colors, so must a perfumer blend his scents.

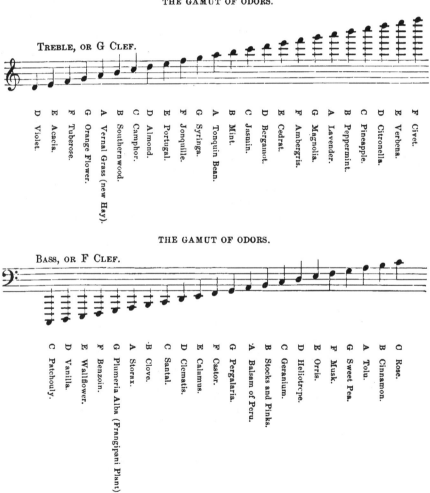

THE GAMUT OF ODORS.

From *The Art of Perfumery*, G. W. Septimus Piesse, 1867

274

Floral Clock

Another exotic invention in the 1800s was the Floral Clock, a planting of flowers in the garden designed to incorporate various plants that would release their fragrance during set hours of the day and night.

To take this one step further, women were encouraged to change their scent regularly to correspond with the correct hours.

Odors sometimes are better used at certain hours of the day, each hour being indicated by the opening of a particular flower. A flower clock can be grown in your garden that would have flowers that opened sequentially depending on the time of day. One could call this a Flower-dial instead of a sundial.

Eugene Rimmel in *The Book of Perfumes* (1865) suggests such a flower dial that he says comes from an even older botanical text:

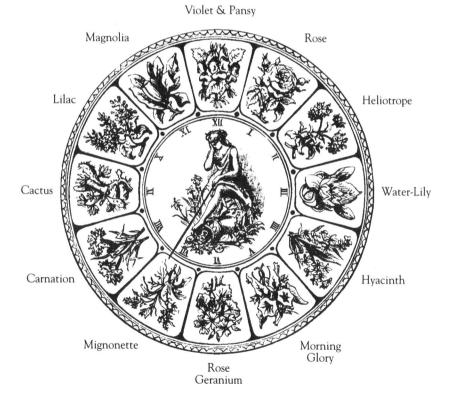

"And the Honeysuckle spices are wafted abroad
And the musk of the Roses blown"

—*The Book of Perfumes*

275

As a final note of fragrance in the garden, the Floral Clock was grown for its decorative use as well as fragrance. These special areas in the garden, called olitories, consisted only of plants with strong-scented foliage or flowers.

There were also many ways to extract fragrance (as outlined in Chapter V), but an early method of distillation was called "the Indian method" and was in use in 1750. This appears in a little book called *Rhodologia: A Discourse on Roses*, by J. Ch. Sawer, F.L.S., 1844.

He opines that the art of distilling Roses originated in Persia and was practiced at a very early date, at least since 810 A.D. Rosewater and Rose oil were used to sprinkle guests as they arrived as a sign of welcome, and when flavoured with Cinnamon and sweetened, it was taken as a beverage. In the Middle Ages Rosewater constituted an important article of commerce, and it was mentioned with other articles such as Balsam of Mecca and Camphor on various customs lists and registers.

The Indian Method of Distillation

About 40 pounds of fresh Roses (including calyces, but with stems cut close) are put into a still with 60 pounds of water, and distillation continued until 30 pounds of water come over (to the receiver), which is generally in about 4–5 hours. This Rosewater is distilled again with a fresh quantity (40 lbs) of Roses, and from 15–20 lbs of Rosewater is drawn over (to the receiver). This is poured into pans either of earthenware or tinned metal, and left exposed to the fresh air for the night. In the morning the otto or attar of Rose is found swimming on the surface. It is then carefully skimmed off with a thin shell and poured into a small flask, and then the water and any impurities and water are distilled again with fresh Roses. The yield of otto is about 1½ drachms from 80 lbs of Roses.

The Egyptians were wild about perfume oils and balsams and used them in excess. The perfumes were mostly oily and fatty to repel bugs as well as to protect against the heat. However, it has been my experience that using something fatty in the sun will only make a person hotter and sweatier.

Here is a favorite Egyptian formula for making scent.

To Make Scented Ox Fat. The Blending of Fats with Scent.

Any fat can have a sweet smell using this method. Remove the blood and skin from the calf or bull fat and pour over it some sweet-smelling wine and simmer it slowly overnight. Add more wine and simmer until the fat has lost its smell and smells like the wine. Skim the fat and add sweet-scented flowers, Rushes, Palma, Cassia, & Calamus, & Aspalathus, & Xylobalsamum, & mix with Cinnamon, Cardamom, Spikenard, of each one ounce. Simmer this altogether. The next day, pour out the old wine and add new and do this until the fat is sweet. Keep the vessels clean and scrubbed between the boilings. Now strain out the sweetened fat and add to it Myrtle, Thyme, and the roots of the Bulrush, as also Aspalathus, all thoroughly beaten. Simmer, strain and put into a new, clean vessel. Cool the fat. But if you would make it to smell sweeter, mix herewithall one ounce of "ye fattest Myrrhe, diluted in wine of many yeares standing."
—from Dioscorides II.91, edited by Robert T. Gunther, facsimile of the 1934 Edition from A.D. 512.

The solid mass of fat is shaped into a cone and placed inside the wig. During the day the fat melts and the fragrance and grease envelope the wig, clothing and body.

Nero, the Wasteful

Nero, ever wasteful of the public's trust and money, practiced every sort of vulgarity and obscenity and at one point built an immense palace. "Parts of the house were overlaid with gold and studded with precious stones and nacre. (!) All the dining rooms had ceilings of fretted ivory, the panels of which could slide back and let a rain of flowers, or of perfume from hidden sprinklers, shower upon his guests."(!)* We can only imagine what the costs were to his people, his guests and to the neighboring countries who had to come up with the extravagant amounts of flowers and perfume these gilded ivory panels let loose. One can only assume that he needed these great displays of scent to cover up the fact that he was described as having a body whose physical characteristic was pustular and malodorous.

---

* *The Twelve Caesars*, by Gaius Suetonius Tranquillus, translated by Robert Graves

The Signature Scent

Some Perfume Formulas to Make at Home

Signature scents can be made using Chapter I to find out the therapeutic value of each fragrance as well as just the pleasure of each scent as it passes through your nose and into your brain. The signature scent is what will always be associated with you and you can use it to scent your body, your clothing, drawers and stationery. An easy rule of thumb is to use 5 drops of a base note to 10 drops of a middle note to 20 drops of a top note. This is easy to remember when you are learning to mix your own scents for personal pleasure. Don't get complicated — in the beginning use only 3–5 scents.

Top Notes	Middle Notes	Base Notes
Basil oil	Clary Sage oil	Frankincense oil
Bergamot oil	Cardamom oil	Patchouli oil
Chamomile oil	Rose Geranium oil	Sandalwood oil
Cedarwood oil	Rose oil	Vanilla oil
Lavender oil	Ylang-Ylang oil	Tolu oil
Anise oil	Jasmine oil	Peru oil
Lemon oil	Neroli oil	Vanilla oil
Mandarin oil	Tuberose oil	Oakmoss oil
Verbena oil		

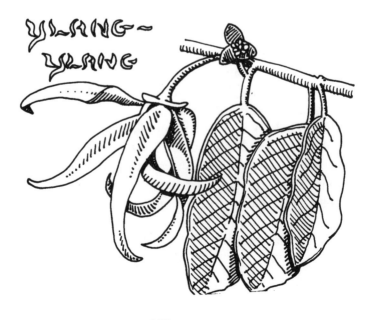

278

Amber's Signature Scent

> 1–2–3 Amber Rose
> for dry, sensitive skin or as a personal scent
> 1 drop Neroli oil
> 2 drops Rose oil
> 3 drops Sandalwood oil
> 7 ml (140 drops) Calendula-infused oil

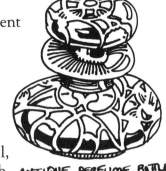

A Man's Citrus Fragrance

Mix together 10 drops each of Grapefruit oil, Bergamot oil and Orange peel oil, 7 drops each ANTIQUE PERFUME BOTTLE of Rose Geranium oil and Sandalwood oil, 4 drops each of Ylang-Ylang oil and Patchouli oil, and 3 drops each of Myrrh oil and Coriander oil, and 2 drops each of Vanilla oil and Oakmoss oil. Let this age at least 2 weeks before using. The scent gets more and more pleasant as the various parts meld.

Use as a base for massage oil, with diluted alcohol as a cologne, on sachets to scent clothing or stationary, or with spring water as a tonic spray after shaving. Ten drops of the mixed oils per ounce of carrier is about right.

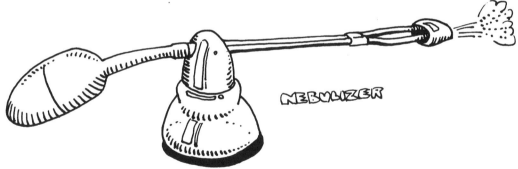

NEBULIZER

A Woman's Scent

Mix together equal quantities of Honeysuckle-infused oil with Carnation- or Wallflower-infused oil. To every 1 ml of this add 5 drops of Spanish Jasmine oil and 5 drops of Violet leaf oil. Let age before using.

A Young Man's Scent

Mix together equal quantities of Vanilla oil, Sandalwood oil and Mandarin oil. Or 5 drops Vanilla oil, 10 drops Sandalwood oil and 20 drops of Mandarin oil.

A Young Girl's Scent

20 drops Clary Sage oil, 10 drops Rose Geranium oil and 5 drops Sandalwood oil.

There are lots of mixtures that can be made. Just use your imagination and sense of smell and remember that you can attract more than birds and bees with your own signature scent.

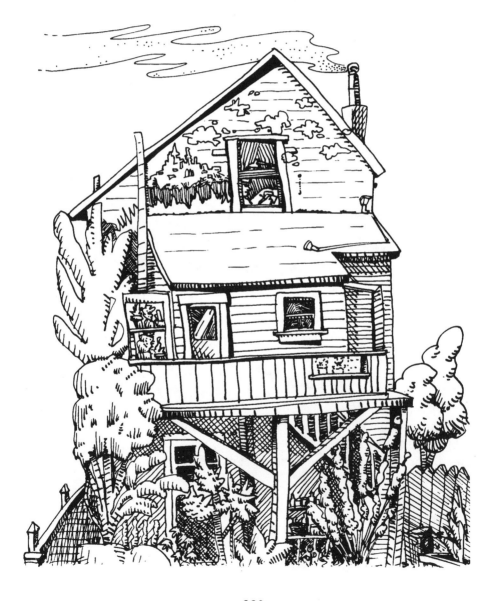

The Origin of the Temezcal
& Fragrant Toltec History*

The River of Floating Flowers & Eternal Beauty
& Origin of the Sauna in the New World

At the time Quetzalcoatl brought the arts to the Toltecs, the Princess Xochitl followed her father on the throne of the great Toltec empire. She had everything a mortal could have. Still, she was not happy because she did not consider herself beautiful.

One day she decided to see the Goddess of Beauty, Xochiquetzal, who was living in the River of Eternal Beauty, the River of the Floating Flowers (Lotus), not far from the Toltec capital. She asked the Goddess for the secret of beauty. Xochiquetzal told her that she could become beautiful only if she crossed the river without becoming wet.

She lost all hope, because no mortal could cross the river without touching the water; only Xochiquetzal was light enough to be able to walk on the floating flowers of the river. The Goddess departed with a malicious smile and the poor princess remained disconsolate, crying on the riverbank.

A little later three figures appeared walking along the river bank; Quetzalcoatl—the Wind God, Tonatinh—the Sun God, and Tlaloc—the Rain God. They tried to console the crying princess and decided to teach a lesson to the jealous Goddess of Beauty. The Rain God stopped the rain and the river started to go down. The Wind God blew harder and harder and the river waters started to dry up. The Sun God shone hotter and hotter and the remaining water started to evaporate. Finally, the princess was able to walk from stone to stone to the opposite bank of the river. The Sun God had caused the flowers to become warm and to scent the air with their dizzying essence. As she went through the aromatic vapors of the floating flowers without touching water, she became the most beautiful woman on earth.

At this moment, the furious Goddess of Beauty returned and with her enchanting song called the waters and the flowers of the river. They started to follow her until they reached the beautiful lake of Xochimilco and here the Goddess formed from the flowers the famous floating gardens of the lake. As the princess saw the waters and the flowers disappear, she again broke into tears.

---

*A little-known Toltec Legend, part of a speech given in San Francisco and Rancho La Puerta Spa during 1975 through 1978, by Jeanne Rose

But the three gods quickly stopped some of the receding waters and flowers by building a small adobe house in the river bed, the *temezcal*. Then the Sun God said to the princess: "The secret of beauty of the Goddess is really the fragrant vapors of the flowers floating on the water under my shining heat. I cannot stay longer to heat these waters since I have to go down the horizon, but I leave with you the stones that I have heated with my rays and whoever exposes her body to these aromatic vapors of the flowers will become as beautiful as yourself. Take some of these flowers and distribute them all over the land; tell your people to build similar stone houses, the *temezcals* (saunas), in every village, so all the Toltec maidens may also become beautiful."

The princess followed his advice and she still lives in the memory of the people as the princess who stole the secret of beauty from the Gods and Goddesses and gave it to mortals. And to this day not far from the old Toltec capital, the dry bed of "the River of Eternal Beauty" that was abandoned by Xochiquetzal is still visible.

Temezcal

The stone houses, or *temezcals*, of the the Toltecs and the Aztecs were small rooms of adobe or stone built adjacent to the temples. The entrances were so tiny that a person could not walk through them while completely upright. In the corner opposite the entrance was a section containing a little lake of hot water and stones, and the lake was covered with fragrant flowers and herbs. Fragrant herbs were continually being thrown on both the hot water and the stones. At the door to the temezcal stood an image of the god of health or maybe of air or sun or water. The Aztecs were quite down-to-earth about their temezcals, and despite the pretty legend you just heard, regarded the use of heat and fragrance in a temezcal as chiefly a health measure. For the sick, the hot, scented air had a stimulating effect on circulation and the metabolism.

The Solomon of the pre-Columbian Aztecs, King Netzahualcoyotl, a great legislator and builder and composer of quite exquisite poetry, gratified his æsthetic instincts by constructing a luxurious temezcal of eight rooms, clustered about a central room. The King passed from one room to another, and in each room different herbs and flowers were vaporized — each for a different part of the body. In the central room he relaxed to receive a massage with fragrant floral oils. The eight-room temezcal became a fixture until the Conquest. Now these large temezcals lie in ruins, but smaller ones still are in use in different parts of Mexico.

Imagine sitting, peacefully, privately, in a small room heated to a comfortable 100° or 110° with warm, healing fragrance permeating the air. The only sound is the bubbling of the water while the herbs and flowers heat enough to release their essence. You lie back and relax and the oils from the plants, transformed into vapor, surround your skin. Your body absorbs the sweet-smelling vapors and your skin and complexion take on an unbelievable softness and clarity. Your mind relaxes through fragrance and tension slips away. Here is the secret that the nose, the sense of smell, shares with the entire body.

You may make a vapor room or temezcal of your own bathroom. You can use a Silex type coffee-maker. Place water in the bottom and cotton that has been saturated in flower oils in the top. Plug into a wall socket and soak in a warm bath or sit in a straight-back wooden chair. The water boils, and turns into a steam that releases the fragrance into the atmosphere. Relax in your private temezcal for at least 20 minutes, letting the fragrant steam and warming waters do their healing work.

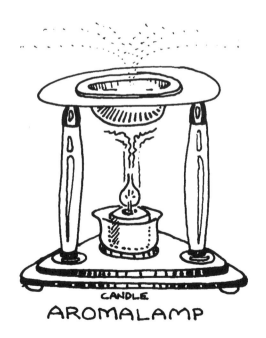

CANDLE

AROMALAMP

The Perfume Vendor

by Gloria Rawlinson—child poet of New Zealand

"Ben Neroli was said by his fellow-merchants to have lost his reason through 'watching the fern' on St. John's Eve."

"He has just returned to the bazaar after a long absence."
Oh! My place is taken I see—
The other Vendors envy me,
The perfume-merchant Neroli.
Ah, well! It does not matter where
I pitch my little stall, for there
I will soon be hemmed about
With buyers—no need for me to shout
Like those who sell their worthless trash—
Beads and bright shawls, and shout for place

I have traveled afar—
To the Valley of the Var,
The Holy River, Arabia, and Peru.
I am come home
To my scent bazaar,
With the rhizome
of Iris Florentina,
(You call it orris-root)—
Gum-resins, myrrh, opoponax,
Tolu, and sandal-wood, storax,
And fifteen ounces of oil of cedar to boot—
Otto of peppermint, lavender, and rose—
Nobody knows
The trouble I have seen in procuring this
Stock of civet and ambergris.

Two months ago, or more, I went
At a Grande Madame's bidding to find out
If the musk had lost its scent,
Well—it has not,
and here is a bouquet I have compounded her,
Of orris, civet, musk, jonquil, and lavender.
Neroli's Narcissi Bouquet—
I shall sell a lot of this,
Sixty-three shillings per one-ounce phial—
A very fine array

Of cut glass bottles for grand ladies—no cheap
Mock perfumes on my shelves I keep.
Upon my silver scales I weigh
My oil and essence, olibanum and bouquet.

"Ben Neroli—Ben Neroli—
Will you please allow me
To dip
My little finger-tip
In the jasmine bowl?"
The Jasmine Bowl!
God bless my soul!
They do not seem to realize
That scent belongs to Paradise.
I give nothing away—but I hope
They note the perfume of my heliotrope.

I talk to myself. Yes, yes, I find
That many scents obscure the mind.
They say that when poor old Neroli dies
He'll mutter perfume praise in Paradise.
Ah, well! Some lives are like the phials of scent I sell,
Until the Holy grass is crushed, who knows what it can tell?
Carefully those little drops of attar I have measured,
Exhaled from what that waiting grass had tasted of and treasured.

On St. John's Eve (the twenty-fourth of June),
I watch the fern in solitude an hour,
For it puts forth, at dusk, a small blue flower,
Which I must gather quickly, ere the moon
Climbs high, and the blossoms disappear.
See I here is the perfume from the Wishing Fern—
A very slight return
For all my fairy work last year.

"Good Ben Neroli, whom everybody knows,
Have you any verbena, wall-flower, or rose?
For I am in love, and I wish for my shawl
One little drop of the scent from your stall."

Oh, Love is like the scents I sell, if sweet and crystal-pure,
It holds the fragrant loveliness of things that will endure.

The Grande Madame has just bought from me
Oil of geranium, bay-leaf, and patchouli.

Her choice is strange? Oh, yes. You know there are
Some very curious folk in this bazaar.
See this sweet child—her weary little feet
Falter towards my stall—I greet
Her with the fairy scent I made
On St. John's Eve, blue flowers from the glade
Where the Wishing Fern grows—
Frangi panni, and wild white rose.
I have known her since—now let me see—
On St. John's Eve, her years were twenty-three—
And it was twenty years ago, last Michaelmas,
When first she smiled
On this same perfume-vendor,
Oh! poor child, poor child!

The promise of her youth is unfulfilled.
"Mad as Old Neroli!" the sharp-folk say,
"'Twas love of beauty made her reason stray,
Or love of Love—Mad as Old Neroli—
A jettatrice! A sorceress is she!"
To me she is like the scents I sell—the promise unfulfilled
Will become the fragrant essence of her Life—in Death distilled.

Gloria Rawlinson is said to be hale and hearty and still living in New Zealand as of April, 1992.

The Perfume Vendor Poems, by Gloria Rawlinson, Hutchinson & Co. Publishers Ltd., London, England, September 1935.

Chapter XI

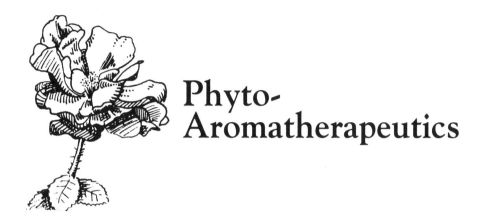

Phyto-
Aromatherapeutics

For Your Favorite Humans & Pets

We see from the chart in Chapter V that essential oils when inhaled affect the body through a psychological process of the brain as well through the circulation of the blood. And when essential oils are applied to the skin they are absorbed dermally and affect muscle tissue that also affects the joints. Via the muscle tissue the essential oils are absorbed into the blood stream and the small intestine, where their chemical components go through the body to affect all the body tissues and organs, finally to be excreted through the skin, kidneys and bladder. Some physicians, particularly those in Europe, inject essential oils into muscle tissue and the blood stream, as well as recommending their use in oral medications. These applications are certainly beyond the scope of this book, and if you are interested in internal uses of the essential oils the primary text would be *The Practice of Aromatherapy* by Jean Valnet, as well as some small booklets produced by Dr. Penoel and Mr. Franchomme (see Bibliography).

There are certain internal uses of essential oils that anyone can practice such as taking a drop of Peppermint oil on a sugar cube and sucking it for relief of indigestion and nausea. Make a mixture of Rosemary oil, Lemongrass oil, Ginger oil and Angelica oil, and use this both by inhalation as well as a drop on the tongue for relief of jet lag.

Certainly there are formulations for essential oil therapy for all sorts of physical conditions including healing deep wounds (see Lavender, Chapter III), arthritis, cancer, infections of the reproductive organs, cystitis, first-aid, etc. I have seen recommendations for uses of massage oil therapy for all these conditions. However, besides deep wounds and the other healing indications as outlined in Chapter III, essential oil therapy has been very important to me in the last five years for respiratory problems and for arthritis.

I have found the following respiratory blend to ease the many problems that are associated with bronchitis and asthma. It seems to work as well on flu and colds.

Respiratory Blend

This is a mixture of oils that has especial use in the diffusor or in the AromaLamp to ease the problems of COPD (chronic obstructive pulmonary disease), bronchitis and asthma. I use it regularly when I have symptoms of "wet" asthma, that is, when there is a lot of mucus and snotty discharge. All of these oils can be purchased from Leydet Oils or from any source of therapeutic-quality essential oils. I originated the formula but Victoria Edwards improved it with certain additions.

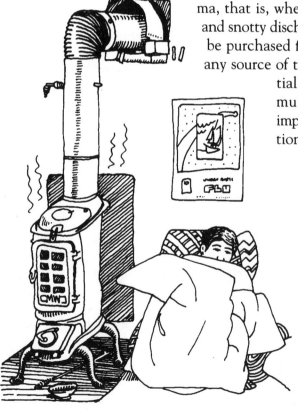

Eucalyptus polybractea	4 parts
Hyssop cineol	1 part
Inula graveolens	1 part
Basil eugenol	2 parts
Lavender	2 parts
Myrrh	2 parts (to stimulate thyroid)
Ammi visnaga	3 parts (to mask mast cell production)
Chamomile, Roman	3 parts (to stimulate adrenal function)
Peppermint, opt.	1 part (uplifting, cooling)

Apply to the chest in a rub containing these oils in a base of Olive oil or Cocoa butter. Use the Respiratory Blend in the diffusor or vaporizer as well.

Respiratory System Remedies

EXPECTORANT : Inhaled :
3 drops Juniper
2 drops Melissa
1 drop Inula
1 drop Sage
                —from Gattefossé

BALSAMIC, Soothing & Restorative: Inhaled :
4 drops Eucalyptus
2 drops each of Thyme, Hyssop and Cubeb

SEDATIVE, Calming & Sleep-Producing : Inhaled
4 drops Marjoram
2 drops Sage
1 drop Peppermint
While drinking 11 ounces of Meadowsweet tea

Regular use of Rosemary oil, Lavender oil, Wild Thyme oil and Cinnamon oil is recommended by Gattefossé for the respiratory system.

For any physical condition that affects the joints and muscles, for athletes and the infirmed, the pain-killing qualities of Chilé and Comfrey root will come in handy. This formulation makes a large quantity of product that can easily be stored for use.

Pain-Killing Formula for Aching Body Parts

Use externally for arthritis, gout, osteoarthritis, aching joints, muscles, sprains and strains, football knees, tennis elbow, etc.

 Ingredients:

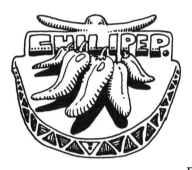

8 oz fresh Cayenne or Habeñero Chilé
    Pepper chopped, or 6 oz dry chopped
    Chilé Pepper
1 quart Olive oil
4 oz fresh Rosemary or 3 oz dry Rosemary
4 oz fresh Comfrey root, finely sliced or
    chopped or 2 oz dry Comfrey root soaked
    in 2 oz boiling water for 20 minutes.

Bring the above ingredients to a low boil, turn down heat and simmer gently for 4 hours. I like to use a copper and ceramic double boiler but a pyrex double boiler or stainless steel bain-marie will also suffice. After simmering for 4 hours turn off heat and cool for 4 hours and repeat this process at least three times. You want to allow enough time for the heat to extract all the active and pain-killing ingredients from the herbs, and intermittent heating and cooling will accomplish this more effectively than one long cooking session. When the oil has gone from yellow to green and then to a nice persimmon-colored red, put the contents into a blender and blend for 20 seconds. Heat again and cool. When cool enough to handle, strain carefully through a sieve that has been lined with silk or a panty hose leg.

Heat together 1 quart of the Chilé Pepper oil and 6 oz beeswax or 8 oz solid Cocoa butter until the solidifier is melted, stir thoroughly, and add 20 drops Lavender oil, 20 drops Marjoram oil, 20 drops Frankincense oil and 20 drops Eucalyptus oil. Stir together and bottle in flat cream-type jars that can hold 4 ounces of cream. Makes 8.

Aromatherapy Cures for Pet Problems

#1 • To heal irritated skin, hot spots, fungal infections

Begin with 2 oz bottle
   10 drops Tea Tree Oil
   10 drops Balsam Tolu
   up to ¼ oz Rose Hip oil
Fill with Calendula-infused oil
Apply freely.

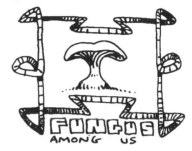

#2 • To Repel Fleas & to Deodorize

Make a strong infusion of Pennyroyal herb in water (1 large handful fresh herb in 2 cups water, bring to gentle boil, turn off heat, cover, and infuse until cool enough to use. Strain through a gold sieve or cheesecloth. Refrigerate for use.

To 4 oz of the Pennyroyal water add
   20 drops Tea Tree oil
   20 drops Rose Geranium oil
   6 drops Lavender oil

This particular mixture is excellent and seems to harmonize with dog smell. Some essential oils make dogs smell nasty, but for a house dog nothing is more complementary than Rose Geranium oil. Some "experts" state that Tea Tree oil will kill fleas. But either their fleas are easy to kill or San Francisco fleas are impossible. I found that even dunking fleas in this mixture did not kill them, although they eventually drowned. But it did *repel* them and it made my stinky smelly dog quite pleasantly fragrant.

I recommend that if you have a particularly difficult flea problem, first have the dog professionally dipped and shampooed. While this is being done spread about 6 lbs of salt/100 ft sq area in your house and leave it sit for several hours and then vacuum carefully using a few drops of Rose Geranium oil in the vacuum bag. You could also spread diatomaceous earth about your rugs. The sharp edges of the earth pierce the fleas, dry them up and then they can be vacuumed. When the dog gets back from the kennel, all nice and clean and the house de-flead, spray the dog from head to toe with this liquid mixture. Make sure you cover the dog's eyes so that the spray won't get into them.

#3 • Cleansing, Deodorizing Foot Wash

One Lemon squeezed into 2 ounces of water to which 10 drops of Lemon oil have been added. With a nonabsorbent pad or your hand or a sprayer, wipe the doggy feet every time he comes in from the outside. (Goes good on funky husband feet also.)

A Coptic Bug Repeller can be made by adding a little Galbanum resin, a little realgar (an orange-red mineral that contains Arsenic sulphide) and a little goat's fat. Put on the fire and add Bayberries. Steep it in the simmering water until it dissolves and then sprinkle the house with this.

—from a Coptic text

You can make this formula at home and it will work just as well by simply mixing Galbanum oil with water, deleting the realgar and goat's fat. Add Bayberry oil and bring to a simmer and then sprinkle on all the rugs and in the corners of the house.

Anti-Parasite Lotions

These are seventy-year-old formulas but still effective. "Anti-parasite lotions and vinegars have always enjoyed a fairly constant market. To popularize such preparations in the colonial civilizations of the Empire would be a very good thing.

In general these preparations consist of alcoholic solutions containing essences, oleoresins or synthetics, the anti-parasite activity of which is known."

#1

Oleoresin of Pyrethrum	0.2 grams
Essence of Artemisia	0.2 grams
Eau-de-cologne essence	0.6 grams
Alcohol 70°	99 grams

#2

Oleoresin of Derris	0.2 grams
Chenopodium oil	0.1 gram
Santalol	0.2 grams
Lavender oil	0.5 grams
Alcohol 70°	99 grams

#3

Ethyl phthalate	1 gram
Ethyl benzoate	1 gram
Tansy oil	0.2 grams
Rosemary oil	0.2 grams
Artificial Rose oil (?)	0.6 grams
Alcohol 75°	97 grams

#4

Oleoresin of Derris	0.2 grams
Benzyl Benzoate	1 gram
Thyme oil	0.3 grams
Lavender oil	0.7 grams
Alcohol 60°	97.8 grams

—after Gattefossé, *Formulary of Cosmetics*, 1928.

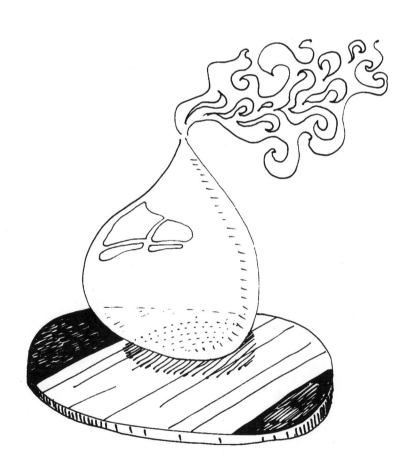

Chapter XII

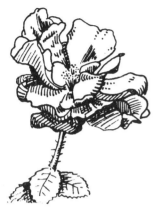

Inhalations for the Mind, Inhalations for Your Home Yummy Fragrance to Eat or Drink

"If one should ask you
What is the heart
of island Yamato;
it is the mountain cherry blossom
Which exhales its perfume
in the morning sun . . ."

—Moto-ori

Surround yourself and your life with scent. Your surroundings are important. The colors, textures, scents of your clothes, accessories and furnishings can create a mood. Together they make a statement, to support or intensify the effect you wish to create in life. Scent has an emotional quality that you can use to create the specific environment or feeling you wish to convey in your home.

Scents have aesthetic, healing qualities. They can be calming to create a relaxed environment, they can be energizing to give you a boost when you need extra energy, they can be purifying to rid the air of germs, they can be warming when the temperature is low or cooling should the weather be warm.

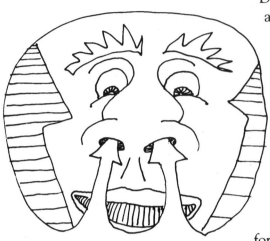

Dabs of oil can be put on light bulbs and will evaporate, wafting about and creating special sensations. A few drops of oil added to steaming bath water can calm a frazzled psyche and relax tense muscles. Use a diffusor—an ingenious device—that allows a fine mist of essential oils to diffuse into the air. It allows the slow dispersion of micro-particles of essential oils into a room. These particles stay suspended in the air for hours, refreshing and cleansing it. One particular combination of scent that I especially like is a soothing, euphoric mixture of Ylang-Ylang oil, Orange oil and Rosewood oil. The sweet, woody scent of the Rosewood blends perfectly with the floral Orange and the voluptuous and exotic Ylang-Ylang, creating a perfect blend that calms, relaxes the frustrated and soothes the angry. This is a perfect combination that can be used as a background for a sophisticated dinner party or a peaceful visit with a friend.

Some Inhalations for the Mind

Each of us is different and each of us has different memories and different scents associated with these memories. Aromemories can be a powerful tool used to ease life or job stress. So certain scents can make you alert, certain others calm and some will leave you refreshed. Generally speaking these aromas can be classified into these three categories, and some companies are using scent to induce states of mind in the work place. The Japanese are on the cutting edge of mood-altering fragrance systems and surely the rest of the mechanized world cannot be far behind.

Use a diffusor, or simply inhale the scents from a bottle.

Some essential oils that will wake you up and keep you *alert* are Eucalyptus, Lemon, Peppermint, Pine, Ginger and Rosemary.

Some essential oils that will *calm* you down are flower scents such as Jasmine, sometimes Lavender, and scents from the woods such as Juniper and Fir. Even Pine scent, which is considered stimulating, also has a calming side to it. When inhaled it keeps you awake but not agitated.

Some essential oils that are very *refreshing* to the psyche are the citrus scents such as Lemon, Grapefruit, Lime, Mandarin and Orange peel.

When using essential oils to work on your brain, inhale them through the nose. For respiratory problems inhale through the mouth and nose, and for circulation inhaling through the mouth is most effective.

General Inhalations for the Mind

To Relieve Aggression . . . Blue Chamomile oil, Bergamot oil, Lavender oil, Marjoram oil

To Soothe and Relieve Anger . . . Blue Chamomile oil, Marjoram oil, Rosemary verbenon oil, Ylang-Ylang oil

To Relieve Depression or a Depressed State . . . Basil oil, Bergamot oil, Chamomile oil, Citrus oil, Frankincense oil, Geranium oil, Jasmine oil, Lavender oil, Neroli oil, Patchouli oil, Peppermint oil, Rose oil, Sandalwood oil, Spearmint oil, Ylang-Ylang oil

To Relieve Anxiety . . . Lavender oil, Chamomile oil, Patchouli oil, Melissa oil, Marjoram oil, Geranium oil, Orange oil, Clary Sage oil, Rosemary oil

Cannot Lie Down or Relax . . . Marjoram oil, Lavender oil, Clary Sage oil, Basil oil

For Panic Attacks, To Relieve Panic . . . Juniper oil, Lavender oil, Geranium oil

To Relieve Grief or an Aching Heart . . . Marjoram oil

Bryan's Anger Oil and To Build Self-Esteem . . . Ylang-Ylang oil 20 drops, Rosemary verbenon oil 10 drops, and Marjoram oil 5 drops. Mix together. Use in a diffusor. Three times per day for at least 20 minutes each time.

Expand the Mental Processes . . . Anise oil, Fennel oil

To Relieve the Memory of a Traumatic Hospital Experience . . . Thyme oil followed by Vanilla oil

To Comfort and Soothe . . . Carnation oil, Chamomile oil, Jasmine oil, Melissa oil

For Those Who Sigh Too Much . . . Marjoram oil, Melilot scent, Marigold flowers

For Those Who Have Lost Their Senses . . . The scent of Hay or Sweet Clover, the scent of Melilot

To Revive Warm Loving Memories . . . Vanilla oil, Spearmint oil

Sedative Lotion . . . 5 grams Neroli water and 3 grams Rose complex to 50° alcohol to make 1 liter. A night's sleep is compensated for by this lotion or by Orange flower water, a teaspoonful of which is used in the wash-basin and somewhat more in a bath.

—after Gattefossé, *Formulary of Cosmetics*, 1928.

An Inhaled Tale
Calming & Relaxing for an Active Household

One Sunday, my children and I along with various friends and babies and two large dogs were in the living room, talking, playing, watching television. The noise level rose and rose, the hysterical quality of conversation became more and more noticeable, my friend and I started to yell at the kids, and the two 14-year-old boys then rode their bikes through the throng. Well, it was just too much. Without asking anybody to go to bed or to go outside and without making any obvious action, I simply added the scent I call Calming (Relaxant) to the diffusor that I keep on top of the television set. The change in the room was quite remarkable. Within 10 minutes, the two large dogs were lying down at two different corners of the room, the two babies were relaxed, one was cooing and chewing its finger and the other was nursing (the mother of course had quieted down and calmed so that baby could nurse), my older daughter started to speak more softly and asked if she might turn off the TV set, and the two boys decided that they were so incredibly exhausted after a full day of play that they were going to bed early.

Aromatherapy works! Aromas have the ability to alter moods through the direct inhalation of the odors. Inhalation affects the mind in a psychological way by acting directly on the mucous membranes of the nose and thereby being absorbed into the brain through the blood circulation.

A calming scent can contain many essential oils, but three potent relaxing fragrances are from the peel of the Sweet Orange, the leaf of the Marjoram herb and the luscious oil from the flower of flowers, Ylang-Ylang.

A Calming Scent for Your Home . . . 5 drops Ylang-Ylang oil, 10 drops Marjoram oil and 20 drops of Orange oil. Chamomile oil could also be added.

Aromatherapeutics for Sleeping . . . Drink a cup of Lemon Verbena tea and inhale the fragrance of Marjoram and Lavender. Sleep on a Hops pillow.

Aromatherapeutics for Waking Up . . . Can't wake up in the morning? Drink a cup of Cowboy Coffee (see formula that follows), take a shower or bath with Rosemary oil, inhale the fragrance of Basil oil and Peppermint oil.

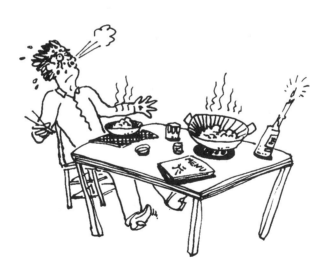

Inhalations for Your Home

Potpourri Green and Golden

When inhaled, this scent is used to stimulate the mind and intellect. Some people, however, have an opposite reaction to the Yellow color and it can create an environment of anger. Once when I had a brilliant yellow and orange kitchen, I could never understand why I was always angry when I cooked. Then I learned about aromatherapy and color therapy and realized that yellow and Lemon scent were an excitable color and aroma. But for the very phlegmatic and those who are extremely slow to show emotion this could be a wonderful potpourri to keep around the home or in pillows. This could also be used when studying to stimulate the mind and memory.

Green color for balance and harmony

> 1 cup dried whole Lemon Verbena leaves, sprinkled with 6 drops of essential oil of Lemon Verbena
> 1 cup dried whole Lemon Balm leaves

Yellow color to stimulate

> 1 cup Chamomile flowers
> 1 peel of 1 Lemon, chopped and dried, sprinkled with 6 drops of essential oil of Lemon peel
> 1 cup yellow Marigold petals, dried
> 1 cup yellow or green whole herb or flower petals, your choice

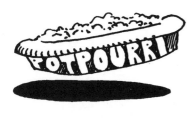

Mix the above together and sprinkle over it ½ cup Orris root powder. Seal in a container and leave to cure for about 6 weeks. It should be kept in a very dry and warm place, out of the light. Shake at least once a week. Then put into pillows or leave in potpourri jars that can be opened when you wish to inhale the aroma and create a special atmosphere.

Easy to Use Smell-Good Drawers . . . (Despite the name this has nothing to do with underpants.) This easy remedy using herbs and essential oils will fragrance clothing, deter wool moths and keep your bureau drawers smelling clean and fresh. Pick or buy small immature Oranges and Lemons. Here in California, citrus trees are a common sight and often the immature fruits simply fall to the ground. However, if you live where there are no citrus trees you can purchase the immature dried fruits by mail order from various herb companies that specialize in potpourri ingredients. So pick or buy 50–100 immature citrus fruits and let them dry thoroughly. Place them in a thick plastic bag or box and sprinkle about 1 ounce of pure Orange oil on them. Seal them up for several weeks. They are now ready to use and can be placed in lingerie bags or bureau drawers, in the pockets of wool suits or in hat bands, in stationery boxes to scent your fine papers, in linen closets and on towel shelves to fragrance and eliminate stale odors.

Another fine formula for use on dried immature Oranges is the fragrance called "A Man's Citrus Fragrance" (see Chapter XI).

This is good inhalation therapy for you as well. The Orange scent will relieve anxiety, calm your nerves and relieve a nervous disposition.

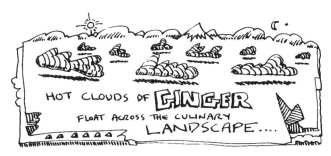

HOT CLOUDS OF GINGER FLOAT ACROSS THE CULINARY LANDSCAPE....

Yummy Fragrance to Eat or Drink

Richard Hilton, who owns Herbal Effect in Monterey, California, likes to add essential oils to food and drink and came up with this remarkable wake-up no-caffeined drink called:

Cowboy Coffee
    1 oz roasted Dandelion root
    ¾ oz roasted Chicory root
    ½ oz Sarsparilla root
    ¼ oz Cinnamon chips
    ¼ oz Licorice root
    A pinch of Cardamom
    1 drop of Anise oil per 2 cups of Espresso style Cowboy Coffee.

For a home or commercial espresso machine: Grind the above combination (minus the Anise oil) to a consistency less fine than Coffee and then brew as you would brew an espresso. Vary the grind until you arrive at an expression which suits you. Add the single drop of Anise oil just after you've "tamped" the grind.

If you have no espresso machine, you can create a fine "Cowboy Coffee Tea" by simmering this mixture (1 teaspoon/cup) lightly for 5–8 minutes and then straining into your cup through a bamboo strainer, or any other preferred device.

More Yummy Fragrance to Eat or Drink

To Relieve the Caffeine Jitter . . . Add 1 teaspoon of Orange flower water to every cup of coffee.

For Delicious Chocolate Drinks . ... Add a drop of Vanilla oil or Cinnamon oil to each cup.

For Extra Basil Flavor in Pasta al Pesto . . . Add 1 drop of Basil oil per serving.

Delicious Orange-Vanilla Ice Cream . . . Add 1 drop of Neroli oil or 1 drop of Orange oil per serving of Vanilla ice cream.

Aphrodisiac Delight . . . Add 1 Tuberose flower per glass of champagne or add 3 drops or Ylang-Ylang oil or Tuberose oil per bottle of Champagne. Let it rest for 20 minutes before drinking.

Special Christmas Ginger Cookies . . . Add 3 drops Ginger oil per batch of cookies. Or spritz the cookies while still warm with Ginger water.

Hollandaise Sauce . . . Add 4 drops Lemon oil per cup for a really lemony taste.

Lamp Chops . . . Love the taste of Spearmint oil on Lamb just as they are served. A drop is all you need.

Orange Wine . . . To sip on a summer evening as an aperitif. Peels from eaten Oranges should be saved and dried. When you have the peels of about 6 Oranges, toast them in 300° oven until the Orange skin is amber and the edges are browned. Let them cool and cut into $\frac{1}{4}$-inch-wide slices. Now rinse a 2-quart bottle with boiling water. Drain the bottle and add the sliced and toasted peels, 1 bottle of Sauvignon Blanc, or Sauvignon Blanc late harvest wine, $\frac{1}{2}$ cup 100° Vodka, and $\frac{3}{4}$ cup sugar. Mix all together and store in refrigerator for one month. Shake carefully daily. Strain and bottle in smaller containers for use. This is a delicious drink, served simply as an aperitif or over crushed ice, half and half with sparkling water as an elegant, lightly alcoholic beverage.

Apple Geranium Apple Sauce

(1) Follow a standard recipe for Applesauce and place 1 Apple Geranium leaf in the bottom of every jar,

or

(2) Wash, core and cut into quarters 2–3 pounds of a firm, tart Apple. Put these into an enamel sauce pan and just cover with water. Add a dash of Cinnamon and simmer until tender but not mooshy.

Add 5 small Apple Geranium leaves to the pot and simmer 3 more minutes. Remove the leaves.

Put Apples through a ricer or blender. Add sugar to taste. Add a little Lemon zest.

Put up in clean, boiled glass jars with an Apple Geranium leaf at the top of each jar. OR serve immediately and garnish with an Apple Geranium leaf.

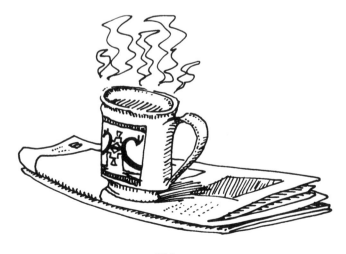

Part **III**

Aromatherapy Magic

. . . The Orchids were large, open, and labial pink. . .
A scandalous scent issued from their florid centers,
   —a stench of strange rapture.
These new Orchids tasted velvety and hot on the tongue
   of the animals
And felt warm, firm, and voluptuous.
The animals became extinct rather than eat them
   —they feared this new vegetation.
                              —J. A. Colón, *Flagrant Fragrance*

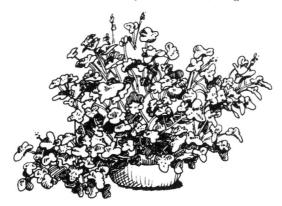

Ordinary Alchemy

by Thomas Norton, 1447 (slightly modernized)

When a substance putrefies
Horrible odors are created
as of dragons, and of men that are long dead,
their stink may cause much death.
It is not wholesome to smell for some
and if a horse smells this stuff, she will cast her foal.
Fishes love sweet smells also it is true
they love not old kettles as they do the new.
all things that is of a good odor has a natural heat
though Camphor, Roses and things cold
have sweet odors as Authors have souls.
No good odor is contrary to another but this is so of stinging smells
For the stink of Garlic avoid the stink of dunghill.
Of odors this doctrine is sufficient
as in alchemy to serve your intent.
Your works to understand thereby,
When things begin to putrefy.
Also by odors this you may learn,
Subtleness and grossness of matters to discern.
A sweet-smelling thing has more purity
and more of spiritual than stinking may be.
As colors change in your sight
So odors change by smelling them at night

The cause of odors to know if you delight
Four things there to be requisite.
First, that subtle matter be obedient to the working of heat.
The working of heat as it shows in the Stone,
Heat makes odors into stink, by reason,
Such as the Dung hills in summer
Do stink more than in winter.
Pleasant odors engendered shall be
Of clear and pure substance for fumigation,
As it appears in Amber, Nard and Myrtle.
Good for a woman for such things do please her,
But of pure substance with a mean in heat
Be temperate odors, in the Violet.
Of mean heat, with substance impure
is odor unpleasant, as Aloes and Sulphur.

You will by smelling learn
Of principal agent truly to declare,
As white and black be colors in extremity,
So of odors sweet and stinking do there be,
But where that slighted know by sight,
Mean colors show that you may be right.
So mean odors shall not by smelling
Be known of you, that is the cause why
The nostrils be as open as in the fishes eye.

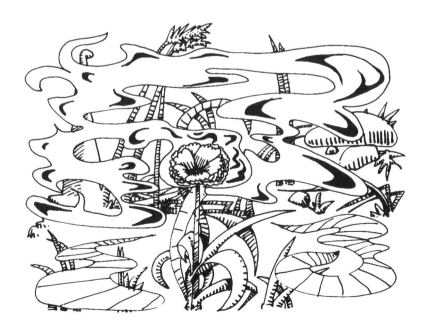

Chapter XIII

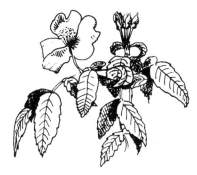

Ritual Aromatics

Ritual Aromatics

Color, scent and taste should be correctly combined, and the body cleaned and perfumed before you enter into a meditative state or before you begin a ritual event. This has been known and practiced in every religion and every spiritual happening. "To show her reverence for the Buddha, she took perfumed baths and spent long hours meditating in front of burning incense at a little shrine" goes a paragraph from a book by a Chinese author. She goes on to describe her grandmother, "She wore no makeup, but was richly scented, as was considered appropriate for a visit to the temple." The grandmother wished to entice a general to be her husband and she plays music for him; "Sitting under a trellis with the scent of Syringa in the air, her performance enchants the general." He does marry her and thus begins the saga of a Chinese woman.

So we use ritual for many events—ritual is an important occasion.

Here is a chart that will help you to combine the various therapies and correlations for healing and ritual.*

---

* The full-color chart is available through North Atlantic Books (2800 Woolsey Street, Berkeley, CA 94705) for $12.00, which includes shipping.

Jeanne Rose Aroma/Color/Plant/

Timing	Aromatherapy	Chromo-therapy	Symbolism	Chakra	Plant Therapy
Day of Week / Planet	Scent	Color / Chakra Color	Symbol / Emotion	Chakra / Element	Herb / Organ/s
Tuesday / TIW's Mars	Rose, Sandalwood, Camphor, Patchouly, Geranium, Jasmine, Pineapple	Red / Yellow	Strength, Vitality, Life / Fear	Root #1 / Earth	Roses, Jasmine, Sandalwood / for the blood and sex organs
Sunday / Sun's Day	Vanilla, Citronella, Bitter Almond, Heliotrope, Violet, Bergamot	Orange / bright Blue	Energy, Courage / Worry	Sacral #2 / Water	Bergamot, Orange juice / for intestines or spleen
Friday / Frigga's Day Venus	Orris, Lemon Verbena, Calamus, Mugwort/Acacia, Lemon	Yellow / golden Orange	Mind, Intellect / Anger	Solar Plexus #3 / Fire	Acacia, Lemons, Camomile / for liver, stomach
Monday / Moon	Tuberose, Narcissus, Jonquil, Musk, Benzoin, Ginger	Green / Pink	Harmony, Balance / Love	Heart #4 / Air	green herbs, Mints, Sage / for heart or headache
Saturday / Saturn	Sweet Pea, Lilac, Orange flower, Magnolia, Myrrh	Blue / Turquoise	Assertion, Serenity, Inspiration, Devotion / Sorrow	Throat #5 / Ether	Violet flowers, Orange flowers, Corn flowers / for throat and gall bladder
Thursday / Thor's Day Jupiter	Balsam Tolu, Lavender, Tonka, Storax, Gardenia, Rosemary	Indigo / blue White	Intuition, Sensitivity, Power of Vision / Brooding	3rd Eye #6	Ginseng, Echinacea, Balsams / for sense organs
Wednesday / Woden Mercury	Peppermint, Cinnamon, Carnation, Clove	Violet / Gold or Silver	Clairvoyance, Spirituality / Pensiveness	Crown #7	Clovers, Carnations, Rosemary / for kidney or bladder

Sound/Crystal Correlations for Healing

Audio-therapy Sound Act	Action of Color/Scent upon Organ/s	Nutrition Therapy Foods	Crystal Therapy
C	stimulates circulation, reduces depression, stimulates and excites, menstrual tonic, used for skin disease (measles, eczema), provides warmth **Sex Organs**	Tomato, Beet, red Pepper, Radish, red wine, Berries, Plums, red Onion, black Cherries	Ruby, Garnet, Spinel
D	body normalizer, used for asthma, improves thyroid, normalizes calcium, releases nervous tension, improves digestion and assimilation **Spleen, Intestine**	Apricots, vitamin A, calcium, Carrots, eggs, Pumpkins, Peaches, Rutabaga, Persimmon	Coral, Fire Opal, Carnelian, Pearl, Agate
E	laxative, stimulates intellect, muscle stimulant, improves bile secretions, builds nerves, heals skin, exhaustion **Adrenal, Pancreas, Stomach, Liver**	Corn, Banana, Lemons, Melons, butter, Pineapples, Yam, Papaya, Grapefruit	Topaz, Citrine, Beryl
F	antiseptic, the master healer, used for all conditions with other colors, soothes entire system, increases vitality, heals burns **Heart, Lungs**	salads, Asparagus, Cucumber, green Peppers, Apples, Kiwi, Celery, green Cabbage, Chives, Leeks, Limes	Emerald, Tsavorite, Peridot, Jade
G	astringent, reduces fever, calming, reduces pain, cooling, reduces hot inflammations, reducing agitation or bleeding (profuse menstruation) **Thyroid, Thymus**	Blueberry, Plum, blue Cornmeal, Grapes, Prunes	Sapphire, Benitoite, Aquamarine, Indicolite, Moonstone
A	anaesthetic, purification, lymph tonic, inflammation of the sense organs, stimulates parathyroid action, rheumatism **Pineal**	blue foods, violet foods, Eggplant, red Cabbage	Lapis Lazuli, Sodalite
B	stimulating, restorative, builds resistance to disease, for bladder and kidneys, stimulates spleen and white cells, helps adrenals, decongestant **Pituitary**	Blackberry, Broccoli, red & blue foods, Plums, dark purple Grapes, Garlic, Beet tops	Amethyst, Tansanite, Iolite

A Bath Oil Mixture to Precede Ritual, for Cleansing, for Calming, for Centering

Mix together 10 drops each of oils of Myrrh, Frankincense, Sandalwood and Ylang-Ylang. Add these to your bath and relax for 20 minutes. If you only take showers, then clean yourself with soap and water, step out of the shower and pat the oils upon your still-damp body. Let yourself air dry—do not towel dry. This mixture of oils is available separately in a wonderful kit produced by C. A. Gregory Aromatics that is carried by Baudelaire, Inc., in New Hampshire. See Chapter VI for complete address.

How to Use the Chart for Healing & Ritual

RITUAL WORKS: Ritual is any practice or system of rites that is done regularly or practiced repeatedly in any set manner so as to satisfy one's sense of rightness. Ritual is the external manifestation of an internal belief. We have ritual ways of gardening, of making tea, rituals of living, rituals of making infusions and tinctures, rituals of worship or honoring goddess or of showing respect for our honored elders. So why appropriate another person's rituals or ritual items? Why not make your own? You can do this by using the chart that precedes this.

You start by determining your problem or situation or which emotion you wish to change or strengthen. At the left you choose the best day to perform your healing ritual, then pick the correct scents, what color of decoration or garment to wear. Next column shows the appropriate symbolic emotion and its opposite and the chakra that will be affected. The chakra is a whirling vortex of energy located at various levels along the spinal cord. Each chakra affects various elements and various organs of the body. The plant therapy column shows the herbs that you should use and the organs of the body upon which the herb will work best as therapy and then the sound or tone of music to affect the healing. Next you will see what action the color/sound/scent will have upon the body and what foods to eat and what crystals or jewels to wear during your ritual or healing. This the true way to correlate the senses for healing or ritual—combining therapies is better than using only one at a time.

Specifically, AROMATHERAPY is the use of essential oils by direct application or inhalation to heal and tend the mind and body. Aromatherapy has a rejuvenating and regenerating effect on the body. It is an ancient method of natural treatment. Marguerite Maury, a magnificent proponent of this art, felt that old age could be conquered through the correct usage of essential oils. Life energy flows through the body, cyclically, along paths called meridians. The best time to use aroma therapeutically is during the lung time or close to it; this is between 3 and 5 A.M.

COLOR THERAPY has also been in use since ancient times to influence human health. It may seem an aesthetic or ethereal form of treatment for some, nevertheless, color can change the way you feel and it can heal. Color therapy is a useful adjunct to herbal and aroma therapies.

Sound therapy or sound medicine has been recognized since ancient times, too. It is known that sound and music have a marked influence upon the human soul and are vital factors in healing and ritual events. Music in the major keys is used for physical problems while music in the minor keys is for emotional or mental states.

USING THE CHART IS EASY: Determine a problem, then use the corresponding therapies to treat any physical or emotional situation. You may also wish to compose a ritual for a special event, and you will know the correct day, color, sound and foods to use.

Examples:

(1) *Mental or Emotional.* If you wish to reduce depression, look first in the horizontal column of the root chakra #1. You will find that red color, the herbs Roses and Sandalwood, the sound of C and such foods as berries and Cherries and the scent of Geranium are known to treat depression. You might make a mixture or potpourri of the herbs and scent them with their own essential oils, sandwich this scented potpourri between red silk cloths and lie in the sun inhaling the scent and letting the light and energy of the sun filter through the red herbed silk onto your body while sleeping on pink or red sheets. You would listen to sound or music in the minor keys such as Vivaldi's Concerto in C minor for flutes, and you could be eating Cherries from a red or clear crystal bowl. This would also be an effective treatment for sexual rejuvenation. I guarantee that this will certainly relieve depression and if you continue the therapy for some days, you may even permanently remove this illness from your life.

(2) *Physical.* Do you have a sore throat and a cold? Use essential oils such as Myrrh for inhalation. Use blue sheets to help you sleep. Listen to music in the major keys. Drink teas of Violet flowers or leaf and eat simple foods such as fruits and Grapes.

(3) *Performing Ritual.* You wish to perform a ritual to Venus, goddess of Love. On a Friday you would rub a yellow candle with oil of Lemon as an inhalation and a flame to burn, drink Camomile tea, sing romantic tunes or hum in the key of E, all the while wearing a citrine or topaz and chanting to your spirit beings.

For more information on color and aromatherapy, read *Jeanne Rose's Modern Herbal* or *Ritual, Creating a Personal Style* by Jeanne Rose.*

A Charm to Bring Your Lover Home

Take an aromatic mixture of Cloves, Cinnamon and Cardamom and place in a large jar. Over this read seven times backward the Yasin chapter of the Koran (or whatever sacred book you believe in). Fill the jar with Rosewater and a shirt of your beloved. Add to this mixture a handmade piece of paper inscribed with the name of the wayward lover and the names of the four angels (according to your faith). Place the jar over the fire (maybe a porcelain pot would have been better); and as soon as the mixture begins to boil, the wandering lover will be on his way home. . . .

—from an ancient Persian formula

An Unpleasant Portent

Should you see the petals fall from a blood-red Rose this means a sudden death for you. This could also occur in a dream

"And here I prophesy; this brawl to-day
Grown to this faction in the Temple garden
Shall send between the Red Rose and White
A thousand souls to death and deadly night."
—Shakespeare, *Henry VI*, Part I
A scene discussing
the Wars of the Roses

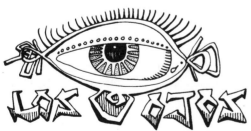

---

* Ritual Works! is the only company in the United States producing correctly made color/sound/aroma products for complete body care and perfect ritual and healing. The address for both is 219 Carl Street, San Francisco, CA 94117. Any questions? Send $3 and an SASE with your query.

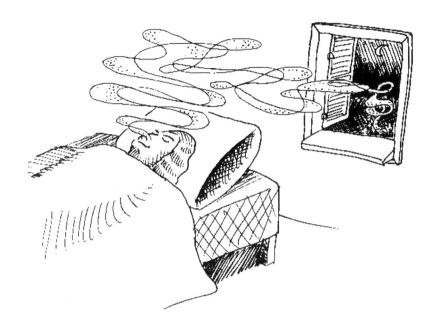

Aromatic Dreaming . . . To Dream in Scent

Dreaming is a particularly psychic event and dreams often do have meanings both past and future. To dream in scent, to dream and be able to comprehend fragrance, is especially propitious.

Recently, I was sleeping peacefully upon my feather bed, my linen sheets were of a salmon color (for lung health), and I had no scents or oils either in my bed or near it. I dreamed—and wafting along an invisible breeze came the scent of a thousand sweet flowers, a living Millefleur Potpourri. My dream was entirely pleasant and relaxing and suddenly I woke up. Sitting straight up, the fragrance still curled around my nostrils, I smiled, and went back to sleep. The next day, my neighbor brought over a small plant and told me that it was fragrant Nicotiana. We planted it and when it bloomed, the fragrance was the same as that which had come whispering through my open window in the months before. This is September, and the Moon of the Blooming Nicotiana, and alongside it blooms also the fragrant yellow Ginger. On these September nights I sleep with the windows wide open and always at 2 A.M. when the Nicotine bursts into full scent and some-times when a new spike of Ginger bursts into yellow bloom my dreams become peaceful, happy and always they bring a smile.

Dreams of scent have various meanings according to *The Dreamer's Dictionary* by Lady Steam Robinson and *The Great Book of Magical Art, Hindu*

315

Magic and Indian Occultism by L. W. deLaurence. Some of the listings are very abstruse and some just make common sense. If you wish to aid your dreams and enhance their odorous appeal, try a crystal CandlEssence Aromatherapy Candle as made by Susan Leigh. Her candles come in soft colors of the spectrum and are enhanced with their correlated scent, and crystal. This unique combination of therapies is all brought together in the candle. You can burn a Creative Essence with Rosemary oil containing a citrine stone that will enhance brain energy, improve memory and facilitate the creative processes. Burn one of these at night when you wish to wake up refreshed and must be ready to tackle that particularly difficult term paper. Your dreams will be enhanced with the scent and you will wake up ready to do whatever needs doing. Some of the other candles that she makes are Dream Essence to calm the mind and enhance intuitive abilities, the Earth Essence to harmonize and balance one's nature, the Energizing Essence, Love Essence and Serene Essence. By the time that you read this she will no doubt have created several more essences for us to use.*

Coincidentally in 1981, I designed the chart that precedes this section, *Aroma/Color/Plant/Sound/Correlations for Healing.* When I compared this chart with the candles, I found that both Susan and I had agreed on all major points. Our correlations were the same, leading me to believe that correlating sound and color, aroma and crystal made sense, what was true thousands of years ago was still true today. That the old adepts and alchemists were correct when they said that to heal one must use all the senses, from smell to sound to touch to taste and even unto the crystal world.

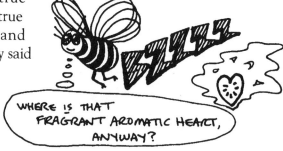

WHERE IS THAT FRAGRANT AROMATIC HEART, ANYWAY?

Aromatic Dreaming
Recipe for Action-Packed Dreams

(1) Take 150 mg of B_6 at bedtime (to recall dreams).
(2) Drink a soothing cup of Lemon Verbena tea (doesn't knock you out, just relaxes you enough to sleep).

---

* See Chapter VI, Oregon, Essence Aromatherapy.

(3) Make sure you are sleeping on natural fabric sheets—100% natural. Linen sheets are luxurious and elegant and help to give you dreams in that realm. Silk sheets are sleek and slippery and tend to the erotic. Cotton sheets are more provincial and the dreams are more in the realm of the normal.

(4) Use a sleep pillow. I would recommend a combination of Mugwort, Marjoram and narrow strips of thin, thin leather that have been massaged with Birch oil 4:4:1. The leather is there for the scent of Russian leather that enhances action. These herbs should be stuffed into pillows whose fabric is either in a plain color such as yellow or maybe a printed fabric with cars, planes or space ships or whatever. There should be at least 8–10 oz of herbs and such in the pillow.

(5) Keep a notebook and pen by the bedside to write down the dreams—and dream you will!

(6) Optional recipe: Drink Mugwort-infused Pernod or Sambuca Romana. Take a large handful of Mugwort and place directly into a large bottle of either of the mentioned liqueurs. Steep for at least three days before drinking. On the night that you want fantastic or action or future dreams, drink $1\frac{1}{2}$ oz just before bed and after #1 & #2 as listed above.

By the way—this formulation is guaranteed.

©1990 Jeanne Rose, an original formulation

Various Meanings of the Scented Dreams

. . . Happy incidents will occur if you dream of inhaling any perfume.

. . . A woman who dreams of using scent on herself predicts an unusual new heart interest; the man who dreams of using scent upon himself shows that he must watch out for misunderstandings in his business and personal affairs.

. . . To dream of perfuming your clothing or your body shows that you will be seeking adulation and will probably obtain what you desire.

. . . Becoming oppressed by the scent of a perfume shows that excesses in joy will impair your mental qualities.

. . . In your dreams if you spill perfume it means that whatever gives you pleasure you will surely lose.

Refer to Rose, Jeanne. Herbs & Things. New York, NY: Grosset & Dunlap, 1969, pages 148–156.

. . . To break a bottle of scent foretells that your cherished wishes and desires will end in a disaster, even while they may promise a happy culmination.

. . . To dream of distilling scent shows that your work and your associations will be of a pleasant character.

. . . For a young woman to add scent and perfume her bath foretells ecstatic experiences.

. . . A young woman who dreams of receiving scent as a gift from a man foretells the experience of fascinating but dangerous pleasures.

. . . In your dreams inhaling sweet odors shows that an intelligent beautiful woman or handsome intelligent man will come into your life and that you will have success in your finances.

. . . In your dream if you can smell disgusting odors it shows that you may have unpleasant disagreements and unreliable servants for help.

. . . To dream and actually wake up with the scent of sweet odors in your nose is to foretell a joyous and happy day.

. . . To dream of smelling a heady and pungent scent but not to wake up forecasts an exciting and passionate new love partner. Dreaming of smelling a very light and delicate scent shows only the stirring of a pleasant not a romantic affair.

. . . To smell the green herbs that come upon the wings of sleep shows that peace and contentment will be your life reward and for the immediate present predicts new and exciting adventures and travel to the land of the herbs that you dreamt of.

. . . In your dreams if the odor is not immediately identifiable it can mean various things depending on your personal reactions; if the scent is pleasant to you the omen is good, if the scent is unpleasant you will have anxieties that could be major or minor depending on the extent of the unpleasantness.

. . . To dream of your head being perfumed or dripping with scented oils or essences signifies great self-esteem and self-pride. If this is a woman dreaming she will glory in the exercise of her power. If she dreams of scent that is in the green to violet range, her power will be beneficent; and if the scents are in the red-yellow range, her power will be on the side of wrong-doing (except for the scents of Roses, Sandalwood, Jasmine and Violet, which never presage any negative effect).

. . . Sometimes to dream of being adorned with sparkling jewels and covered with fragrant oil and scents and bouquets of flowers can have opposite meanings: if the jewels are dirty, the scent spoiled and the flowers withered means misfortune; if the jewels are clean and sparkling, the scent fresh or sweet and flowers upright and freshly cut means fortune and happiness.

. . . To be adorned with jewels and flowers and to feel that you look your best speaks of "Look out, danger nears." The danger can be a physical attack or an illness. Be careful now, be aware!

. . . To dream of being lightly and freshly scented means that we are respected by our neighbors and cared for by others.

. . . If you dream that you smell bad or that there is a bad odor about you you will prove hateful to others. (In this case it would be wise to bathe in fragrant herbs and take zinc tablets to correct the odor whether it be real or imagined.)

. . . The one who dreams that s/he has been presented with aromatic or scented waters will have good news in proportion to the quality and extent of the gifts received in sleep; s/he will make substantial gain and acquire honors.

. . . The one who dreams of giving out scents and essential oils to one's friends will receive news that is advantageous to the dreamer as well as the receivers of the scents.

"Nothing so swiftly creates an
   atmosphere of happiness as fragrance.
   The mind insensibly forgets its cares, and the soul dreams—

> As when a box of essences
> Is broken on the air.

—The Romance of Perfume
by Richard Le Gallienne,
published by Richard Hudnut, 1928.

319

Death by Fine Fragrance—A Well-Smelt Tale

My great-uncle Joe (Edmund Laramée) once showed me our Laramée family lineage, charted on a piece of parchment, that said we were directly related to Gabrielle d'Estrées, the consort to the French King Henry IV about 1592. Gabrielle and Henry had three children, and a grandchild who was thought to be the "Man in the Iron Mask." When Uncle Joe told me this I was 20 years old, and I was visiting him at his "little" cabin in the Laurentian mountains. "Little" was a euphemism for a large beautiful log house that had 5 bedrooms and a large and lovely kitchen with a wood-burning stove where he made Buckwheat pancakes every morning, and a huge basement where he would hang game and where he taught me to make handmade wooden dowels for furniture. Uncle Joe had very little love for Americans and once for sport took me snowshoeing around his lake where we apparently got lost. Hah! He was teasing me and as the sun began to set and the temperature dipped to 20° below zero, he "found" the little cabin, and when we got warm again told me the story of my French heritage. It was 30 years later that I found out that Gabrielle died of subterfuge having been poisoned by aromatherapy. So I think it fitting that I write a book in which I may be a little part of the legacy of this interesting woman.

The lovely Gabrielle d'Estrées was descended on her mother's side from a family of which some thirty women were notorious for their love affairs. One had been mistress of the French King Francis I, one of Emperor Charles V and another mistress of Pope Clement VII. Gabrielle had five sisters and a brother and she was called "La Belle Gabrielle," and with her sisters and brother were known in Paris as the Seven Deadly Sins. She was twenty when the King saw her and was struck with her beauty. He managed to get her married to an obliging old widower, then later had the marriage annulled when the old man would not claim his marital rights. He then established Gabrielle as his, the King's, official mistress. Henry was 38 at this time. In 1593 she became pregnant and César was born in 1594. In January when the marriage was annulled she was given the title of Marchioness of Monceaux and eventually Duchesse de Beaufort and César was legitimized. It was one of his sons who was thought to be the "Man in the Iron Mask."

Gabrielle was popular in court, had a gentle nature, a brilliant mind, and supported Henry's notion of freedom of worship and political equality for Protestants. She rode horseback like a man and played tennis well. Henry, the King of France and Navarre, loved her dearly and continually sent her love letters. They had two other children, Alexandre de Bourbon and Catherine. She was pregnant with a fourth when she died in April of 1599.

Henry had arranged for Gabrielle to dine at the house of Sebastien Zamet (Zametti), a wealthy Italian banker of Jewish descent from whom Henry often borrowed money and in whose house he frequently gambled and fornicated. Zamet had originally come to France as part of the household of Catherine d'Medici. It was thought that many in the household of Catherine were skilled in the dark ways of poison made with herbs. Now Zamet lived in great luxury in a magnificently furnished palace when Gabrielle was sent at Henry's request for a visit.

Gabrielle and Henry were loving parents and Gabrielle was always reluctant to leave her children—especially so this time having had a premonition of evil. She begged Henry to let her stay with him. But they (Henry and Gabrielle) had " . . . a tender farewell and she embarked in a royal barge, which was attended by a flotilla of boats decorated with flags and streamers in the Venetian style."

She arrived in Paris on April 6 and was met by her host Zamet and a number of his retainers. She had a bite to eat. Possibly her pregnancy made her nauseous, but the food may have disagreed with her. On Wednesday, April 7, she still felt ill and dizzy but wished to attend Mass in a nearby church. Before leaving the Palace, Zamet "presented her with an exquisitely decorated scent-bottle containing a strong perfume."[1] During the service she fainted. The fragrance of the scent was all about her, and as it was quite hot in the church she asked to be taken to the house of a relative nearby, an aunt. She went to bed complaining of a headache but the next morning, April 8, she felt well enough to go to church and take the Sacrament. By 2 P.M. she was distinctly unwell, very thirsty and labor pains were followed by convulsions that continued into the night. On Good Friday she was hemorrhaging and endured an embryotomy. In the hands of the physicians she underwent the modern medical techniques of the time, cupping[2] and clistering[3] and other fashionable forms of timely medical torture. The pain distorted her features and limbs. By evening she was unable to speak, hear, see or move

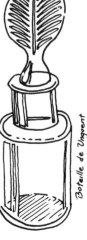

Boteille de Unguent

and finally on Saturday April 10, 1599 death released her.

While she lay in the home of her aunt she "lay with her eyes opened and turned upward, her face livid and her mouth distorted." She called for the King but he was unable to reach her before death. She was given the funeral of a Queen.

If you analyze the written complications surrounding Gabrielle's death—that is, pregnancy, eating some food, nausea, dizziness, a poisonously strong fragrance, fainting, thirst, labor pains, convulsions, hemorrhaging, fashionable medical interventions, pain, distortion of face and limbs, face livid, finally unable to speak, hear, move or see, and death—it seems rather obvious that a combination of Datura, Belladonna, possibly Bufo skin and maybe even puffer fish was mixed together to cause these problems. Combinations of these ingredients have been used for centuries to cause any number of deaths and even zombification in Haiti. A distillation of the Datura flower when inhaled as a perfume is more or less toxic depending on the amount inhaled. If the Datura were mixed with other strong scents a perfume could be formulated that would be very poisonous both inhaled and applied as a perfume. Toad skin (Bufo) and puffer fish have been used by evil-doers to create the effect of flying; the side effect of course is often a paralysis followed by death. These ingredients are effective whether inhaled, ingested or simply rubbed on the surface of the skin. And Gabrielle was subjected to all these plus cupping and clistering. All in all, a very unpleasant albeit fragrant way to die.*

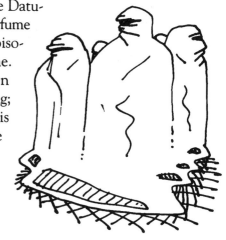

---

[1]C. J. S. Thompson. *The Mystery and Lure of Perfume.* p. 103.

[2]Cupping is a technique used for drawing blood to the surface, employing counterirritation with a glass cup applied to the skin and heating, thus creating a vacuum in the glass.

[3]Clistering or clystering is a powerful purging enema.

*Other references include Britannica Library Research Service, *The Life of Gabrielle d'Estrées* and the Hesketh Pearson book *Henry of Navarre* published in London by Heinemann, 1963. Supplementary reading includes:

Edwards, Samuel. *Lady of France, A Biography of Gabrielle d'Estrées, Mistress of Henry the Great.* London: Alvin Redman, 1964.

Sedwick, Henry D. *Henry of Navarre.* Indianapolis: Bobbs:Merrill Company, 1930.

Part **IV**

The Fragrance Foundation Survey on the Sense of Smell

Age: ❏ 10-20 ❏ 41-60 Sex: ❏ M Present Residence (city & state)
❏ 21-40 ❏ over 60 ❏ F _____

Cigarette smoker: ❏ yes ❏ no
If yes: ❏ less than 1 pack daily ❏ 1-2 packs daily ❏ more than 2 packs daily

Cigar smoker: ❏ yes ❏ no *Pipe* smoker: ❏ yes ❏ no
If yes: ❏ less than 6 per day ❏ 6-12 per day ❏ more than 12

1. Do you consider yourself to have a keen sense of smell? ❏ yes ❏ no
    If yes, explain:

    _____

    _____

2. Are you concerned about the sense of smell of anyone in your family?
    ❏ yes ❏ no If yes, explain:

    _____

    _____

3. Can you identify people close to you by their odor? ❏ yes ❏ no

4. As a child were you made aware of the sense of smell? ❏ yes ❏ no

If yes, by whom and/or by what?

_____

_____

5. If you have children, do you make the sense of smell a learning experience for them? ☐ yes ☐ no If yes, please explain:

_____

_____

6. On a range of 1–10 (highest is 10) how important is smell in your relationship with the opposite sex? _____

7. Does smell play an important part in your daily relationships or activities? ☐ yes ☐ no Please explain:

_____

_____

8. Does your home have an odor that pleases you? Please explain:

_____

_____

9. Do you alter household odors with fragrance products? ☐ yes ☐ no On what occasions? What type of products do you use? What rooms in the house are involved?

_____

_____

10. Has there ever been a period in your life when your sense of smell was not keen? ☐ yes ☐ no If yes:
    Was it due to a cold? ☐ yes ☐ no   To an allergy? ☐ yes ☐ no
    To a bump on the head? ☐ yes ☐ no
    To another cause? ☐ yes ☐ no   If other, describe:

_____

_____

_____

If yes, how long did this period last?
  ❑ days ❑ weeks ❑ months ❑ years
If yes, is it present now? ❑ yes ❑ no

11. Has there ever been a period in your life when your sense of smell was distorted? ❑ yes ❑ no
If yes, how long did this period last?
  ❑ days ❑ weeks ❑ months ❑ years
If yes, is it present now? ❑ yes ❑ no

12. Have you ever noticed any change in your ability to smell throughout the day? ❑ yes ❑ no
If yes, when do your think your sense of smell is most acute?
❑ morning ❑ afternoon ❑ evening

13. Have you ever noticed any lessening in your ability to smell as you have gotten older? ❑ yes ❑ no

14. Have you ever had a nasal polyp? ❑ yes ❑ no

15. Have you ever had hay fever or asthma? ❑ yes ❑ no

16. Do you blow your nose every day? ❑ yes ❑ no
If yes, does this affect your ability to smell? ❑ yes ❑ no

17. Do your eyes tear when you peel an onion? ❑ yes ❑ no

18. How often do you use fragrance? ❑ once daily ❑ more than once daily
❑ less than twice a week ❑ 2 times a month ❑ never
If never, please explain:

_____

_____

19. What characteristics do you look for when you buy a fragrance?
❑ heaviness ❑ lightness ❑ woodsy ❑ muskiness ❑ spiciness
❑ floweriness ❑ sweetness ❑ other _____

20. Do you use one type of fragrance in the morning and another in the evening? ❑ yes ❑ no
    If yes, what type of fragrance do you prefer:
    in the morning? _____
    in the evening? _____

21. Can you smell better through one side of your nose than another?
    ❑ yes ❑ no
    If yes, which side is better? ❑ left ❑ right
    If unsure, sniff a fragrance, first with your right nostril, then with your left.

Send this form to:
    Fragrance Foundation
    145 East 32nd Street
    New York, NY 10016

or to:
    Dr. Robert I Henkin, Director
    Center for Molecular Nutrition & Sensory Disorders
    Georgetown Medical Center, Georgetown University
    3800 Reservoir Road, Washington, D.C. 20007

Part V

The End

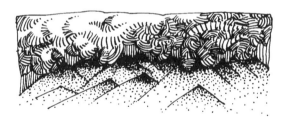

HEADWATERS
...ARE GOOD FOR YOUR HEAD

QUESTION THE
SOURCE

(OF EVERYTHING YOU USE)

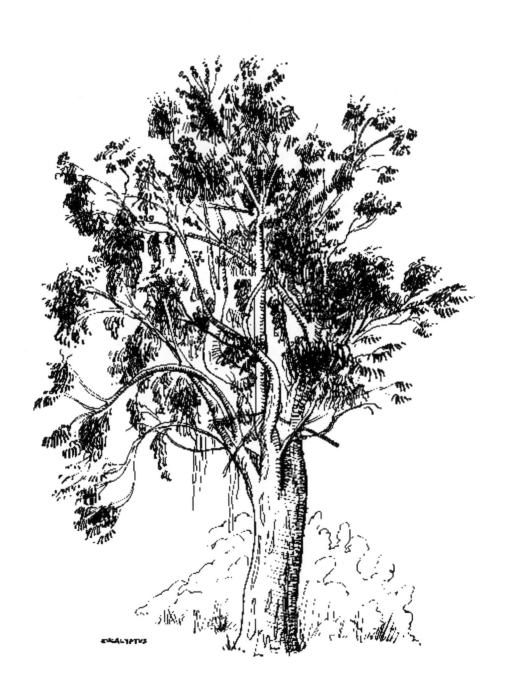

EUCALYPTUS

BIBLIOGRAPHY

I have always liked to say that a bibliography is a map whereby the reader can follow the progression of the author's research, showing how the author arrived at the conclusions that the text conveys.

This is especially true in aromatherapy, a subject that only begins to be seen in bibliographies around 1937 with the publication of Gattefossé's seminal work *Aromatherapy*. He began his work in 1910 and published continually after that. Marguerite Maury's *Guide to Aromatherapy* was published in 1961 as *Le Capital "Jeunesse,"* a ground-breaking text, but she told no secrets, only alluding to the magical and rejuvenating effects of the essential oils. In 1975, I flew to New York to give a presentation to the Fragrance Foundation and immediately my luggage was stolen, including an original manuscript called *Aromatherapy, Inhalations for the Mind*. This was such a blow that it is only fifteen years later that I have been able to recompile and update my original work. In the meantime, dozens of books have been published on the subject.

This work is new. The bibliographical map is more convoluted. If you pursue my bibliographical path, then you will indeed see how I arrived at some rather unique conclusions in this subject matter. The most telling may be the last section of the book. Read well . . . Enjoy!

Ackerman, Diane. *A Natural History of the Senses*. New York, NY: Random House, 1990.

Arctander, Steffen. *Perfume and Flavor Materials of Natural Origin*. Elizabeth, NJ: S. Arctander, 1960.

Bailes, Edith. *An Album of Fragrance*. Richmond, Maine: Cardamom Press, 1983.

Bernadet, Marcel. *La Phyto-Aromatherapie Pratique*. St.-Jean-de-Braye, France: Editions D'Angles, 1983.

Bienfang, Ralph. *The Subtle Sense, Key to the World of Odors*. Oklahoma: University of Oklahoma Press, 1946.

Brownlow, Margaret. *Herbs and the Fragrant Garden*. London, England: Darton, Longman and Todd, 1957.

Clifford, F. S., *A Romance of Perfume Lands, or, The Search for Capt. Jacob Cole with interesting facts about perfumes and articles used in the toilet*. Boston, Mass: Clifford and Company, 1881.

THE END

Cooley, Arnold J. *A Complete Practical Treatise on Perfumery: Being a Handbook of Perfumes, Cosmetics, and Other Toilet Articles, including Instructions and Cautions . . . Their Preparation.* Philadelphia, Penn: Henry Carey Baird, 1874.

Cunningham, Scott. *Magical Aromatherapy.* St. Paul, Minn: Llewellyn Publications, 1989.

Davis, Patricia. *Aromatherapy: An A to Z.* Essex, England: Saffron Walden, 1988.

Deite, Dr. C. *A Practical Treatise on the Manufacture of a Perfumer: Comprising Directions. . . for Making . . . Cosmetics, Etc., Etc., with a Full Account of . . . Purity.* from the German by William T. Brannt. Philadelphia, Penn: Henry Carey Baird & Co., 1892.

Dorrance, Anne. *Fragrance in the Garden.* Garden City, NY: Doubleday, Doran and Company, Inc., 1937.

Dugdale, Rose Sydenham. *Fragrant Herbs.* Birmingham, England: The Weather Oak Press, 1936.

Duraffourd, Paul. *En Forme Tous Les Jours, Grace Aux Vertus Des Huiles Essentielles.* Perigny, France: La Vie Claire, 1982.

Farkas, Alexander. *Perfume thru the Ages.* New York, NY: Psychological Library, 1951.

Fox, Helen Morgenthau. *Gardening with Herbs for Flavor & Fragrance.* New York, NY: The Macmillan Company, 1933.

Fragrance Foundation. *Fragrance & Olfactory Dictionary & Directory.* New York, NY: Fragrance Foundation, 1981.

Franchomme, Pierre. *Phytoguide N.°1 Aromatherapy, Advanced Therapy for Infectious Illnesses.* La Courtete, France: International Phytomedical Foundation.

Gaborit, Jean-Yves. *Perfumes, The Essences and Their Bottles.* New York, NY: Rizzoli International Publications, Inc., 1985.

Gattefossé, R. M. *Aromatherapie.* Paris, France: Librairie des Sciences, 1937.

———. *Aromatherapy: Essential Oils, Plant Hormones,* a translation of *Aromatherapie.* San Francisco, CA: Herbal Studies Library, 1990.

———. *Esthetique Physiologique et Cosmetique Moderne.* Paris, France: Librairie des Sciences, 1938.

———. *Formulaire du Chemiste-Parfumeur et du Savonnier*. Paris, France: Librairie des Sciences, 1932.

———. *Theorie de la Chevelure*. Paris, France: Librairie des Sciences, 1947.

Genders, Roy. *A History of Scent*. London, England: Hamish Hamilton, 1972.

———. *Scented Flora of the World*. New York, NY: St. Martin's Press, 1977.

Gruenberg, Louise. *Potpourri, the Art of Fragrance Crafting*. Norway, Iowa: Frontier Cooperative Herbs, 1984.

Gumbel, Dietrich. *Principles of Holistic Skin Therapy with Herbal Essences*. Heidelberg, Germany: Karl F. Haug Publ., 1986.

Hampton, F. A. *The Scent of Flowers and Leaves, Its Purpose and Relation to Man*. Great Britain: Dulau & Company, Ltd., 1925.

Heriteau, Jacqueline. *Potpourris and Other Fragrant Delights*, New York, NY: Simon and Schuster, 1973.

Hunt, Roland. *Fragrant and Radiant Healing Symphony*. [no publisher listed] 1937. First use of the word "aromo-therapy."

Jackson, Judith. *Scentual Touch, Aromatherapy—The Time-Honored Art of Massage*. New York, NY: Fawcett Columbine, 1986.

James, Ronald W. *Fragrance Technology: Synthetic and Natural Perfumes*. Park Ridge, NJ: Noyes Data Corp., 1975.

Jessee, Jill. *Perfume Album*. New York, NY: Beauty Data, 1951.

Karpilow, Shelley. *Sachets and Dry Perfumes*. San Francisco, Cal: [publisher unknown], 1960.

Killian, Emily Hart. *Perfume Bottles Remembered*. Chelsea, Mich: BookCrafters, 1989.

Lavabre, Marcel. *Aromatherapy Workbook*. Rochester, Vermont: Healing Arts Press, 1990. (The original was called *The Handbook of Aromatherapy or How to Cure Yourself*. circa 1986.)

Le Gallienne, Richard. *The Romance of Perfume*. New York, NY: Richard Hudnut, 1928.

Leyel, Mrs. C. F. *The Magic of Herbs: A Modern Book of Secrets*. London, England: Jonathan Cape, 1926.

MacDonell, Anne, editor. *The Closet of Sir Kenelm Digby Knight Opened*, 1669. London, England: Philip Lee Warner, 1910. Newly edited, with introduction, notes and glossary.

McKenzie, Dan. *Aromatics and the Soul: A Study of Smells*. New York, NY: Paul B. Hoeber, Inc., 1926.

Manniche, Lise. *An Ancient Egyptian Herbal*. Austin, Tex.: University of Texas Press, 1989.

Maple, Eric. *The Magic of Perfume: Aromatics and Their Esoteric Significance*. New York, NY: Samuel Weiser, 1973.

Martin, Hazel. *A Collection of Figural Perfume & Scent Bottles*. Lancaster, Cal: Hazel Martin, 1982.

Maury, Marguerite. *The Secret of Life and Youth*. London, England: Mac-Donald, 1964. [recently republished by C. W. Daniel]

Ohrbach, Barbara Milo. *The Scented Room*. New York, NY: Crown Publ., 1986.

Paltz, J. *Le fascinant Pouvoir des Huiles Essentielles*. Publisher unknown, 1984.

Parry, Ernest J. *Cyclopedia of Perfumery*, in 2 volumes. Philadelphia, Penn: P. Blakiston's Son & Co., 1925.

Piesse, G. W. Septimus. *The Art of Perfumery and the Methods of Obtaining the Odors of Plants* . . . Philadelphia, Penn: Lindsay & Blakiston, 1867.

Pollard, H. B. C. *The Mystery of Scent*. London, England: Eyre and Spottiswoode, 1937.

Popov, Ivan. *Stay Young*. New York, NY: Grosset & Dunlap, 1975.

Poucher, W. A. *Perfumes & Cosmetics*. New York, NY: D. Van Nostrand Company, 1923.

Price, Shirley. *Everyday Aromatherapy*. [publisher unknown]

———. *Practical Aromatherapy: How to Use Essential Oils to Restore Vitality*. Northamptonshire, England: Thorsons Publ. Group, 1983.

Rimmel, Eugene. *The Book of Perfumes*. London, England: Chapman and Hall, MDCCCLXV

Rose, Jeanne. *Herbs & Things*. New York, NY: Grosset & Dunlap, 1969.

———. *Jeanne Rose's Herbal Body Book*. New York, NY: GD/Perigee, 1976.

———. *Kitchen Cosmetics*. Berkeley, Cal.: North Atlantic Books, 1988.

———. *Jeanne Rose's Modern Herbal*. New York, NY: GD/Perigee, 1987.

———. The Herbal Studies Course. Chapter 32. San Francisco, CA: Herbal Studies Course Library, 1988.

Ryman, Daniele. *The Aromatherapy Handbook*. Essex, England: C. W. Daniel Co., Ltd., 1984.

Sagarin, Edward. *The Science and Art of Perfumery*. New York, NY: Greenberg, 1945.

Sawer, J. Ch. *Rhodologia: A Discourse on Roses and the Odour of Rose*. Brighton, England: W. J. Smith, 1844.

Schnaubelt, Kurt. *Aromatherapy Course*. San Rafael, Cal: Kurt Schnaubelt, 1985. Relies heavily on the work of Pierre Franchomme (see Franchomme in Bibliography).

Suskind, Patrick. *Perfume: The Story of a Murderer*. New York, NY: Pocket Books, 1985. Originally published in Germany.

Szekely, Edmond Bordeaux. *The Golden Door Book of Beauty and Health*. Los Angeles, Cal: Ward Ritchie Press, 1961.

Thompson, C. J. S. *The Mystery and Lure of Perfume*. Philadelphia, Penn: J. B. Lippincott Company, 1927.

Tisserand, Maggie. *Aromatherapy for Women*. Wellingborough, England: Thorsons Publ. Group, 1985.

Tisserand, Robert. *Aromatherapy to Heal and Tend the Body*. Santa Fe, NM: Lotus Press, 1988.

——. *The Art of Aromatherapy*. New York, NY: Inner Traditions, 1977.

Tolkien, J. R. R. *The Return of the King*. New York, NY: Ballantine Books, 1954. The authorized edition of *The Lord of the Rings*, Part Three.

Valnet, Jean. *The Practice of Aromatherapy*. New York, NY: Destiny Books, 1980. An English translation of the French *Aromatherapie*, 1964.

Von Buddenbrock, Wolfgang. *The Senses*. Ann Arbor, Mich: University of Michigan Press, 1958.

Wilder, Louise Beebe. *The Fragrant Path*. New York, NY: Macmillan Company, 1932.

Wilson, Helen Van Pelt and Leonie Bell. *The Fragrant Year*. London, England: J. M. Dent & Sons Ltd., 1967.

Worwood, Valerie Ann. *Aromantics*. London, England: Pan Books, 1987.

Magazine Articles prior to 1975

"Aromatherapy: Could There Be More to Perfume than Meets the Nose?" *Vogue*, May 1969.

"Smell: The Next Erogenous Zone?" *Viva*, October 1973.

"Scent and the Sexual Object" — Fitzherbert, Joan. *British Journal of Medical Psychology*. 1959.

"Some Observations of the Sense of Smell" — Friedman, Paul. *Psychoanalytic Quarterly.* 1959.

"Contribution to the Development of Smell and Feeling" — Peto, Andrew. *British Journal of Medical Psychology.* 1936.

"The Sense of Smell in Neuroses and Psychoses" — Brill, A. A. *Psychoanalytic Quarterly.* 1932.

Givaudan Company—Series of articles currently running, beginning with issue #1, 1974. Jellinek, Paul.

Journals and Quarterlies

Aroma Notes — A Monthly Newsletter • New Century Press, P. O. Box 63, Boulder Creek, CA 95006.

Aromatherapy Quarterly • edited by Tricia Davis, 5, Ranelagh Avenue, London SW13 OBY, England.

The International Journal of Aromatherapy • edited by Robert Tisserand, P. O. Box 746, Hove, E. Sussex, BN3 3XA, England.

Scentsitivity • c/o NAHA, P. O. Box 17622, Boulder, CO 80308.

The Quintessence Aromatherapy Newsletter • P. O. Box 4996, Boulder, CO 80306.

Zia Cosmetic Newsletter • 300 Brannan Street, San Francisco, CA 94107.

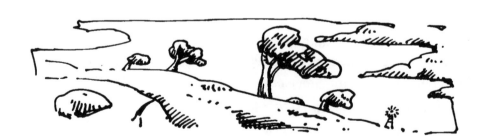

ADDENDUM

An Aromatherapy Afterthought

Preface to the Jeanne Rose English Translation of *Aromatherapie* by R. M. Gattefossé, 1937

My Search for Gattefossé

In 1969, while doing the writing for the book that ultimately came to be called *Herbs & Things, Jeanne Rose's Herbal*, I found occasional mention of a subject called aromatherapy. Aromatherapy seemed to be the use of essential oils for mental and physical healing through the process of inhalation as well as external applications of these oils. It struck an immediate chord of recognition as I had always been very specifically affected by certain scents. So I wrote a bit about the uses of essential oils in *Herbs & Things* (original title, *The Urban Herbalist)* in dream use and massage oils, and began to carry around a small leather case with 6–8 separate oils for specific purposes. I called this kit "Aromatherapy First-Aid, Inhalations for the Mind." I carried Jasmine oil, Rose, Peppermint, Rosemary, Lavender, Eucalyptus, Carnation and sometimes Camomile and Basil oils. I still have this kit, although I stopped carrying it about 1982.

My publishers thought so little of the subject that it is not even listed in the Index to *Herbs & Things* (pub. date 1972). But in my own personal records I began a file called aromatherapy. The file grew very slowly and in 1972 I found a book published in 1937 called *Fragrant and Radiant Healing Symphony*. This book written by Roland Hunt is the first one in which I actually saw mentioned the subject of aromatherapy. It was mentioned so subtly and so casually, that it became immediately apparent that as early as 1930 (ignoring ancients' use as mentioned by Budge and others in Egyptian anthologies), essential oils had been in common use for healing. Roland Hunt says, " . . . This is the important principle that is employed in aromo-therapy, or treatment by perfumes. [For] Into the subject's atmosphere is sprayed a perfume keyed to the opposite trait or emotion from which he is suffering."

For years I thought that Roland Hunt might have actually coined the word aromatherapy, in spite of the fact that by 1972 I occasionally heard the name Gattefossé mentioned as originator of both the word and the subject of aromatherapy.

By 1972 I was teaching my students at the University of California Extension the use of essential oils and giving aromatherapy demonstrations. At the UCSF Medical Center Library I came across the mention of a person named Gattefossé and an article in *La Perfumerie Moderne*. The reference was to another article or book that was stored at the Public Library in New York city. Letters to New York regarding the book or articles were fruitless. I continued my personal experimentation with inhalations and public demonstrations and continued to teach and research herbal cosmetic use while writing the *Herbal Body Book*, which was dedicated in the summer of 1973 and published in 1976. Still, my own personal bibliography does not mention Gattefossé because I had not actually seen his work (I was following the lead of Pliny the Elder (A.D. 50), whose main gift to scientific scholarship was *citing his reference works by title and author*). I already had had aromatherapy facials at Rancho La Puerta in Tecate, Mexico, and at The Essential Salon in Beverly Hills as well. The latter was so far ahead of its time here in the United States that few knew what they were advocating, and unfortunately it had closed its doors due to lack of customers by 1975. In the *Herbal Body Book* I mention André Virel, a psychoanalyst, and Knutt Larrson, a Swedish doctor, who were both working and studying the effects of odor and trauma.

Around the same time I came into possession of the French work by Docteur J. Valnet, *Aromatherapie* (published 1964) and in his bibliography is mentioned R. M. Gattefossé, *Aromatherapie*, with a publishing date of 1928. The work was of course in French, and struggling to read it I could find little mention of René Maurice Gattefossé, only his name and "L'ecole lyonnaise, de son cote, heritiere des traditions de R. M. Gattefossé, a qui nous devons le terme d'Aromatherapie, continue les travaux de ce precurseur." [The school at Lyons for its part, as inheritor of the traditions of R. M. Gattefossé—to whom we owe the term Aromatherapy itself—carries on the work of its predecessor.]

In 1975, I spoke before the Fragrance Foundation at the invitation of Annette Green, executive director, now a long-time friend and ally in the field. My thought was to come to New York and go to the Public Library and find the elusive Gattefossé book, occasionally mentioned but never quoted or correctly referenced. I carried along a hand-tooled leather briefcase in which I carried all my aromatherapy notes and the speech to be given to the Fragrance Foundation, *Aromatherapy, Modern Techniques and Ancient Indian Remedy*.

My traveling companion was Penelope, then wife to Terence Hallinan who was the attorney in the (in)famous Patty Hearst hold-up case. Penelope and I were incredibly excited to be going to New York together. We were also basking in the reflected glitter of that case. Our plane came in during a lightning storm, lightning striking near the plane. We were reading all about the Patty Hearst case and discussing it with nearby passengers while landing, holding onto each other during the storm and overwhelmed at being invited to stay (all expenses paid) at the Plaza Hotel. By the time we arrived at the Plaza I made the unfortunate discovery that my briefcase containing all my original notes on aromatherapy, my manuscript and all my records was missing.

On a piece of The Plaza stationary dated 9-21-75, I note the following:

Lost Briefcase Contents
> mss Kitchen Cosmetics, illustrated and marked
> contract and letters, K.C. and HBB
> Aromatherapy, Inhalations for Mind & Body, orig. mss
> original pb with notes, letters and herb inserts
> 3 8x10 glossies of me, Valerie, etc.
> Bienfang book, U of OK, 1946, *Sense of Odor*
> Original copy *Fragrant and Color Symphony*, by Hunt
> *entire* aromatherapy file
>> all letters
>> all news clippings
>> letters
>> 4 years of student reactions to essential oils, collated (approx. 500 references)
>> Gattefossé reference
>> yellow pad and original Fragrance Foundation speech
>> original material on the temezcal or room of vapors (Golden Door)
>> pages from personal diary about color and fragrance
>> file cards from personal aromata file listing imp. people,
>> herbs including Jasmine, Carnation, Rose, Camomile.

Whew!

I was devastated at this horrible loss, gave an impromptu speech at the Fragrance Foundation, came home, put aside my research into aromatherapy and pretty much neglected the subject for five years.

But I kept a file including answers from various people regarding my requests for aromatherapy information. I have a letter from Virginia Castleton and one from Daniele Ryman regarding Marguerite Maury's work. Both of these women were working in the field of aromatherapy, keeping it alive, the latter by her practice at her salon at the Park Lane Hotel in London and the former by her writings in *Prevention* magazine. Me? I had only the oils and a few books that I had wisely kept at home that had not been lost in the fated briefcase.

So my search for Gattefossé came to a temporary end.

By 1977, Robert Tisserand's fine book *The Art of Aromatherapy* had been published. It was a book of library study and research rather than actual hands-on work, but it proved to be a seminal work in the study of aromatherapy and excited many future students of the field. His bibliography mentions that all the books he referred to are listed in chronological order and that the 13th and 15th century books "can all be found in the library of Trinity College, Cambridge." He mentions R. M. Gattefossé, *Aromatherapie*. This was a very exciting find and I immediately called a friend in England who went to that very library, but nowhere could he find mentioned or referenced the Gattefossé book. Another dead end!

Subsequently, in early 1990 having casually met Robert, I asked him about this seeming mystery. He said that he had never actually seen the Gattefossé book, that part of the bibliography of his *Art of Aromatherapy* should probably have been listed more accurately as a reading list. Our letters read as follows:

January 27, 1990

Dear Robert . . . Is Aromatherapie by Gattefossé a ghost book? I too have seen it mentioned in bibliographies. And no, I have never known anyone to have actually seen the book. Does it exist? Did it ever exist? I have had it on file in rare book shops since 1972 and no one has ever found one. Actually, the first time that I ever saw that word (aromatherapy) mentioned was in Roland Hunt's book . . . published in 1937. Maybe Roland Hunt made up the name. Do you have any ideas on the subject? . . .

And Robert answers:

9 February 1990

Dear Jeanne . . . I do not know if Gattefossé's book is a ghost book, but I do have a series of three articles published by him in 1937. It is interesting that he makes no mention of his book on aromatherapy in these articles. This would certainly seem to indicate that the book was not published before that date although Dr. Valnet gives a publications date of 1928. Many years ago I put in an application for an international library loan to the British library, and during twelve months they were unable to obtain a copy of Gattefossé's book. If a library copy existed anywhere in the UK or France they should have been able to get hold of one. I have never actually seen a copy of the book, although it is very possible that only a very few copies were printed and hardly any actually survive.

So although he had requested this book he had been unable to obtain it.

By this time I figured that the book was most definitely a ghost book, that possibly in Gattefossé's lifetime he had desired to write such a book and might have mentioned it in his writings and that others reading this might then have concluded that there was actually such a work.

In the early '80s I had a visit from Marcel Lavabre, who left with me a prototype of the aromatic diffusor that I used with great effect in my home and my classes. I met him again in 1986 and he left me with a copy of *The Handbook of Aromatherapy* in manuscript form (published in 1990 as *The Aromatherapy Workbook*). While reading it I saw that "modern aromatherapy was born at the turn of the century from the works of the French chemist R. M. Gattefossé." Looking in the bibliography—sure enough—the elusive book is mentioned. I wasn't able to get back to Marcel until the latter part of 1989, when I asked him about the book. He, too, said that he had never actually seen the Gattefossé book and that he had mentioned it in his bibliography because it was important. But he said that he knew someone who had a copy.

Soon after I received in the mail from a rare book collector the title *Formulaire due Chimiste-Parfumeur et du Savonnier* by R. M. Gattefossé, published date 1932. He mentions his work at the back of the book but not the so-called *Aromatherapie* that was supposedly published in 1928. I was at this point 80% convinced that the book was in fact a ghost book, a hoax, or really just an article that had been written and at some point been accidentally turned into a book by a careless bibliographer.

In 1982 the English translation of Dr. Jean Valnet's book was available and I was able to read more thoroughly his ideas and confirm that his mention of Gattefossé is brief (as previously mentioned). But still I could not find the book, and my interlibrary loan requests and calls to various library's research staff proved fruitless.

In December 1989, I started up my search in earnest for the book. I really wanted to use it as a reference in my own work *Cosmetic Aromatherapy*. I was determined to get to the bottom of the mystery. I wrote to Booknoll Farm, which had in the past supplied me with many books that had to do with herbs, botany and related subjects. The answer came on 1/11/90, "Regret to say . . . cannot supply." A letter to my antiquarian friend at Bernard Quaritch, Ltd. was sent and on 1/22/90 a letter to Ancient House Bookshop, also in England. These provided my first clue that the book actually existed and I would be able to get a copy.

I wrote, "I am anxious to locate a copy of the following book and articles or information—to learn at least if they exist or not!"

Bernard Quaritch, an antiquarian bookshop in London, immediately responded and indeed my joy at the answer was phenomenal. The Ancient House Bookshop in Reigate also immediately responded and my joy doubled. All of sudden the search was getting hot!

Bernard Quaritch:

"Your book, 1937, One copy in library at U. of Iowa, and one in N.Y. Public Library. Your *L'Aromatherapie En Amerique* is held possibly by USNL of Med. and U. of Texas, Austin."

Ancient House Bookshop:

"This book out of print . . . very much regret we cannot help you . . . might we suggest that you try Natl. Congress Library or look in the National Union Catalogue to see where a copy might be located."

Dear me, had I been hiding out in the dark ages? And for what reason did I not know that the libraries were all computerized and any good research librarian could have found me this information years ago.

At this point I asked Scott Cunningham to check the New York Public Library as he would soon be there for a lecture. We had also been corresponding about the book and had compared our notes and titles with each other. He had some physical troubles and was unable to do so.

I wrote to the three libraries in question and immediately received a call from the National Medical Library saying that not only did they have the *Aromatherapie* book but several others by Gattefossé as well. She said, "Would

I care for the call numbers?" and that in order to be sent the book it would have to be requested by interlibrary loan.

A private detective located here in San Francisco, and wily in the ways of obtaining information, suggested that I use my Mechanic Library card, the same card that he had insisted that I get sometime before. I had had that card for months for just such an eventuality. A quick phone call later and I was assured that the book that I had so ardently pursued for 20 years would be in my hands within six weeks. Two weeks later, the reference librarian called me and said I could pick up the book and the others that had been sent as well. The next day I received a package from the University of Iowa and there was a second copy of the book. And the next day after that the New York Public Library called and asked if I would like to see their copy as well, and a week later I had word from the University of Texas.

An amazing plethora of riches had dropped into my hands. The arrival of these three copies of *Aromatherapie* by R. M. Gattefossé was in March. What was so interesting to me was that the books all arrived within a short time of one another and most especially that the books, each from a different library, had not ever been checked out—I was the first person to lay eyes on *Aromatherapie* by R. M. Gattefossé (in the United States).

AND so my search ended!

—*Jeanne Rose*, August 1990

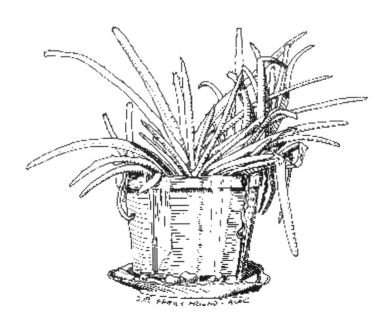

INDEX

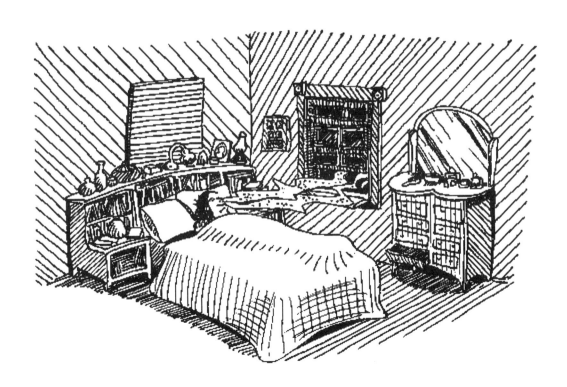

BIOGRAPHY

Jeanne Rose

This California native daughter is an international authority on the therapeutic uses of herbs, both medicinal and cosmetic, and a well-known teacher of aromatherapy. The author of eight herbal books and an Herbal Studies Course by Correspondence, Ms. Rose has a rich familial and ethnic background in plant use. Jeanne's mother, Aline Lalancette, a beautiful French-Canadian woman, met Arsenio Colón through the love-lorn column of a New York newspaper in 1936. Ms. Lalancette boarded a transcontinental train just six weeks after their first letters were exchanged and married Mr. Colon in May 1936. Jeanne was born just eight months later. She grew up in the fertile valley of Contra Costa county on an Apricot orchard and from the first her days were filled with the natural experiences of country living and plant use. Jeanne graduated from the local schools, earned a degree in zoology at San Jose State College and received a scholarship to the Marine Laboratory in Coral Gables, Florida. She worked in herbal and pesticide research at the Agricultural Experiment Stations in Florida, eventually relocating to her home state of California where she continued her private and public research into the medicinal uses of herbs and therapeutic values of essential oils. Jeanne is an academic enthusiast and pursues her studies continually by personal and library research. She has a world-class personal library containing most of the important volumes in herbal studies and aromatherapy and is an inveterate reader.

This book has been in the works since 1975 and will add a distinguished note to the aromatherapy literature of the world.